Clinical Pharmacology

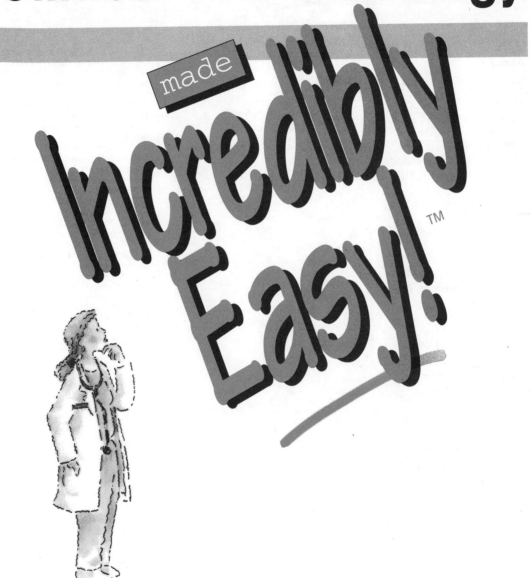

made Incredibly Easy!™

Springhouse Corporation
Springhouse, Pennsylvania

Staff

Publisher
Judith A. Schilling McCann, RN, MSN

Design Director
John Hubbard

Editorial Director
Michael Shaw

Clinical Manager
Joan M. Robinson, RN, MSN, CNS, CCRN

Clinical Editors
Collette Bishop Hendler, RN, CCRN (clinical project manager); Marcy S. Caplin, RN, MSN, CS

Senior Associate Editor
Brenna H. Mayer

Editors
Ty Eggenberger, Kevin Haworth, Jacqueline Mills, Stephen Page, Kirk Robinson, Frank Thakuria

Copy Editors
Jaime Stockslager (supervisor), Jeri Albert, Virginia Baskerville, Priscilla DeWitt, Tom DeZego, Mary T. Durkin, Amy Furman, Kimberly A.J. Johnson, Judith Orioli, Pamela Wingrod

Designers
Arlene Putterman (associate design director), Mary Ludwicki (art director), Joseph John Clark, Lynn Foulk

Illustrators
Bot Roda, Bob Neumann, Gary Welch, Julie Devito-Kruk

Electronic Production Services
Diane Paluba (manager), Joyce Rossi Biletz

Manufacturing
Deborah Meiris (director), Patricia K. Dorshaw (manager), Otto Mezei (book production manager)

Projects Coordinator
Liz Schaeffer

Editorial and Design Assistants
Tom Hasenmayer, Beverly Lane, Beth Janae Orr, Elfriede Young

Indexer
Ellen Brennan

Printed in the United States of America.

CPIE- D N O S A J J M A M F J
04   10 9 8 7 6

Library of Congress Cataloging-in-Publication Data

Clinical pharmacology made incredibly easy.
   p. ; cm.
   Includes bibliographical references and index.
   1. Clinical pharmacology—Handbooks, manuals, etc. I. Springhouse Corporation
   [DNLM: 1. Pharmacology, Clinical—methods—Handbooks. QV 39 C6417 2001]
RM301.28 .C556 2001
615'.1—dc21   00-041972
ISBN 1-58255-042-5 (alk. paper)

Contents

Contributors and consultants

Stephen C. Adams, RPh, PharmD, DABFE, DABFM, FACFE
Director of Drug Information and Clinical Services
St. Luke's Episcopal Hospital — Texas Heart Institute
Houston

Carol L. Beck, RPh, PharmD, PhD
Assistant Professor
Department of Biochemistry and Molecular Pharmacology
Thomas Jefferson University
Jefferson Medical College
Philadelphia

Tricia M. Berry, PharmD
Assistant Professor, Department of Pharmacy Practice
St. Louis College of Pharmacy

James M. Camano, PharmD
Clinical Specialist for Medication Information and Policy
Development
University Medical Center Corp.
Tucson, Ariz.

Lawrence Carey, PharmD
Clinical Pharmacy Supervisor
Jefferson Home Infusion Service
Philadelphia

Joseph L. DuFour, RN, MS, CS, FNP
Lecturer
State University of New York at New Paltz
Nurse Practitioner, Family Practice
Glen Falls, N.Y.

William A. Kehoe, PharmD, MA, FCCP, BCPS
Professor of Clinical Pharmacology and Psychology
School of Pharmacy and Health Sciences
University of the Pacific
Stockton, Calif.

Tara Kukuschkin, PharmD
Clinical Pharmacist
Kosciusko Community Hospital
Warsaw, Ind.

David J. Lash, PA-C, MPAS
Department Head, Medical Annex
Camp H.M. Smith, U.S. Navy
Pearl Harbor, Hawaii

Stephanie M. Levine, MD
Associate Professor of Medicine
Division of Pulmonary Diseases and Critical Care Medicine
University of Texas Health Science Center
San Antonio

Norma Mann, RN, MSN, NPC
Nurse Practitioner
Private Practice
Sewell, N.J.

Keith M. Olsen, PharmD, FCCP
Associate Professor of Pharmacy
University of Nebraska Medical Center
Omaha

David Pipher, RPh, PharmD
Director of Pharmacy
Forbes Regional Hospital
Monroeville, Pa.

Barbara Barnes Rogers, CRNP, MN, AOCN
Adult Oncology Nurse Practitioner
Fox Chase Cancer Center
Philadelphia

Paul Keith Small, PhD
Professor of Biology
Eureka (Ill.) College

Foreword

Pharmacology is a subject that intimidates most students, and not without reason. Learning long lists of drugs, mechanisms, and adverse reactions can be intimidating and can appear irrelevant to the practice of medicine. Yet, the same students recognize the value of pharmacologic knowledge when they see it applied in a clinical situation. This book fills the gap for students learning pharmacology who are unsure of its relevance as well as health professionals who may not remember the scientific details underlying drug usage.

Pharmacology stands at the center of the medical sciences. It relates the mechanism of drug action to the treatment of disease. In addition to being a discipline in its own right, pharmacology interacts with biochemistry, cell biology, genetics, physiology, immunology, and pathology. As our understanding of medicine becomes more and more an understanding of all the molecular components that underlie physiologic function, the knowledge of how drugs interact with these components becomes more important. New targets for drug action are characterized every week. Thus, it has become a daunting task to keep track of where and how drugs act and interact with each other.

The goal of this book is to make the study and review of pharmacology entertaining and simple to understand. It succeeds admirably at this task. As students read this book, their constant companion is Nurse Joy, who explains the fine points, emphasizes the important aspects, and warns against the dangers. Nurse Joy is aided by her friends Mr. Pill, Mr. I.V. Bag, Mr. Liver, Mr. Heart, and Mr. Neuron, among others. These characters liven up the text and keep the important messages up front for the reader. Marginal notes also emphasize and further explain the text. These include *Clinical controversy*, *Advice from the experts*, *Pharm fact*, and *Now I get it!*, which provide detailed explanations of the science behind drugs.

This is a book that a wide variety of health professionals will find useful, including physical therapists, respiratory therapists, radiologic technologists, nurses, nursing students, and medical students. It begins with an overview of pharmacology that explains and demystifies the basis of pharmacokinetics, pharmacodynamics, routes of administration, and drug interactions. With deftly entertaining treatment of these issues, the book introduces students to the foundations of pharmacology as the basis for cutting edge research and therapy. The overview is followed by chapters devoted to specific types of drugs organized by their sites of action or the disorders they're used to treat. Not only the therapeutic applications but also the mechanisms of action of drugs are reviewed.

Throughout the book, the material is presented in a lighthearted but informative manner. In its charming way, *Clinical Pharmacology Made Incredibly Easy* serves as an important reference, ensuring that the facts important for high quality health care remain fresh in the mind of the health care professional in this changing world of drug therapy.

Gary Rudnick, PhD
Professor of Pharmacology
Yale University School of Medicine
New Haven, Conn.

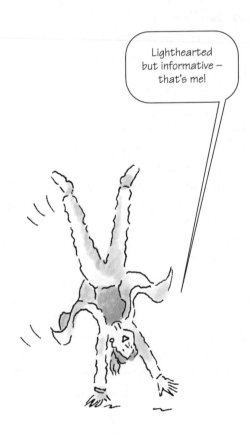

Lighthearted but informative — that's me!

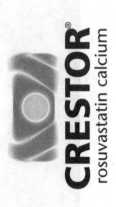

CRESTOR®
rosuvastatin calcium

www.crestor.com

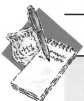

①

Fundamentals of clinical pharmacology

Just the facts

In this chapter, you'll review:

♦ pharmacology basics

♦ routes by which drugs are administered

♦ key concepts of pharmacokinetics

♦ key concepts of pharmacodynamics

♦ key concepts of pharmacotherapeutics

♦ key types of drug interactions and adverse reactions.

Pharmacology basics

This chapter focuses on the fundamental principles of pharmacology. It discusses basic information, such as how drugs are named and how they are created. It also discusses the different routes by which drugs can be administered.

Kinetics, dynamics, therapeutics

The chapter also discusses what happens when a drug enters the body. This involves three main areas:

☝ pharmacokinetics (the absorption, distribution, metabolism, and excretion of a drug)

✌ pharmacodynamics (the biochemical and physical effects of drugs and the mechanisms of drug actions)

✌ pharmacotherapeutics (the use of drugs to prevent and treat diseases).

In addition, the chapter provides an introduction to adverse drug reactions.

What's in a name?

Drugs have a specific kind of nomenclature—that is, a drug can go by three different names:
• The *chemical name* is a scientific name that precisely describes its atomic and molecular structure:
• The *generic*, or nonproprietary, name is an abbreviation of the chemical name.
• The *trade name* (also known as the brand name or proprietary name) is selected by the drug company selling the product. Trade names are protected by copyright. The symbol ® after the trade name indicates that the name is registered by and restricted to the drug manufacturer.

To avoid confusion, it's best to use a drug's generic name because any one drug can have a number of trade names.

In 1962, the federal government mandated the use of official names so that only one official name would represent each drug. The official names are listed in the United States Pharmacopeia and National Formulary.

This is confusing! Each drug has at least three names: a chemical name, a generic name, and a trade name.

Family dynamics

Drugs that share similar characteristics are grouped together as a *pharmacologic class* (or family). Beta-adrenergic blockers are an example of a pharmacologic class.

A second grouping is the *therapeutic classification*, which groups drugs by therapeutic use. Antihypertensives are an example of a therapeutic class.

Where drugs come from

Traditionally, drugs derived from *natural* sources, such as:
• plants
• animals
• minerals.

Today, however, laboratory researchers have used traditional knowledge, along with chemical science, to develop *synthetic* drug sources. One advantage of chemically developed drugs is that they're free from the impurities found in natural substances.

Also, researchers and drug developers can manipulate the molecular structure of substances such as antibiotics so that a slight change in the chemical structure makes the drug effective against different organisms. The first-, second-, third-, and fourth-generation cephalosporins are an example.

Old-fashioned medicine

The earliest drug concoctions from plants used everything: the leaves, roots, bulb, stem, seeds, buds, and blossoms. Subsequently, harmful substances often found their way into the mixture.

As the understanding of plants as drug sources became more sophisticated, researchers sought to isolate and intensify *active components* while avoiding harmful ones.

Power plant

The active components consist of several types and vary in character and effect:

• *Alkaloids*, the most active component in plants, react with acids to form a salt that is able to dissolve more readily in body fluids. The names of alkaloids and their salts usually end in "-ine;" examples include atropine, caffeine, and nicotine.

• *Glycosides* are another active components found in plants. Names of glycosides usually end in "-in" such as *digoxin*.

• *Gums* constitute another group of active components. Gums give products the ability to attract and hold water. Examples include seaweed extractions and seeds with starch.

• *Resins*, of which the chief source is pine tree sap, commonly act as local irritants or as laxatives and caustic agents.

• *Oils*, thick and sometimes greasy liquids, are classified as volatile or fixed. Examples of volatile oils include peppermint, spearmint, and juniper. Fixed oils, which aren't easily evaporated, include castor oil and olive oil.

> Drugs can be derived from just about any substance on earth!

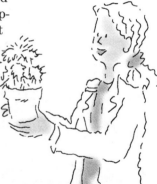

Animal magnetism

The body fluids or glands of animals can also be drug sources. The drugs obtained from animal sources include:

• *hormones*, such as insulin
• *oils* and *fats* (usually fixed), such as cod-liver oil

> *Pharm fact*
>
> ## Old McDonald had a pharm
>
> In the near future, traditional barnyard animals might also be small, organic pharmaceutical factories. Some animals have already been genetically altered to produce pharmaceuticals, and their products are being tested by the Food and Drug Administration. Here are a few examples of the possibilities:
> • a cow that produces milk containing lactoferrin, which can be used to treat human infections
> • a goat that produces milk containing antithrombin III, which can help prevent blood clotting in humans
> • a sheep that produces milk containing alpha-antitrypsin, which is used to treat cystic fibrosis.

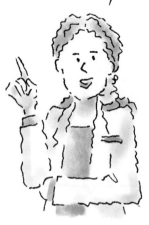

Hmmm...farm fresh pharmaceuticals? That is an unusual idea.

• *enzymes*, which are produced by living cells and act as catalysts, such as pancreatin and pepsin
• *vaccines*, which are suspensions of killed, modified, or attenuated microorganisms. (See *Old McDonald had a pharm.*)

Mineral springs

Metallic and nonmetallic minerals provide various inorganic materials not available from plants or animals. The mineral sources are used as they occur in nature or are combined with other ingredients. Examples of drugs that contain minerals are iron, iodine, and Epsom salts.

Down to DNA

Today, most drugs are produced in laboratories and can be:
• natural (from animal, plant, or mineral sources)
• synthetic
• a combination of the two.
   Examples of drugs produced in the laboratory include thyroid hormone (natural), cimetidine (synthetic), and anistreplase (a combination of natural and synthetic).
   Recombinant deoxyribonucleic acid (DNA) research has led to another chemical source of organic compounds. For example, the reordering of genetic informa-

tion enables scientists to develop bacteria that produce insulin for humans.

New drug development

In the past, drugs were found by trial and error. Now, they're developed primarily by systematic scientific research. The Food and Drug Administration (FDA) carefully monitors new drug development, which can take many years to complete.

Only after reviewing extensive animal studies and data on the safety and effectiveness of the proposed drug will the FDA approve an application for an Investigational New Drug (IND). (See *Phases of new drug development.*)

Exceptions to the rule

Although most INDs undergo all four phases of clinical evaluation mandated by the FDA, a few can receive expedited approval. For example, because of the public health threat posed by acquired immunodeficiency syndrome

Now I get it!

Phases of new drug development

When the Food and Drug Administration (FDA) approves the application for an investigational new drug, the drug must undergo clinical evaluation involving human subjects. This clinical evaluation is divided into four phases.

Phase I
The drug is tested on healthy volunteers in phase I.

Phase II
Phase II involves trials with human subjects who have the disease for which the drug is thought to be effective.

Phase III
Large numbers of patients in medical research centers receive the drug in phase III. This larger sampling provides information about infrequent or rare adverse effects. The FDA will approve a new drug application if phase III studies are satisfactory.

Phase IV
Phase IV is voluntary and involves postmarket surveillance of the drug's therapeutic effects at the completion of phase III. The pharmaceutical company receives reports from doctors and other health care professionals about the therapeutic results and adverse reactions of the drug. Some medications, for example, have been found to be toxic and have been removed from the market after their initial release.

(AIDS), the FDA and drug companies have agreed to shorten the IND approval process for drugs to treat the disease. This allows doctors to give qualified AIDS patients "Treatment INDs," which are not yet approved by the FDA.

Sponsors of drugs that reach phase II or III clinical trials can apply for FDA approval of Treatment IND status. When the IND is approved, the sponsor supplies the drug to doctors whose patients meet appropriate criteria. (See *Cheaper and easier.*)

Pharmacokinetics

Kinetics refers to movement. Pharmacokinetics deals with a drug's actions as it moves through the body. Therefore, pharmacokinetics discusses how a drug is:

- absorbed (taken into the body)
- distributed (moved into various tissues)
- metabolized (changed into a form that can be excreted)
- excreted (removed from the body).

This branch of pharmacology is also concerned with a drug's onset of action, peak concentration level, and duration of action.

Absorption

Drug absorption covers the progress of a drug from the time it's administered, through the time it passes to the tissues, until it becomes available for use by the body.

On a cellular level, drugs are absorbed by several means — primarily through active or passive transport.

The lazy way

Passive transport requires no cellular energy because the drug moves from an area of higher concentration to one of lower concentration. It occurs when small molecules diffuse across membranes. Diffusion (movement from a higher concentration to a lower concentration) stops when drug concentration on both sides of the membrane is equal.

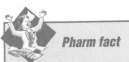

Pharm fact

Cheaper and easier

In the past, only a few drugs for acute conditions (such as headaches and colds) have been available without prescription. The Food and Drug Administration is currently considering a move that would make more drugs available over the counter, making the drugs much less expensive to consumers. Some of the drugs that might one day be available without prescription include birth control pills as well as treatments for chronic disorders, such as high blood pressure, diabetes, and osteoporosis.

Using muscle

Active transport requires cellular energy to move the drug from an area of lower concentration to one of higher concentration. Active transport is used to absorb electrolytes, such as sodium and potassium, as well as some drugs such as levodopa.

Taking a bite

Pinocytosis is a unique form of active transport that occurs when a cell engulfs a drug particle. Pinocytosis is commonly employed to transport fat-soluble vitamins (vitamins A, D, E, and K).

Watch the speed limit!

If only a few cells separate the active drug from the systemic circulation, absorption will occur rapidly and the drug will quickly reach therapeutic levels in the body. Typically, drug absorption occurs within seconds or minutes when administered sublingually, I.V., or by inhalation.

Not so fast

Absorption occurs at a slower rate when drugs are administered by the oral, I.M., or subcutaneous routes because the complex membrane systems of GI mucosal layers, muscle, and skin delay drug passage.

At a snail's pace

At the slowest absorption rates, drugs can take several hours or days to reach peak concentration levels. A slow rate usually occurs with rectally administered or sustained-release drugs.

Not enough time

Other factors can affect how quickly a drug is absorbed. For example, most absorption of oral drugs occurs in the small intestine. If a patient has had large sections of the small intestine surgically removed, drug absorption decreases because of the reduced surface area and the reduced time a drug is in the intestine.

Look to the liver

Drugs absorbed by the small intestine are transported to the liver before being circulated to the rest of the body. The liver may metabolize much of the drug before it en-

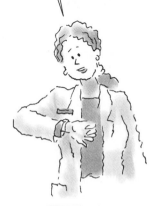

Drugs given under the tongue, I.V., or by inhalation are quickly absorbed…

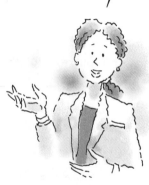

…while those administered orally, I.M., or subcutaneously require more time to be absorbed.

ters circulation. This mechanism is referred to as the first-pass effect. Liver metabolism may inactivate the drug; if so, the first-pass effect lowers the amount of active drug released into the systemic circulation. Therefore, higher drug dosages must be administered to achieve the desired effect.

More blood, more absorption

Increased blood flow to an absorption site improves drug absorption, while reduced blood flow decreases absorption. More rapid absorption leads to a quicker onset of drug action.

For example, the muscle area selected for I.M. administration can make a difference in the drug absorption rate. Blood flows faster through the deltoid muscle (in the upper arm) than through the gluteal muscle (in the buttocks). The gluteal muscle, however, can accommodate a larger volume of drug than the deltoid muscle.

Slowed by pain and stress

Pain and stress can decrease the amount of drug absorbed. This may be due to a change in blood flow, reduced movement through the GI tract, or gastric retention triggered by the autonomic nervous system response to pain.

High fat doesn't help

High-fat meals and solid foods slow the rate at which contents leave the stomach and enter the intestines, delaying intestinal absorption of a drug.

Dosage form factors

Drug formulation (such as tablets, capsules, liquids, sustained-release formulas, inactive ingredients, and coatings) affects the drug absorption rate and the time needed to reach peak blood concentration levels.

Interactions increase? Or decrease?

Combining one drug with another drug, or with food, can cause interactions that increase or decrease drug absorption, depending on the substances involved.

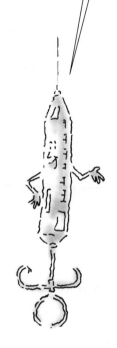

A drug injected into muscle of the buttock is absorbed more slowly than one injected into the upper arm.

Distribution

Drug distribution is the process by which the drug is delivered to the tissues and fluids of the body. Distribution of an absorbed drug within the body depends on several factors:

- blood flow
- solubility
- protein binding.

Quick to the heart

After a drug has reached the bloodstream, its distribution in the body depends on blood flow. The drug is quickly distributed to organs with a large supply of blood. These organs include the:

- heart
- liver
- kidneys.

Distribution to other internal organs, skin, fat, and muscle is slower.

Lucky lipids

The ability of a drug to cross a cell membrane depends on whether the drug is water- or lipid- (fat-) soluble. Lipid-soluble drugs easily cross through cell membranes, while a water-soluble drug can't.

Lipid-soluble drugs can also cross the blood-brain barrier and enter the brain.

Free to work

As a drug travels through the body, it comes in contact with proteins such as the plasma protein albumin. The drug can remain free or bind to the protein. The portion of a drug that is bound to a protein is inactive and can't exert a therapeutic effect. Only the free, or unbound, portion remains active.

A drug is said to be highly protein-bound if it's more than 80% bound to protein.

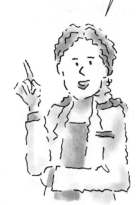

Only free drugs, not those bound to protein, can produce a therapeutic effect.

Metabolism

Drug metabolism, or biotransformation, refers to the body's ability to change a drug from its dosage form to a more water-soluble form that can then be excreted. Drugs can be metabolized in several ways:

• Most commonly, a drug is metabolized into inactive metabolites (products of metabolism), which are then excreted.

• Other drugs can be converted to metabolites that are active, meaning they're capable of exerting their own pharmacologic action. Metabolites may undergo further metabolism or may be excreted from the body unchanged.

• Still other drugs can be administered as inactive drugs, called prodrugs, and don't become active until they're metabolized.

Where metabolism happens

The majority of drugs are metabolized by enzymes in the liver; however, metabolism can also occur in the plasma, kidneys, and membranes of the intestines. In contrast, some drugs inhibit or compete for enzyme metabolism, which can cause the accumulation of drugs when they're given together. This accumulation increases the potential for an adverse reaction or drug toxicity.

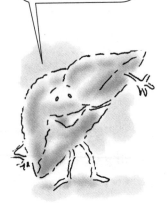

If I'm not working right, a drug doesn't get metabolized normally.

Conditional considerations

Certain diseases can reduce metabolism. These include cirrhosis (liver disease) and heart failure, which reduces circulation to the liver.

Gene machine

Genetics can allow some people to metabolize drugs rapidly, while others metabolize them more slowly.

Stress test

Environment, too, can alter drug metabolism. For example, if a person is surrounded by cigarette smoke, the rate of metabolism of some drugs may be affected; a stressful environment can also change how a person metabolizes drugs.

The age game

Developmental changes can also affect drug metabolism. For instance, infants have immature livers that reduce the rate of metabolism, and elderly patients experience a decline in liver size, blood flow, and enzyme production that also slows metabolism.

Excretion

Drug excretion refers to the elimination of drugs from the body. Most drugs are excreted by the kidneys and leave the body through urine. Drugs can also be excreted through the lungs, exocrine glands (sweat, salivary, or mammary glands), skin, and intestinal tract.

Half-life = half the drug

The half-life of a drug is the time it takes for half of the drug to be eliminated by the body. Factors that affect a drug's half-life include its rate of absorption, metabolism, and excretion. Knowing how long a drug remains in the body helps determine how frequently a drug should be taken.

A drug that is given only once is eliminated from the body almost completely after five half-lives. A drug that is administered at regular intervals, however, reaches a steady concentration (or steady state) after about five half-lives. Steady state occurs when the rate of drug administration equals the rate of drug excretion.

Because some drugs are excreted in breast milk, a breast-feeding mother should check with her health care provider before taking any drug.

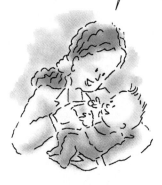

Onset, peak, and duration

In addition to absorption, distribution, metabolism, and excretion, three other factors play important roles in a drug's pharmacokinetics:
• onset of action
• peak concentration
• duration of action.

Lights, camera...action!

Onset of action refers to the time interval that starts when the drug is administered and ends when the therapeutic effect actually begins. Rate of onset varies depending on the route of administration and other pharmacokinetic properties.

A drug with a long half-life can take days to reach therapeutic blood levels.

Peak performance

As the body absorbs more drug, blood concentration levels rise. The peak concentration level is reached when the absorption rate equals the elimination rate. However, the time of peak concentration isn't always the time of peak response.

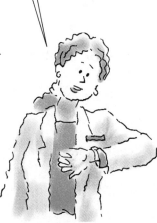

Sticking around

The duration of action is the length of time the drug produces its therapeutic effect.

Pharmacodynamics

Pharmacodynamics is the study of the drug mechanisms that produce biochemical or physiologic changes in the body. The interaction at the cellular level between a drug and cellular components, such as the complex proteins that make up the cell membrane, enzymes, or target receptors, represents drug action. The response resulting from this drug action is the drug effect.

It's the cell that matters

A drug can modify cell function or the rate of function, but a drug can't impart a new function to a cell or to target tissue. Therefore, the drug effect depends on what the cell is capable of accomplishing.

A drug can alter the target cell's function by:
• modifying the cell's physical or chemical environment
• interacting with a receptor (a specialized location on a cell membrane or inside a cell).

Agonist drugs

Many drugs work by stimulating or blocking drug receptors. A drug attracted to a receptor displays an affinity (attraction) for that receptor. When a drug displays an affinity for a receptor and stimulates it, the drug acts as an *agonist*. The drug's ability to initiate a response after binding with the receptor is referred to as *intrinsic activity*.

Antagonist drugs

If a drug has an affinity for a receptor but displays no intrinsic activity (in other words, it doesn't stimulate the receptor), it's called an *antagonist*. The antagonist prevents a response from occurring.

Reversible or irreversible

Antagonists can be competitive or noncompetitive.
• A *competitive antagonist* competes with the agonist for receptor sites. Because this type of receptor binds

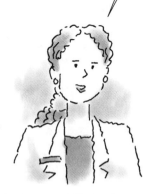

A drug that enhances or stimulates a receptor is called an agonist...

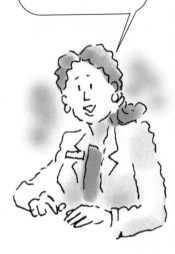

...while a drug that occupies a receptor and prevents the actions of an agonist is called an antagonist.

reversibly to the receptor site, giving larger doses of an agonist can overcome the antagonist's effects.
• A *noncompetitive antagonist* binds to receptor sites and blocks the effects of the agonist. Giving larger doses of the agonist can't reverse its action.

Regarding receptors

If a drug acts on a variety of receptors, it's said to be non-selective and can cause multiple and widespread effects. In addition, some receptors are classified further by their specific effects. For example, beta receptors typically produce increased heart rate and bronchial relaxation as well as other systemic effects.

Beta receptors, however, can be further divided into $beta_1$ receptors (which act primarily on the heart) and $beta_2$ receptors (which act primarily on smooth muscles and gland cells).

Potent power

Drug potency refers to the relative amount of a drug required to produce a desired response. Drug potency is also used to compare two drugs. If drug X produces the same response as drug Y but at a lower dose, then drug X is more potent than drug Y.

As its name implies, a dose-response curve is used to graphically represent the relationship between the dose of a drug and the response it produces. (See *Dose-response curve*, page 14.)

Maximum effect

On the dose-response curve, a low dose usually corresponds with a low response. At a low dose, an increase in dose produces only a slight increase in response. With further increases in dose, there is a marked rise is drug response. After a certain point, an increase in dose yields little or no increase in response. At this point, the drug is said to have reached maximum effectiveness.

Margin of safety

Most drugs produce multiple effects. The relationship between a drug's desired therapeutic effects and its adverse effects is called the drug's *therapeutic index*. It's also referred to as its *margin of safety*.

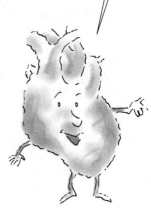

Stimulate beta receptors, and I'm likely to speed up.

When a drug has a narrow margin of safety, there is a very small difference between a therapeutic dose and a lethal one.

CAUTION!

14

Now I get it!

Dose-response curve

This curve shows the drug-response curve for two different drugs. As you can see, at low doses of each drug, a dosage increase results in only a small increase in drug response (for example, from point A to point B). At higher doses, an increase in dosage produces a much greater response (from point B to point C). As the dosage continues to climb, an increase in dose produces very little increase in response (from point C to point D).

This graph also shows that drug X is more potent than drug Y because it results in the same response, but at a lower dose (compare point A to point E).

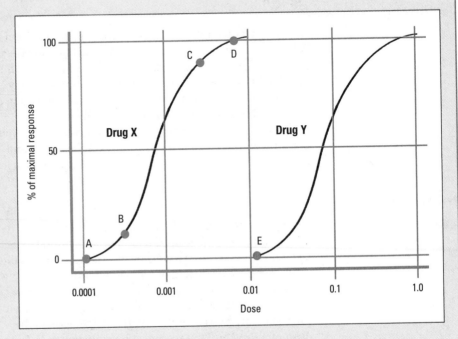

The therapeutic index usually measures the difference between:

- an effective dose for 50% of the patients treated
- the minimal dose at which adverse reactions occur.

Low index = potential danger

Drugs with a low therapeutic index have a narrow margin of safety. This means that there is a narrow range of safety between an effective dose and a lethal one. On the other hand, a drug with a high therapeutic index has a large margin of safety and less risk of toxic effects.

Pharmacotherapeutics

Pharmacotherapeutics is the use of drugs to treat disease. When choosing a drug to treat a particular condition, health care providers consider not only the drug's effectiveness but also other factors such as the type of therapy the patient will receive.

Not all therapy is the same

The type of therapy a patient receives depends on the severity, urgency, and prognosis of the patient's condition and can include:
• *acute therapy*, if the patient is critically ill and requires acute intensive therapy
• *empiric therapy*, based on practical experience rather than on pure scientific data
• *maintenance therapy*, for patients with chronic conditions that don't resolve
• *supplemental* or *replacement therapy*, to replenish or substitute for missing substances in the body
• *supportive therapy*, which doesn't treat the cause of the disease but maintains other threatened body systems until the patient's condition resolves
• *palliative therapy*, used for end-stage or terminal diseases to make the patient as comfortable as possible.

I can only be myself

A patient's overall health as well as other individual factors can alter that patient's response to a drug. Coinciding medical conditions and personal lifestyle characteristics must be considered when selecting drug therapy. (See *Factors affecting a patient's response to a drug.*)

Decreased response...

In addition, it's important to remember that certain drugs have a tendency to create drug tolerance and drug dependence in patients. *Drug tolerance* occurs when a patient has a decreased response to a drug over time. The patient then requires larger doses to produce the same response.

...and increased desire

Tolerance differs from *drug dependence*, in which a patient displays a physical or psychological need for the drug. Physical dependence produces withdrawal symptoms when the drug is stopped, while psychological dependence results in drug-seeking behaviors.

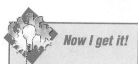
Now I get it!

Factors affecting a patient's response to a drug

Because no two people are alike physiologically or psychologically, patient response to a drug can vary greatly, depending upon such factors as:
• age
• cardiovascular function
• diet
• disease
• drug interactions
• GI function
• hepatic function
• infection
• renal function
• sex.

Drug interactions

Drug interactions can occur between drugs or between drugs and foods. They can interfere with the results of a laboratory test or produce physical or chemical incompatibilities. The more drugs a patient receives, the greater the chances are that a drug interaction will occur.

Potential drug interactions include:
- additive effects
- potentiation
- antagonistic effects
- decreased or increased absorption
- decreased or increased metabolism and excretion.

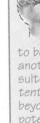

Memory jogger

When a drug is said to be potentiated by another drug, the results are more potent — the drug goes beyond its original potential.

Adding it all up

An *additive* effect can occur when two drugs with similar actions are administered to a patient. The effects are equivalent to the sum of the effects of either drug administered alone in higher doses.

Giving two drugs together such as two analgesics (painkillers) has several potential advantages: lower doses of each drug, decreased probability of adverse reaction, and greater pain control than from one drug given alone (probably because of different mechanisms of action).

Potent problem

A synergistic effect, also called *potentiation*, occurs when two drugs that produce the same effect are given together and one drug potentiates (enhances the effect) of the other drug. This produces greater effects than each drug taken alone.

Fighting it out

An *antagonistic* drug interaction occurs when the combined response of two drugs is less than the response produced by either drug alone.

An absorbing problem

Two drugs given together can change the absorption of one or both of the drugs:
- Drugs that change the acidity of the stomach can affect the ability of another drug to dissolve in the stomach.
- Some drugs can interact and form an insoluble compound that can't be absorbed.

Bound and determined

After a drug is absorbed, the blood distributes it through-out the body as a free drug or one that is bound to plasma protein.

When two drugs are given together, they can com-pete for protein-binding sites, leading to an increase in the effects of one drug as that drug is displaced from the protein and becomes a free, unbound drug.

Toxic waste

Toxic drug levels can occur when a drug's metabolism and excretion are inhibited by another drug. Some drug interactions affect excretion only.

Back to the lab

Drug interactions can also alter laboratory tests and can produce changes seen on a patient's electrocardiogram.

Menu planning

Interactions between drugs and food can alter the therapeutic effects of the drug. Food can also alter the rate and amount of drug absorbed from the GI tract, af-fecting bioavailability — that is, the amount of a drug dose available to the systemic circulation. Drugs can also impair vitamin and mineral absorption.

Some drugs stimulate enzyme production, increas-ing metabolic rates and the demand for vitamins that are enzyme cofactors (which must unite with the en-zyme in order for the enzyme to function). Dangerous in-teractions can also occur. For instance, when food that contains tyramine (such as aged cheddar cheese) is eaten by a person taking a monoamine oxidase inhibitor, hyper-tensive crisis can occur.

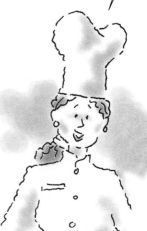

Review a patient's diet carefully — drug interactions with food can reduce absorption or even produce dangerous changes.

Adverse drug reactions

A drug's desired effect is called the expected therapeutic response. An adverse drug reaction, on the other hand (also called a side effect or adverse effect) is a harmful, undesirable response. Adverse drug reactions can range from mild ones that disappear when the drug is discontin-ued to debilitating diseases that become chronic.

Dosage dilemma

Adverse drug reactions can be classified as dose-related or patient sensitivity–related. Most adverse drug reactions result from the known pharmacologic effects of a drug and are typically dose-related. These types of reactions can be predicted in most cases.

Dose-related reactions include:

- secondary effects
- hypersusceptibility
- overdose
- iatrogenic effects.

Extra effects

A drug typically produces not only a major therapeutic effect but also additional, secondary effects that can be beneficial or adverse. For example, morphine used for pain control can lead to two undesirable secondary effects: constipation and respiratory depression. Diphenhydramine used as an antihistamine is accompanied by the adverse reaction of sedation and is sometimes used as a sleep aid.

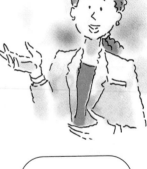

For an allergic reaction to occur, the patient must have received the drug before...

Enhanced action

A patient can be hypersusceptible to the pharmacologic actions of a drug. Even when given a usual therapeutic dose, a hypersusceptible patient can experience an excessive therapeutic response or secondary effects.

Hypersusceptibility typically results from altered pharmacokinetics (absorption, metabolism, and excretion), which leads to higher-than-expected blood concentration levels. Increased receptor sensitivity also can increase the patient's response to therapeutic or adverse effects.

...but a toxic reaction can occur in anyone, if the dose is high enough.

Oh no! Overdose

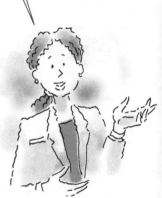

A toxic drug reaction can occur when an excessive dose is taken, either intentionally or by accident. The result is an exaggerated response to the drug and can lead to transient changes or more serious reactions, such as respiratory depression, cardiovascular collapse, and even death. To avoid toxic reactions, chronically ill or elderly patients often receive lower drug doses.

Iatrogenic issues

Some adverse drug reactions, known as iatrogenic effects, can mimic pathologic disorders. For example, drugs, such as antineoplastics, aspirin, corticosteroids, and indomethacin, commonly cause GI irritation and bleeding. Other examples of iatrogenic effects include induced asthma with propranolol, induced nephritis with methicillin, and induced deafness with gentamicin.

You're so sensitive

Patient sensitivity–related adverse reactions aren't as common as dose-related reactions. Sensitivity-related reactions result from a patient's unusual and extreme sensitivity to a drug. These adverse reactions arise from a unique tissue response rather than from an exaggerated pharmacologic action. Extreme patient sensitivity can occur as a drug allergy or an idiosyncratic response.

Immunity misidentification

A *drug allergy* occurs when a patient's immune system identifies a drug, a drug metabolite, or a drug contaminant as a dangerous foreign substance that must be neutralized or destroyed. Previous exposure to the drug or to one with similar chemical characteristics sensitizes the patient's immune system, and subsequent exposure causes an allergic reaction (hypersensitivity).

An allergic reaction not only directly injures cells and tissues but also produces broader systemic damage by initiating cellular release of vasoactive and inflammatory substances.

Inconsequential...or critical?

The allergic reaction can vary in intensity from an immediate, life-threatening anaphylactic reaction with circulatory collapse and swelling of the larynx and bronchioles to a mild reaction with a rash and itching.

Idiosyncratic response

Some sensitivity-related adverse reactions don't result from pharmacologic properties of a drug or from allergy but are specific to the individual patient. These are called idiosyncratic responses. A patient's idiosyncratic response sometimes has a genetic cause.

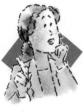

Quick quiz

1. While teaching a patient about drug therapy for diabetes, you review the absorption, distribution, metabolism, and excretion of insulin and oral antidiabetic agents. Which principle of pharmacology are you describing?

    A.   Pharmacokinetics

    B.   Pharmacodynamics

    C.   Pharmacotherapeutics

Answer: A. Pharmacokinetics discusses the movement of drugs through the body and involves absorption, distribution, metabolism, and excretion.

2. Which type of drug therapy is used for patients who have a chronic condition that can't be cured?

    A.   Empiric therapy

    B.   Palliative therapy

    C.   Maintenance therapy

Answer: C. Maintenance therapy seeks to maintain a certain level of health in patients who have chronic conditions.

3. Which branch of pharmacology studies the way drugs work in living organisms?

    A.   Adverse reactions

    B.   Pharmacokinetics

    C.   Pharmacodynamics

Answer: C. Pharmacodynamics studies the mechanisms of action of drugs and seeks to understand how drugs work in the body.

Scoring

☆☆☆   If you answered all three questions correctly, excellent! You've absorbed this chapter in a hurry.

☆☆   If you answered two questions correctly, terrific! You've reached therapeutic levels of this chapter in a flash.

☆   If you answered fewer than two questions correctly, no need for concern. Sometimes food enhances absorption — so grab a quick snack and come back for a review.

2

Autonomic nervous system drugs

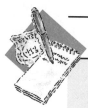

Just the facts

In this chapter, you'll review:

♦ functions of the autonomic nervous system

♦ classes of drugs that affect the autonomic nervous system

♦ uses and varying actions of these drugs

♦ how these drugs are absorbed, distributed, metabolized, and excreted

♦ drug interactions and adverse reactions to these drugs.

Cholinergic drugs

Cholinergic drugs promote the action of the neurotransmitter *acetylcholine*. These drugs are also called parasympathomimetic drugs because they produce effects that imitate parasympathetic nerve stimulation.

Mimickers and inhibitors

There are two major classes of cholinergic drugs:
• *Cholinergic agonists* mimic the action of the neurotransmitter acetylcholine.
• *Anticholinesterase drugs* work by inhibiting the destruction of acetylcholine at the cholinergic receptor sites. (See *How cholinergic drugs work*, page 22.)

> Cholinergic drugs enhance the action of acetylcholine, stimulating the parasympathetic nervous system.

Now I get it!

How cholinergic drugs work

Cholinergic drugs fall into one of two major classes: cholinergic agonists and anticholinesterase drugs. Here is how these drugs achieve their effects.

Cholinergic agonists

When a neuron in the parasympathetic nervous system is stimulated, the neurotransmitter acetylcholine is released. Acetylcholine crosses the synapse and interacts with receptors in an adjacent neuron. Cholinergic agonist drugs work by stimulating cholinergic receptors, mimicking the action of acetylcholine.

Anticholinesterase drugs

After acetylcholine stimulates the cholinergic receptor, it's destroyed by the enzyme acetylcholinesterase. Anticholinesterase drugs produce their effects by inhibiting acetylcholinesterase. Acetylcholine isn't broken down and begins to accumulate; therefore, the effects of acetylcholine are prolonged.

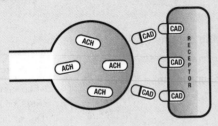

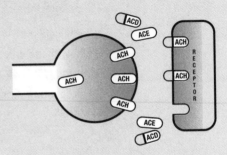

Key:

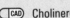 Acetylcholine   ⬭CAD Cholinergic agonist drug   ⬭ACE Acetylcholinesterase   ⬭ACD Anticholinesterase drug

Cholinergic agonists

By directly stimulating cholinergic receptors, cholinergic agonists mimic the action of the neurotransmitter acetylcholine. They include such drugs as:
- acetylcholine (rarely used clinically)
- bethanechol
- carbachol
- pilocarpine.

Pharmacokinetics (how drugs circulate)

The action and metabolism of the cholinergic agonists vary widely. Acetylcholine poorly penetrates the central nervous system (CNS), and its effects are primarily peripheral, with a widespread action. The drug is rapidly destroyed in the body.

Avoid injections

The cholinergic agonists rarely are administered by I.M. or I.V. injection because they're almost immediately broken down by cholinesterases in the interstitial spaces between tissues and inside the blood vessels. Moreover, they begin to work rapidly and can cause a cholinergic crisis (a drug overdose resulting in extreme muscle weakness and possible paralysis of the muscles used in respiration).

Topically, orally, or under the skin

Cholinergic agonists are usually administered:
- topically, with eye drops
- orally (P.O.)
- by subcutaneous (S.C.) injection.
    S.C. injections begin to work more rapidly than oral doses. In addition, their response is often more effective.

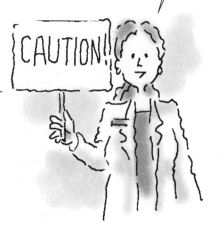

Cholinergic agonists administered by injection are rapidly broken down and could cause a cholinergic crisis.

Metabolism and excretion

All cholinergic agonists are metabolized by cholinesterases:
- at the muscarinic and nicotinic receptor sites
- in the plasma (the liquid portion of the blood)
- in the liver.
    All drugs in this class are excreted by the kidneys.

Pharmacodynamics (how drugs act)

Cholinergic agonists work by mimicking the action of acetylcholine on the neurons in certain organs of the body, called target organs. When they combine with receptors on the cell membranes of target organs, they stimulate the muscle and produce:
- salivation
- bradycardia (a slow heart rate)
- dilation of blood vessels
- constriction of the bronchioles of the lungs
- increased activity of the GI tract
- increased tone and contraction of the muscles of the bladder
- constriction of the pupils of the eye.

Pharmacotherapeutics (how drugs are used)

Cholinergic agonists are used to:

• treat atonic (weak) bladder conditions and postoperative and postpartum urine retention
• treat GI disorders, such as postoperative abdominal distention and GI atony
• reduce eye pressure in patients with glaucoma and during eye surgery
• treat salivary gland hypofunction caused by radiation therapy and Sjögren's syndrome.

Drug interactions

Cholinergic agonists have specific interactions with other drugs. Here are some examples:
• Other cholinergic drugs, particularly anticholinesterase drugs (such as ambenonium, edrophonium, neostigmine, physostigmine, and pyridostigmine), boost the effects of cholinergic drugs and increase the risk of cholinergic toxicity.
• Cholinergic blocking drugs (such as atropine, belladonna, homatropine, methantheline, methscopolamine, propantheline, and scopolamine) reduce the effects of cholinergic drugs.
• Quinidine also reduces the effectiveness of cholinergic agonists. (See *Adverse reactions to cholinergic agonists.*)

Anticholinesterase drugs

Anticholinesterase drugs block the action of the enzyme acetylcholinesterase (which breaks down acetylcholine) at cholinergic receptor sites, preventing the breakdown of the neurotransmitter acetylcholine. As acetylcholine builds up, it continues to stimulate the cholinergic receptors. (See *One day at a time: Recognizing toxic response.*)

Anticholinesterase drugs are divided into two categories — reversible and irreversible.

These you can reverse...

Reversible anticholinesterase drugs have a short duration of action and include:
• ambenonium
• donepezil
• edrophonium
• neostigmine

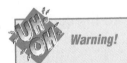

Adverse reactions to cholinergic agonists

Because they bind with receptors in the parasympathetic nervous system, cholinergic agonists can produce adverse effects in any organ innervated by the parasympathetic nerves. These adverse effects can include:
• nausea and vomiting
• cramps and diarrhea
• blurred vision
• decreased heart rate and low blood pressure
• shortness of breath
• urinary frequency
• increased salivation and sweating.

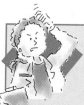

Clinical controversy

One day at a time: Recognizing toxic response

It's difficult to predict adverse reactions to anticholinesterase drugs in a patient with myasthenia gravis because the therapeutic dose varies from day to day. Increased muscle weakness can result from:
- resistance to the drug
- receiving too little anticholinesterase drug
- receiving too much anticholinesterase drug.

Enter edrophonium
Deciding whether a patient is experiencing a toxic drug response (too much drug) or a myasthenic crisis (extreme muscle weakness and severe respiratory difficulties) can be difficult. Edrophonium can be used to distinguish between a toxic drug effect or a myasthenic crisis. When edrophonium is used, suction, oxygen, mechanical ventilation, and emergency drugs (such as atropine) must be readily available in case a cholinergic crisis occurs.

- physostigmine salicylate
- pyridostigmine
- tacrine.

...these you can't

Irreversible anticholinesterase drugs have long-lasting effects and are used primarily as toxic insecticides and pesticides or as nerve gas in chemical warfare. Only one has therapeutic usefulness: echothiophate.

Pharmacokinetics

Here is a brief rundown of how anticholinesterase drugs move through the body.

Generally GI

Many of the anticholinesterase drugs are readily absorbed from the GI tract, S.C., and mucous membranes.

Because neostigmine is poorly absorbed from the GI tract, the patient needs a higher dose when taking this drug orally. Because the duration of action for an oral dose is longer, however, the patient doesn't need to take it as frequently. When a rapid effect is needed, the drug should be given by the I.M. or I.V. route.

Distribution

Of all the anticholinesterase drugs, only physostigmine is able to cross the blood-brain barrier (a protective barrier

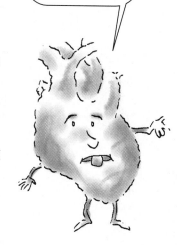

Easy does it. Overstimulation of the parasympathetic nervous system can send me into cardiac arrest!

between the capillaries and brain tissue that prevents harmful substances from entering the brain). Donepezil is highly bound to plasma proteins, while tacrine is about 55% bound to plasma proteins.

Metabolism and excretion

Most anticholinesterase drugs are metabolized in the body by enzymes in the plasma and excreted in the urine. Donepezil and tacrine are metabolized in the liver.

Pharmacodynamics

Anticholinesterase drugs, like cholinergic agonists, promote the action of acetylcholine at receptor sites. Depending on the site and the drug's dose and duration of action, they can produce a stimulant or depressant effect on cholinergic receptors.

From minutes to weeks

Reversible anticholinesterase drugs block the breakdown of acetylcholine for minutes to hours, while the blocking effect of the irreversible anticholinesterase drugs lasts for days or weeks.

Pharmacotherapeutics

Anticholinesterase drugs have a variety of therapeutic uses. They're used:
• to reduce eye pressure in patients with glaucoma and during eye surgery
• to increase bladder tone
• to improve tone and peristalsis (movement) through the GI tract in patients with reduced motility and paralytic ileus (paralysis of the small intestine)
• to promote muscular contraction in patients with myasthenia gravis
• to diagnose myasthenia gravis (neostigmine and edrophonium are used for this purpose)
• as an antidote to cholinergic blocking drugs (also called anticholinergic drugs), tricyclic antidepressants, belladonna alkaloids, and narcotics
• to treat mild to moderate dementia of the Alzheimer's type.

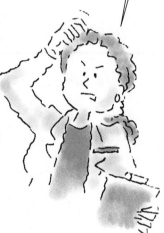

Depending on the dosage, anticholinesterase drugs can produce a stimulant or a depressant effect on receptors.

Drug interactions

These interactions can occur with anticholinesterase drugs:

• Other cholinergic drugs, particularly cholinergic agonists (such as bethanechol, carbachol, and pilocarpine), increase the risk of a toxic effect when taken with anticholinesterase drugs.

• Carbamazepine, dexamethasone, rifampin, phenytoin, and phenobarbital may increase the rate of elimination of donepezil.

• Aminoglycoside antibiotics, anesthetics, cholinergic blocking drugs (such as atropine, belladonna, propantheline, and scopolamine), magnesium, corticosteroids, and antiarrhythmic drugs (such as procainamide and quinidine) can reduce the effects of anticholinesterase drugs and can mask early signs of a cholinergic crisis. (See *Adverse reactions to anticholinesterase drugs.*)

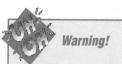 *Warning!*

Adverse reactions to anticholinesterase drugs

Most of the adverse reactions caused by anticholinesterase drugs are the result of increased action of acetylcholine at receptor sites. Adverse reactions associated with these drugs include:
• nausea and vomiting
• diarrhea
• shortness of breath, wheezing, or tightness in the chest
• seizures.

Cholinergic blocking drugs

Cholinergic blocking drugs interrupt parasympathetic nerve impulses in the central and autonomic nervous systems. These drugs are also referred to as anticholinergic drugs because they prevent acetylcholine from stimulating cholinergic receptors.

Not all receptors are receptive

Cholinergic blocking drugs don't block all cholinergic receptors, just the muscarinic receptor sites. Muscarinic receptors are cholinergic receptors that are stimulated by the alkaloid muscarine and blocked by atropine.

First come the belladonna alkaloids

The major cholinergic blocker drugs are the belladonna alkaloids:
• atropine (the prototype cholinergic blocking drug)
• belladonna
• homatropine
• hyoscyamine sulfate
• scopolamine hydrobromide.

Next come their synthetic sisters

Synthetic derivatives of these drugs (the quaternary ammonium drugs) include:
- clidinium
- glycopyrrolate
- propantheline.

In third are the tertiary amines

The tertiary amines include:
- benztropine
- dicyclomine
- ethopropazine
- oxybutynin
- trihexyphenidyl.

Let's talk about it later

Because benztropine, ethopropazine, and trihexyphenidyl are almost exclusively treatments for parkinsonism, they're discussed fully in chapter 3, "Neurologic and neuromuscular drugs."

Pharmacokinetics

Here is how cholinergic blockers move through the body.

Absorption

The belladonna alkaloids are absorbed from the:
- eyes
- GI tract
- mucous membranes
- skin.

The quaternary ammonium drugs and tertiary amines are absorbed primarily through the GI tract, although not as readily as the belladonna alkaloids.

If you want it fast, go I.V.

When administered I.V., cholinergic blockers such as atropine begin to work immediately.

Distribution

The belladonna alkaloids are distributed more widely throughout the body than the quaternary ammonium derivatives or dicyclomine. The alkaloids readily cross the blood-brain barrier; the other drugs in this class don't.

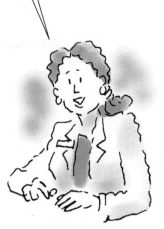

Belladonna alkaloids are less likely to bind with serum proteins. More drug remains available to produce a therapeutic effect.

Metabolism and excretion

The belladonna alkaloids have low to moderate binding with serum proteins. This means that a moderate to high amount of the drug is active and available to produce a therapeutic response. The belladonna alkaloids are metabolized in the liver and excreted by the kidneys as unchanged drug and metabolites.

The quaternary ammonium drugs are a bit more complicated. Hydrolysis occurs in the GI tract and the liver; excretion is in feces and urine. Dicyclomine's metabolism is unknown, but it's excreted equally in feces and urine.

Pharmacodynamics

Cholinergic blockers can have paradoxical effects on the body, depending on the dosage and condition being treated.

Dual duty

The cholinergic blockers can produce a stimulating or depressing effect, depending on the target organ. In the brain, they do both — low drug levels stimulate and high drug levels depress.

Conditional considerations

The effects of a drug in your patient are also determined by the patient's disorder. Parkinsonism, for example, is characterized by low dopamine levels that intensify the stimulating effects of acetylcholine. Cholinergic blockers, however, depress this effect. In other disorders, these same drugs stimulate the CNS.

Pharmacotherapeutics

Cholinergic blockers are often used to treat GI disorders and complications:
• All cholinergic blockers are used to treat spastic or hyperactive conditions of the GI and urinary tracts because they relax muscles and decrease GI secretions. The quaternary ammonium compounds, such as propantheline, are the drugs of choice for these conditions because they cause fewer adverse reactions than the belladonna alkaloids.
• The belladonna alkaloids are used with morphine to treat biliary colic (pain caused by stones in the bile duct).

Overdose of cholinergic blockers causes excessive stimulation of the central nervous system.

• Cholinergic blocking drugs are given by injection before such diagnostic procedures as endoscopy or sigmoidoscopy to relax the GI smooth muscle.

Before surgery

Cholinergic blockers such as atropine are given before surgery to:
• reduce oral and gastric secretions
• reduce secretions in the respiratory system
• prevent a drop in heart rate caused by vagal nerve stimulation during anesthesia.

Brainy belladonna

The belladonna alkaloids can affect the brain in several ways:
• Scopolamine, given with the pain medications morphine or meperidine, causes drowsiness and amnesia in the patient having surgery.
• Scopolamine is used in treating motion sickness.
• Cholinergic blockers can be used to treat extrapyramidal (Parkinson–like) symptoms caused by drugs and in treating Parkinson's disease.

And the beat goes on

The belladonna alkaloids also have important therapeutic effects on the heart. Atropine is the drug of choice to treat:
• symptomatic sinus bradycardia — when the heart beats too slow, causing low blood pressure or dizziness (See *How atropine speeds the heart rate.*)
• arrhythmias resulting from anesthetics, choline esters, or succinylcholine.

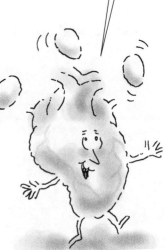

Cholinergic blocking drugs can help me regain my rhythm!

An eye on the problem

Cholinergic blockers also are used as cycloplegics. That means that they:
• paralyze the ciliary muscles of the eye (used for fine focusing)
• alter the shape of the lens of the eye.
    Moreover, cholinergic blockers act as mydriatics to dilate the pupils of the eye, making it easier to measure refractive errors during an eye examination or to perform surgery on the eye.

Now I get it!

How atropine speeds the heart rate

To understand how atropine affects the heart, first consider how the heart's electrical conduction system functions.

Without the drug

When the neurotransmitter acetylcholine is released, the vagus nerve stimulates the sinoatrial (SA) node (the heart's pacemaker) and atrioventricular (AV) node, which controls conduction between the atria and ventricles of the heart. This inhibits electrical conduction and causes the heart rate to slow down.

With the drug

When a patient receives atropine, a cholinergic blocking drug, it competes with acetylcholine for binding with the cholinergic receptors on the SA and AV nodes. By blocking acetylcholine, atropine speeds up the heart rate.

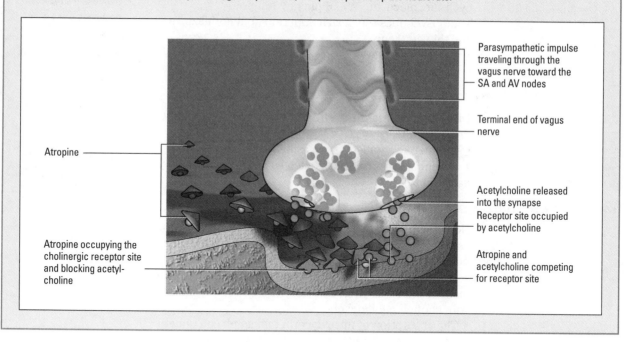

Atropine

Atropine occupying the cholinergic receptor site and blocking acetylcholine

Parasympathetic impulse traveling through the vagus nerve toward the SA and AV nodes

Terminal end of vagus nerve

Acetylcholine released into the synapse

Receptor site occupied by acetylcholine

Atropine and acetylcholine competing for receptor site

Punishing pesticides

The belladonna alkaloids, particularly atropine and hyoscyamine, are effective antidotes to cholinergic and anticholinesterase drugs. Atropine is the drug of choice to treat poisoning from organophosphate pesticides. Atropine and hyoscyamine also counteract the effects of the neuromuscular blocking drugs by competing for the same receptor sites.

Drug interactions

Because cholinergic blockers slow the passage of food and drugs through the stomach, drugs remain in prolonged contact with the mucous membranes of the GI tract. This increases the amount of the drug that is absorbed and, therefore, increases the risk of adverse effects.

Increased effect...

Drugs that increase the effects of cholinergic blocking drugs include:
- disopyramide, tricyclic and tetracyclic antidepressants
- antidyskinetics (such as amantadine)
- antiemetics and antivertigo drugs (such as buclizine, cyclizine, meclizine, and diphenhydramine)
- antipsychotics (such as haloperidol, phenothiazines, and thioxanthenes)
- cyclobenzaprine
- orphenadrine.

...or decreased effect

Drugs that decrease the effects of cholinergic blocking drugs include:
- cholinergic agonists (such as bethanechol)
- anticholinesterase drugs (such as neostigmine and pyridostigmine).

Mixing it up some more

Here are other drug interactions that can occur:
- The risk of digoxin toxicity increases when digoxin is taken with a cholinergic blocker.
- Opiate-like analgesics further enhance the slow movement of food and drugs through the GI tract when taken with cholinergic blockers.
- The absorption of nitroglycerin tablets placed under the tongue is reduced when taken with a cholinergic blocker. (See *Adverse reactions to cholinergic blockers.*)

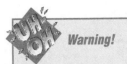 *Warning!*

Adverse reactions to cholinergic blockers

Adverse reactions of cholinergic blockers are closely related to the drug dose. The difference between a therapeutic and a toxic dosage is small with these drugs.

Dried up
Adverse reactions may include:
- dry mouth
- reduced bronchial secretions
- increased heart rate
- decreased sweating.

Adrenergic drugs

Adrenergic drugs are also called sympathomimetic drugs because they produce effects similar to those produced by the sympathetic nervous system.

Classified by chemical...

Adrenergic drugs are classified into two groups based on their chemical structure — catecholamines (both naturally occurring as well as synthetic) and noncatecholamines.

...or by action

Adrenergic drugs are also divided by how they act. They can be:
• *direct-acting*, in which the drug acts directly on the organ or tissue innervated (supplied with nerves or nerve impulses) by the sympathetic nervous system
• *indirect-acting*, in which the drug triggers the release of a neurotransmitter, usually norepinephrine
• *dual-acting*, in which the drug has both direct and indirect actions. (See *Understanding adrenergics*, page 34.)

Which receptor does it affect?

Therapeutic use of adrenergic drugs, catecholamines as well as noncatecholamines, depend on which receptors they stimulate and to what degree. Adrenergic drugs can affect:
• alpha-adrenergic receptors
• beta-adrenergic receptors
• dopamine receptors.

Mimicking norepinephrine and epinephrine

Most of the adrenergic drugs produce their effects by stimulating alpha receptors and beta receptors. These drugs mimic the action of norepinephrine or epinephrine.

Doing it like dopamine

Dopaminergic drugs act primarily on receptors in the sympathetic nervous system stimulated by dopamine.

Catecholamines

Because of their common basic chemical structure, catecholamines share certain properties — they stimulate the nervous system, constrict peripheral blood vessels, increase heart rate, and dilate the bronchi. They can be manufactured in the body or in a laboratory. Common catecholamines include:
• dobutamine

Memory jogger

A drug that is direct-acting has a direct effect on a target organ.

A drug that is indirect-acting triggers a neurotransmitter, and the transmitter takes over from there.

Dual-acting drugs work both ways.

Now I get it!

Understanding adrenergics

Adrenergic drugs are distinguished by how they achieve their effect. The illustrations below show the action of direct-, indirect-, and dual-acting adrenergics.

Direct-acting adrenergic action
Direct-acting adrenergic drugs directly stimulate adrenergic receptors.

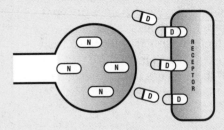

Indirect-acting adrenergic action
Indirect-acting adrenergic drugs stimulate the release of norepinephrine from nerve endings into the synapse.

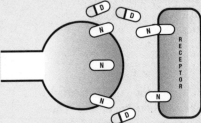

Dual-acting adrenergic action
Dual-acting adrenergic drugs stimulate both adrenergic receptor sites and the release of norepinephrine from nerve endings.

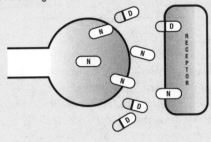

Key:
(N) Norepinephrine   (D) Adrenergic drug

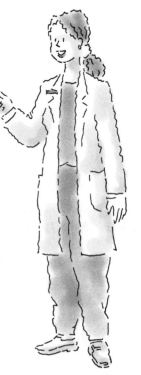

Adrenergic drugs can be direct-acting, indirect-acting, or both.

- dopamine
- epinephrine, epinephrine bitartrate, and epinephrine hydrochloride
- norepinephrine (levarterenol)
- isoproterenol hydrochloride and isoproterenol sulfate.

Pharmacokinetics

Catecholamines can't be taken orally because they're destroyed by digestive enzymes. In contrast, when these drugs are given sublingually (under the tongue), they're rapidly absorbed through the mucous membranes. Any sublingual drug not completely absorbed is rapidly metabolized by swallowed saliva.

Subcutaneously slow

S.C. absorption is slowed because these drugs cause the blood vessels around the injection site to constrict.

I.M. absorption is more rapid because there is less constriction of local blood vessels.

Distribution and metabolism

Catecholamines are widely distributed in the body. They're metabolized and inactivated predominantly in the liver but can also be metabolized in the:

- GI tract
- lungs
- kidneys
- plasma
- other tissues.

Excretion

Catecholamines are excreted primarily in the urine; however, a small amount of isoproterenol is excreted in the feces and some epinephrine is excreted in breast milk.

Pharmacodynamics

Catecholamines are primarily direct-acting. When catecholamines combine with alpha receptors or beta receptors, they cause either an excitatory or inhibitory effect. Typically, activation of alpha receptors generates an excitatory response except for intestinal relaxation. Activation of the beta receptors mostly produces an inhibitory response except in the cells of the heart, where norepinephrine produces excitatory effects.

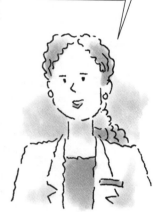

Catecholamines are ineffective when taken orally because they're destroyed by digestive enzymes.

Memory jogger

To help you remember the effects of catecholamines on alpha and beta receptors, remember that A stands for alpha (and *activation*, suggesting an excitatory response), and B stands for beta (or *banished*, which suggests an inhibitory effect).

How heartening

The clinical effects of catecholamines depend on the dosage and the route of administration. Catecholamines are potent inotropes — they make the heart contract more forcefully. As a result, the ventricles of the heart empty more completely with each heart beat, increasing the workload of the heart and the amount of oxygen it needs to do this harder work.

Catecholamines increase my workload.

Rapid rates

Catecholamines also produce a positive chronotropic effect, which means they cause the heart to beat faster. That is because the pacemaker cells in the sinoatrial (SA) node of the heart depolarize at a faster rate. As catecholamines cause blood vessels to constrict and blood pressure to rise, the heart rate can fall as the body tries to prevent an excessive rise in blood pressure.

Fascinating rhythm

Catecholamines can cause the Purkinje fibers (an intricate web of fibers that carry electrical impulses into the ventricles of the heart) to fire spontaneously, possibly producing abnormal heart rhythms, such as premature ventricular contractions and fibrillation. Epinephrine is more likely than norepinephrine to produce this spontaneous firing.

Pharmacotherapeutics

The therapeutic use of catecholamines depends on the particular receptor activity that is activated. Of the catecholamines:
- norepinephrine has the most nearly pure alpha activity
- dobutamine and isoproterenol have only beta-related therapeutic uses
- epinephrine stimulates alpha receptors and beta receptors
- dopamine primarily exhibits dopaminergic activity.

Boosting blood pressure

Catecholamines that stimulate alpha receptors are used to treat low blood pressure (hypotension). As a rule,

catecholamines work best when used to treat hypotension caused by:
• relaxation of the muscles of the blood vessels (also called a loss of vasomotor tone)
• blood loss (such as from hemorrhage).

Restoring the rhythm

Catecholamines that stimulate $beta_1$ receptors are used to treat:
• bradycardia
• heart block (a delay or interruption in the conduction of electrical impulses between the atria and ventricles)
• low cardiac output
• paroxysmal atrial or nodal tachycardia (bursts of rapid heart rate).

It's electric

Because they're believed to make the heart more responsive to defibrillation (using an electrical current to terminate a deadly arrhythmia), $beta_1$-adrenergic drugs are used in treatment of:
• ventricular fibrillation (quivering of the ventricles resulting in no pulse)
• asystole (no electrical activity in the heart)
• cardiac arrest.

Better breathing

Catecholamines that exert $beta_2$ activity are used to treat:
• acute and chronic bronchial asthma
• emphysema
• bronchitis
• acute hypersensitivity (allergic) reactions to drugs.

Kind to the kidneys

Dopamine, which stimulates the dopaminergic receptors, is used in low doses to improve blood flow to the kidneys because it dilates the renal blood vessels.

Synthetic vs. natural

The effects of catecholamines produced by the body differ somewhat from the effects of manufactured catecholamines. Manufactured catecholamines have a short duration of action, which can limit their therapeutic usefulness.

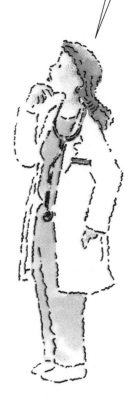

Catecholamines have a wide variety of therapeutic uses but the adverse effects can impact almost all body systems.

Drug interactions

Drug interactions involving catecholamines can be serious, causing hypotension, hypertension (high blood pressure), arrhythmias, seizures, and high blood glucose levels in diabetic patients. Some drugs can cause serious interactions when taken with catecholamines:

• Alpha blockers, such as phentolamine, can produce hypotension.
• Insulin and oral antidiabetic drugs can result in high blood glucose levels.
• Beta blockers, such as propranolol, can lead to hypertension, bronchial constriction, or asthma.
• Sympathomimetics can produce additive, or double, effects, such as hypertension and arrhythmias, as well as enhance adverse effects.
• Tricyclic antidepressants can lead to hypertension.
(See *Adverse reactions to catecholamines.*)

Noncatecholamines

Noncatecholamine adrenergic drugs have a variety of therapeutic uses because of the many effects these drugs can have on the body, including:

• local or systemic constriction of blood vessels (mephentermine, metaraminol, methoxamine, and phenylephrine)
• nasal and eye decongestion and dilation of the bronchioles (albuterol, ephedrine, isoetharine hydrochloride, isoetharine mesylate, metaproterenol, and terbutaline)
• smooth-muscle relaxation (ritodrine hydrochloride and terbutaline).

Pharmacokinetics

While these drugs are all excreted through the urine, they're absorbed in different ways.

Absorption and distribution

Absorption of the noncatecholamine adrenergic drugs depends on the route of administration:

• Inhaled drugs, such as albuterol, are gradually absorbed from the bronchi of the lungs and result in lower drug levels in the body.

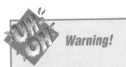

Warning!

Adverse reactions to catecholamines

Adverse reactions to catecholamines can include:
• restlessness
• anxiety
• dizziness
• headache
• palpitations
• cardiac arrhythmias
• hypotension
• hypertension and hypertensive crisis
• stroke
• angina
• increased blood glucose levels
• tissue necrosis and sloughing (if any catecholamine given I.V. leaks into the surrounding tissue).

• Oral drugs are absorbed well from the GI tract and are distributed widely in the body fluids and tissues.
• Some noncatecholamine drugs (such as ephedrine) cross the blood-brain barrier and can be found in high concentrations in the brain and cerebrospinal fluid (fluid that moves through and protects the brain and spinal canal).

Metabolism

Metabolism and inactivation of noncatecholamines occur primarily in the liver but can also occur in the lungs, GI tract, and other tissues.

Excretion

Noncatecholamine drugs and their metabolites are excreted primarily in the urine. Some, such as inhaled albuterol, are excreted within 24 hours; others, such as oral albuterol, within 3 days. Acidic urine increases excretion of many noncatecholamines; alkaline urine slows excretion.

Pharmacodynamics

Noncatecholamines can be direct-acting, indirect-acting, or dual-acting (unlike catecholamines, which are primarily direct-acting):
• Direct-acting noncatecholamines that stimulate alpha activity include methoxamine and phenylephrine. Those that selectively exert beta$_2$ activity include albuterol, isoetharine, metaproterenol, ritodrine, and terbutaline.
• Indirect-acting noncatecholamines include phenylpropanolamine.
• Dual-acting noncatecholamines include ephedrine, mephentermine, and metaraminol.

Pharmacotherapeutics

Noncatecholamines stimulate the sympathetic nervous system and produce a variety of effects in the body. Metaraminol, for example, causes vasoconstriction and is used to treat hypotension in cases of severe shock. Ritodrine is used to stop preterm labor.

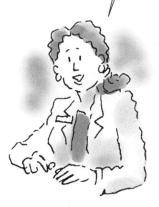

Unlike catecholamines, noncatecholamines aren't destroyed by digestive enzymes and can be given orally.

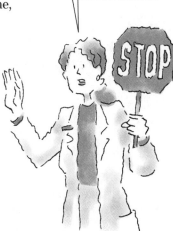

Monoamine oxidase inhibitors interact dangerously with noncatecholamine drugs — possibly resulting in death.

Drug interactions

Here are a few examples of drugs that interact with non-catecholamines:

• Anesthetics (general), cyclopropane, and halogenated hydrocarbons can cause arrhythmias. Hypotension can also occur if taken with noncatecholamines that have predominantly beta$_2$ activity, such as ritodrine and terbutaline.

• Monoamine oxidase inhibitors can cause severe hypertension and even death.

• Oxytocic drugs that stimulate the uterus to contract can be inhibited when taken with terbutaline or ritodrine. When taken with other noncatecholamines, oxytocic drugs can cause hypertensive crisis or a stroke.

• Tricyclic antidepressants can cause hypertension and arrhythmias.

• Urine alkalizers, such as acetazolamide and sodium bicarbonate, slow excretion of noncatecholamine drugs, prolonging their action. (See *Adverse reactions to noncatecholamines.*)

Adrenergic blocking drugs

Adrenergic blocking drugs, also called sympatholytic drugs, are used to disrupt sympathetic nervous system function. These drugs work by blocking impulse transmission (and thus sympathetic nervous system stimulation) at adrenergic neurons or adrenergic receptor sites. Their action at these sites can be exerted by:

• interrupting the action of sympathomimetic (adrenergic) drugs

• reducing available norepinephrine

• preventing the action of cholinergic drugs.

Classified information

Adrenergic blocking drugs are classified according to their site of action as:

• alpha-adrenergic blockers

• beta-adrenergic blockers.

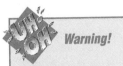

Warning!

Adverse reactions to noncatecholamines

Adverse reactions to noncatecholamine drugs may include:

• headache
• restlessness
• anxiety or euphoria
• irritability
• trembling
• drowsiness or insomnia
• light-headedness
• incoherence
• seizures
• hypertension or hypotension
• palpitations
• bradycardia or tachycardia
• irregular heart rhythm
• cardiac arrest
• cerebral hemorrhage
• tingling or coldness in the arms or legs
• pallor or flushing
• angina
• changes in heart rate and blood pressure in a pregnant woman and fetus.

Alpha-adrenergic blockers

Alpha-adrenergic blocking drugs work by interrupting the actions of the catecholamines epinephrine and norepinephrine at alpha receptors. This results in:
- relaxation of the smooth muscle in the blood vessels
- increased dilation of blood vessels
- decreased blood pressure.
    Drugs in this class include:
- ergoloid mesylates
- ergotamine
- phenoxybenzamine
- phentolamine
- prazosin.

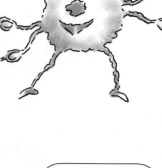

Adrenergic blocking drugs block stimulation of the sympathetic nervous system.

A mixed bag

Ergotamine is a mixed alpha agonist and antagonist; at high doses, it acts as an alpha blocker.

Pharmacokinetics

The action of alpha blockers in the body isn't well understood. Most of these drugs are absorbed erratically when administered orally and more rapidly and completely when administered sublingually. The various alpha blockers vary considerably in their onset of action, peak concentration levels, and duration of action.

Pharmacodynamics

Alpha blockers work in one of two ways:
- They interfere with or block the synthesis, storage, release, and reuptake of norepinephrine by neurons.
- They antagonize epinephrine, norepinephrine, or adrenergic (sympathomimetic) drugs at alpha receptor sites.

Not very discriminating

Although alpha receptor sites are either $alpha_1$ or $alpha_2$ receptors, alpha blockers include drugs that block stimulation of $alpha_1$ receptors and that may block $alpha_2$ stimulation.

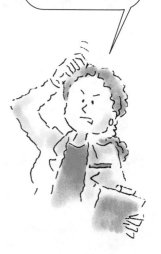

Let's face it — the action of alpha-adrenergic blockers is a bit puzzling.

Now I get it!

How alpha-adrenergic blockers affect peripheral blood vessels

By occupying alpha receptor sites, alpha-adrenergic blocking drugs cause the blood vessel walls to relax. This leads to dilation of the blood vessels and reduced peripheral vascular resistance (the pressure that blood must overcome as it flows in a vessel).

One result: Orthostatic hypotension
These effects can cause orthostatic hypotension, which is a drop in blood pressure that occurs when changing position from lying down to standing. Redistribution of blood to the dilated blood vessels of the legs causes hypotension.

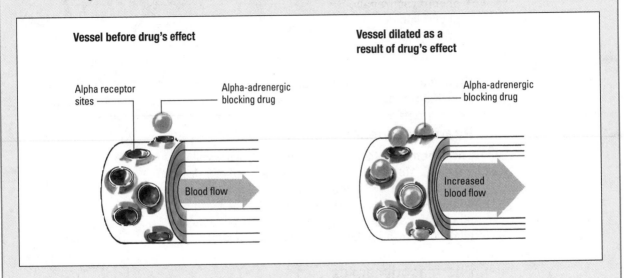

Reducing resistance

Alpha blockers occupy alpha receptor sites on the smooth muscle of blood vessels. (See *How alpha-adrenergic blockers affect peripheral blood vessels*.)

This prevents catecholamines from occupying and stimulating the receptor sites. As a result, blood vessels dilate, increasing local blood flow to the skin and other organs. The decreased peripheral vascular resistance (resistance to blood flow) helps to decrease blood pressure.

Sympathetic response?

The therapeutic effect of an alpha blocker depends on the sympathetic tone (the state of partial constriction of blood vessels) in the body before the drug is administered. For instance, when the drug is given with the patient lying down, only a small change in blood pressure occurs. In this position, the sympathetic nerves release very little norepinephrine.

Patient stands up, blood pressure goes down

On the other hand, when a patient stands up, norepinephrine is released to constrict the veins and shoot blood back up to the heart. If the patient receives an alpha blocker, however, the veins can't constrict and blood pools in the legs. Because blood return to the heart is reduced, blood pressure drops. This drop in blood pressure that occurs when a person stands up is called *orthostatic hypotension.*

Alpha-adrenergic blockers produce only a small change in blood pressure if your patient is lying down but...

Pharmacotherapeutics

Because alpha blockers cause smooth muscles to relax and blood vessels to dilate, they increase local blood flow to the skin and other organs and reduce blood pressure. As a result, they're used to treat:
• hypertension
• peripheral vascular disorders (disease of the blood vessels of the extremities), especially those in which spasm of the blood vessels causes poor local blood flow such as Raynaud's disease (intermittent pallor, cyanosis, or redness of fingers), acrocyanosis (symmetrical mottled cyanosis [bluish color] of the hands and feet), and frostbite
• pheochromocytoma (a catecholamine-secreting tumor causing severe hypertension).

...when the patient stands, the drug prevents her veins from constricting — causing a drastic drop in blood pressure.

Drug interactions

Many drugs interact with alpha-adrenergic blocking drugs, producing a synergistic or exaggerated effect. The most serious include severe hypotension or vascular collapse.

The following interactions can occur when these drugs are taken with ergoloid mesylates and ergotamine:
• Caffeine and macrolide antibiotics can increase the effects of ergotamine.
• Dopamine increases the pressor (rise in blood pressure) effect.

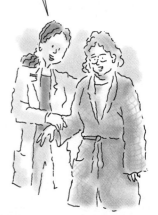

• Nitroglycerin can produce hypotension due to excessive dilation of blood vessels.
• Sympathomimetics, including many over-the-counter drugs, can increase the stimulating effects on the heart. Hypotension with rebound hypertension can occur. (See *Adverse reactions to alpha-adrenergic blocking drugs.*)

Beta-adrenergic blockers

Beta-adrenergic blockers, the most widely used adrenergic blockers, prevent stimulation of the sympathetic nervous system by inhibiting the action of catecholamines at beta-adrenergic receptors. These drugs are commonly referred to as "beta blockers."

From not so selective...

Beta-adrenergic drugs are selective or nonselective. Nonselective beta-adrenergic drugs affect:
• beta$_1$ receptor sites (located mainly in the heart)
• beta$_2$ receptor sites (located in the bronchi, blood vessels, and uterus).

Nonselective beta-adrenergic blocking drugs include carvedilol, labetalol, levobunolol hydrochloride, penbutolol sulfate, pindolol, sotalol, nadolol, propranolol, and timolol.

...to highly discriminating

Selective beta-adrenergic blockers primarily affect the beta$_1$-adrenergic sites only. They include acebutolol, atenolol, betaxolol, bisoprolol, esmolol, and metoprolol tartrate.

The not so beta blockers

Some beta-adrenergic blockers, such as pindolol and acebutolol, have intrinsic sympathetic activity. This means that instead of attaching to beta receptors and blocking them, these beta blockers attach to beta receptors and stimulate them. These drugs are sometimes classified as partial agonists.

Pharmacokinetics

Beta-adrenergic blockers are usually absorbed rapidly and well from the GI tract and are protein-bound to some extent. Food doesn't inhibit their absorption and can en-

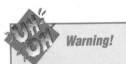

Warning!

Adverse reactions to alpha-adrenergic blocking drugs

Most adverse reactions associated with alpha blockers are caused primarily by dilation of the blood vessels. They include:
• orthostatic hypotension or severe hypertension
• bradycardia or tachycardia
• edema
• difficulty breathing
• light-headedness
• flushing
• arrhythmias
• angina
• heart attack
• spasm of the blood vessels in the brain
• a shocklike state.

hance absorption of some drugs. Some beta-adrenergic blockers are absorbed more completely than others.

Peak by I.V.

The onset of action of beta-adrenergic blockers is primarily dose- and drug-dependent. The time it takes to reach peak concentration levels depends on the route of administration. Beta blockers given I.V. reach peak levels much more rapidly than when given by mouth.

Distribution
Beta-adrenergic blockers are distributed widely in body tissues, with the highest concentrations found in the:
- heart
- liver
- lungs
- saliva.

Metabolism and excretion
With the exception of nadolol and atenolol, beta-adrenergic blockers are metabolized in the liver. They're excreted primarily in the urine, as metabolites or in unchanged form, but can also be excreted in feces and bile with some secretion in breast milk.

Pharmacodynamics
Beta-adrenergic blockers have widespread effects in the body because they produce their blocking action not only at adrenergic nerve endings but also in the adrenal medulla. Here are some of the specific effects this can create.

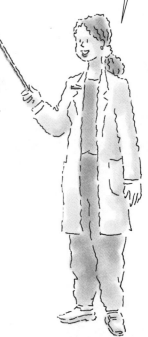

The onset and peak of beta blockers varies widely, depending on the route of administration.

A matter of the heart

Effects on the heart include increased peripheral vascular resistance, decreased blood pressure, decreased force of the contractions of the heart, decreased oxygen consumption by the heart, slowed conduction of impulses between the atria and ventricles of the heart, and decreased cardiac output (the amount of blood pumped by the heart each minute). (See *How beta-adrenergic blockers work*, page 46.)

Selective and nonselective effects

Some of the effects of beta-adrenergic blocking drugs depend on whether the drug is classified as selective or nonselective.

Now I get it!

How beta-adrenergic blockers work

By occupying beta receptor sites, beta-adrenergic blockers prevent catecholamines (norepineph-rine and epinephrine) from occupying these sites and exerting their stimulating effects. This illus-tration shows the effects of beta-adrenergic blockers on the heart, lungs, and blood vessels.

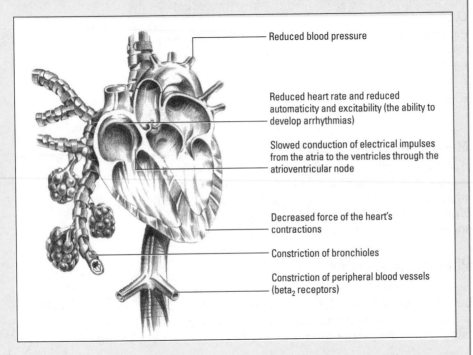

Reduced blood pressure

Reduced heart rate and reduced automaticity and excitability (the ability to develop arrhythmias)

Slowed conduction of electrical impulses from the atria to the ventricles through the atrioventricular node

Decreased force of the heart's contractions

Constriction of bronchioles

Constriction of peripheral blood vessels (beta$_2$ receptors)

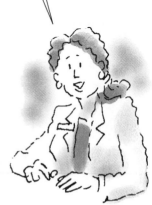

Beta blockers typically cause few adverse reactions but...

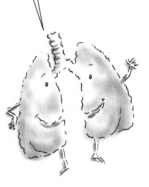

...because of the potential for bronchospasm, they should be used with extreme care in patients suffering from respiratory disorders.

Selective beta-adrenergic blockers, which preferen-tially block beta$_1$ receptor sites, reduce stimulation of the heart. They're often referred to as cardioselective beta-adrenergic blockers.

Nonselective beta-adrenergic blockers, which block both beta$_1$ and beta$_2$ receptor sites, not only reduce stim-ulation of the heart but also cause the bronchioles of the lungs to constrict. For instance, nonselective beta-adrenergic blockers can cause bronchospasm in patients with chronic obstructive lung disorders. This adverse effect isn't seen when cardioselective drugs are given at lower doses.

Pharmacotherapeutics

Beta blockers are used to treat many conditions and are under investigation for use in many more. As mentioned earlier, their clinical usefulness is based largely (but not exclusively) on how they affect the heart. (See *Are beta-adrenergic blockers underused in the elderly?*)

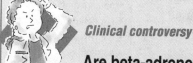

Helping the heart

Beta-adrenergic blockers can be prescribed after a heart attack to prevent another heart attack or to treat:
- angina (chest pain)
- hypertension
- hypertrophic cardiomyopathy (a disease of the heart muscle)
- supraventricular arrhythmias (irregular heartbeats that originate in the atria, SA node, or atrioventricular node).

Jack of all trades

Beta-adrenergic blockers are also used to treat:
- anxiety
- cardiovascular symptoms associated with thyrotoxicosis (overproduction of thyroid hormones)
- essential tremor

Clinical controversy

Are beta-adrenergic blockers underused in the elderly?

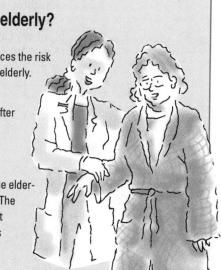

Research has clearly shown that beta-adrenergic blocker use after a heart attack reduces the risk of death and another heart attack. Even so, these drugs aren't being prescribed for the elderly.

What one study found

One study found that only 34% of patients were prescribed a beta-adrenergic blocker after discharge from the hospital following a heart attack. The least likely patients to receive beta-adrenergic blockers included very sick patients, blacks, and the elderly.

Why?

The chief investigator of a study that looked at the use of beta-adrenergic blockers in the elderly believes that many doctors fear the adverse effects of these drugs on older patients. The study suggested that a beta-adrenergic blocker can be given safely to an elderly patient after a heart attack if the lowest effective dose of a selective beta-adrenergic blocker is prescribed.

- migraine headaches
- open-angle glaucoma
- pheochromocytoma.

Drug interactions

Many drugs can interact with beta-adrenergic blocking drugs to cause potentially dangerous effects. Some of the most serious effects include cardiac depression, arrhythmias, respiratory depression, severe bronchospasm, and severe hypotension that can lead to vascular collapse. Here are some others:

• Increased effects or toxicity can occur when digoxin, calcium channel blockers (primarily verapamil), and cimetidine are taken with beta-adrenergic blockers.

• Decreased effects can occur when antacids, calcium salts, barbiturates, anti-inflammatories (such as indomethacin and salicylates), and rifampin are taken with beta blockers.

• Potential lidocaine toxicity can occur when it's taken with beta blockers.

• The requirements for insulin and oral antidiabetic drugs can be altered when taken with beta-adrenergic blockers.

• The ability of theophylline to produce bronchodilation is impaired by nonselective beta-adrenergic blockers.

• Clonidine taken with a nonselective beta-adrenergic blocker can result in life-threatening hypertension during clonidine withdrawal.

• Sympathomimetics and nonselective beta-adrenergic blockers can cause hypertension and reflex bradycardia. (See *Adverse reactions to beta-adrenergic blockers.*)

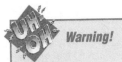

Warning!

Adverse reactions to beta-adrenergic blockers

Beta-adrenergic blockers generally cause few adverse reactions; the adverse reactions that do occur are drug- or dose-dependent and include:

• hypotension
• bradycardia
• peripheral vascular insufficiency
• atrioventricular block
• heart failure
• bronchospasm
• diarrhea or constipation
• nausea and vomiting
• abdominal discomfort
• anorexia
• flatulence
• rash
• fever with sore throat
• spasm of the larynx
• respiratory distress (allergic response).

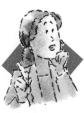

Quick quiz

1. During bethanechol therapy, which common adverse reactions do you expect to observe?
   A. Dry mouth, flushed face, and constipation
   B. Fasciculations, dysphagia, and respiratory distress
   C. Nausea, vomiting, diarrhea, and intestinal cramps

Answer: C. Bethanechol is a cholinergic agonist. Common adverse reactions to cholinergic agonists include such GI symptoms as nausea, vomiting, diarrhea, and intestinal cramps.

2. Your patient is scheduled for hip replacement surgery. The cholinergic blocker atropine to is be given I.M. 1 hour before surgery. This medication is given before surgery to:
   A. reduce reflexes during surgery.
   B. minimize the risk of abdominal problems after surgery.
   C. dry up oral and gastric secretions.

Answer: C. The cholinergic blocker atropine is typically given 1 hour before surgery to dry up oral and gastric secretions.

3. Like the other catecholamines, epinephrine isn't administered orally. Why?
   A. Catecholamines are destroyed by digestive enzymes.
   B. Catecholamine absorption after oral administration is delayed and unpredictable.
   C. Normal intestinal flora block catecholamine absorption from the GI tract.

Answer: A. Because catecholamines are destroyed by digestive enzymes, they aren't administered orally. They're absorbed slowly when administered S.C. but rapidly when administered sublingually or I.M.

4. Catecholamines act as potent inotropes. That means that they:
- A.   cause the heart to contract forcefully.
- B.   slow the heart rate.
- C.   lower blood pressure.

Answer: A. Catecholamines cause the heart to contract forcefully, increasing the heart's workload. They also cause the heart to beat faster and raise blood pressure.

5. Noncatecholamines can interact with monoamine oxidase inhibitors to cause:
- A.   arrhythmias.
- B.   severe hypertension.
- C.   seizures.

Answer: B. Noncatecholamines can interact very dangerously with monoamine oxidase inhibitors, causing severe hypertension and even death.

6. Beta-adrenergic blockers have widespread effects because they produce their blocking action in the:
- A.   hypothalamus.
- B.   adrenal medulla.
- C.   pituitary gland.

Answer: B. Beta-adrenergic blockers have widespread effects in the body because they produce their blocking action not only at adrenergic nerve endings but also in the adrenal medulla.

Scoring

☆☆☆   If you answered all six questions correctly, fabulous! You're automatic with the autonomic nervous system.

☆☆   If you answered four or five questions correctly, great! You've had nothing but positive interactions with these drugs.

☆   If you answered fewer than four questions correctly, don't worry. Like the nervous system, you have a lot of information to coordinate. Just review the chapter and try again.

3

Neurologic and neuromuscular drugs

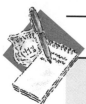

Just the facts

In this chapter, you'll review:

♦ classes of drugs used to treat neurologic and neuromuscular disorders

♦ uses and varying actions of these drugs

♦ how these drugs are absorbed, distributed, metabolized, and excreted

♦ drug interactions and adverse reactions to these drugs.

Skeletal muscle relaxants

Skeletal muscle relaxants relieve musculoskeletal pain or spasm and severe musculoskeletal spasticity (stiff, awkward movements). They're used to treat acute, painful musculoskeletal conditions and the muscle spasticity associated with multiple sclerosis (MS) (a progressive demyelination of the white matter of the brain and spinal cord causing widespread neurologic dysfunction), cerebral palsy (a motor function disorder caused by neurologic damage), stroke (reduced oxygen supply to the brain resulting in neurologic deficits), and spinal cord injuries (injuries to the spinal cord that can result in paralysis or death).

This chapter discusses:
• the two main classes of skeletal muscle relaxants — centrally acting and peripherally acting
• baclofen and diazepam, two other drugs used to manage musculoskeletal disorders.

Cycling problems

Exposure to severe cold, lack of blood flow to a muscle, or overexertion can send sensory impulses from the posterior sensory nerve fibers to the spinal cord and the higher levels of the central nervous system (CNS). These sensory impulses can cause a reflex (involuntary) muscle contraction or spasm from trauma, epilepsy, hypocalcemia (low calcium levels), or muscular disorders. The muscle contraction further stimulates the sensory receptors to a more intense contraction, establishing a cycle. Centrally acting muscle relaxants are believed to break this cycle by acting as CNS depressants.

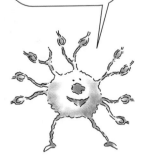

Spasticity can be caused by a cyclical pattern of impulses...

Centrally acting skeletal muscle relaxants

Centrally acting skeletal muscle relaxants, which act on the central nervous system, are used to treat acute spasms, caused by such conditions as:
- anxiety
- inflammation
- pain
- trauma.

Not for chronic disease

Centrally acting skeletal muscle relaxants aren't very effective in treating the patient with spasticity caused by a chronic neurologic disease such as cerebral palsy.

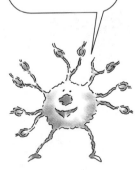

...and skeletal muscle relaxants help to break the pattern.

Options for acute spasms

A patient with acute muscle spasms may receive one of the following drugs:
- carisoprodol
- chlorphenesin
- chlorzoxazone
- cyclobenzaprine
- metaxalone
- methocarbamol
- orphenadrine.

Pharmacokinetics (how drugs circulate)

There is still a lot we don't know about how centrally acting skeletal muscle relaxants circulate within the body. In general, these drugs are absorbed from the GI tract, widely distributed in the body, metabolized in the liver, and excreted by the kidneys.

Cyclobenzaprine sticks around

When these drugs are administered orally, it can take from 30 minutes to 1 hour for effects to be achieved. While the duration of action of most of these drugs varies from 4 to 6 hours, cyclobenzaprine has the longest duration of action at 12 to 25 hours.

Pharmacodynamics (how drugs act)

The centrally acting drugs don't relax skeletal muscles directly or depress neuronal conduction, neuromuscular transmission, or muscle excitability. While the precise mechanism of action of centrally acting drugs is unknown, these drugs are known to be CNS depressants. Skeletal muscle relaxant effects can be related to their sedative effects.

Pharmacotherapeutics (how drugs are used)

Patients receive centrally acting skeletal muscle relaxants to treat acute, painful musculoskeletal conditions. They're usually prescribed along with rest and physical therapy.

Drug interactions

The centrally acting skeletal muscle relaxants interact with other CNS depressants (including alcohol, narcotics, barbiturates, anticonvulsants, tricyclic antidepressants, and antianxiety drugs), causing increased sedation, impaired motor function, and respiratory depression. In addition, some of these drugs have other interactions:
• Cyclobenzaprine interacts with monoamine oxidase (MAO) inhibitors and can result in a high body temperature, excitation, and seizures.
• Cyclobenzaprine can decrease the antihypertensive effects of the blood pressure-lowering drugs guanethidine and clonidine.
• Orphenadrine and cyclobenzaprine sometimes enhance the effects of cholinergic blocking drugs.
• Methocarbamol can antagonize the cholinergic effects of the anticholinesterase drugs used to treat myasthenia gravis.

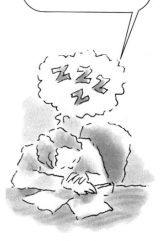

Centrally acting skeletal muscle relaxants should be used to treat painful musculoskeletal conditions along with physical therapy and plenty of rest.

- Orphenadrine can reduce the effects of phenothiazines.
- Orphenadrine and propoxyphene taken together can cause additive CNS effects, including mental confusion, anxiety, and tremors. (See *Adverse reactions to centrally acting skeletal muscle relaxants*.)

Peripherally acting skeletal muscle relaxants

Dantrolene sodium is the most common peripherally acting skeletal muscle relaxant. Although dantrolene has a similar therapeutic effect to the centrally acting drugs, it works through a different mechanism of action. Because its major effect is on the muscle, dantrolene has a lower incidence of adverse CNS effects; high therapeutic doses, however, are toxic to the liver.

In the head

Dantrolene seems most effective for spasticity of cerebral origin. Because it produces muscle weakness, dantrolene is of questionable benefit in patients with borderline strength.

Pharmacokinetics

Although the peak drug concentration of dantrolene occurs within about 5 hours after it's ingested, the patient may not notice any therapeutic benefit for a week or more.

Absorption

Dantrolene is absorbed poorly from the GI tract and is highly plasma protein–bound. This means that only a small portion of the drug is available to produce a therapeutic effect.

Metabolism and excretion

Dantrolene is metabolized by the liver and excreted in the urine. Its elimination half-life in healthy adults is about 9 hours. Because dantrolene is metabolized in the liver, its half-life can be prolonged in patients with impaired liver function.

Pharmacodynamics

Dantrolene is chemically and pharmacologically unrelated to the other skeletal muscle relaxants.

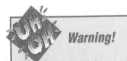
Warning!

Adverse reactions to centrally acting skeletal muscle relaxants

A patient can develop physical and psychological dependence after long-term use of these drugs. Abruptly stopping any of these drugs can cause severe withdrawal symptoms. Other adverse reactions can also occur.

Common reactions
- Dizziness
- Drowsiness

Occasional reactions
- Abdominal distress
- Ataxia
- Constipation
- Diarrhea
- Heartburn
- Nausea and vomiting

Dantrolene works by acting on the muscle itself. It interferes with calcium ion release from the sarcoplasmic reticulum and weakens the force of contractions. At therapeutic concentrations, dantrolene has little effect on cardiac or intestinal smooth muscle.

Pharmacotherapeutics

Dantrolene helps manage all types of spasticity but is most effective in patients with:
- cerebral palsy
- MS
- spinal cord injury
- stroke.

Anesthesia antidote

Dantrolene is also used to treat and prevent malignant hyperthermia. This rare but potentially fatal complication of anesthesia is characterized by skeletal muscle rigidity and high fever. (See *How dantrolene reduces muscle rigidity.*)

Drug interactions

CNS depressants can increase the depressive effects of dantrolene and result in sedation, lack of coordination, and respiratory depression.

Estrogens, when given with dantrolene, can increase the risk of liver toxicity.

Other skeletal muscle relaxants

Two other drugs used as skeletal muscle relaxants are diazepam and baclofen. Diazepam, however, is primarily an antianxiety drug. (See *Diazepam as a skeletal muscle relaxant,* page 56.) This section discusses baclofen only.

Pharmacokinetics

Baclofen is absorbed rapidly from the GI tract. It's distributed widely (with only small amounts crossing the blood-brain barrier), undergoes minimal liver metabolism, and is excreted primarily unchanged in the urine.

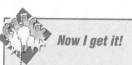
Now I get it!

How dantrolene reduces muscle rigidity

Dantrolene appears to decrease the number of calcium ions released from the sarcoplasmic reticulum (a structure in muscle cells involved in muscle contraction and relaxation by releasing and storing calcium). The lower the calcium level in the muscle plasma or myoplasm, the less energy produced when calcium prompts the muscle's actin and myosin filaments (responsible for muscle contraction) to interact. Less energy means a weaker muscle contraction.

Reducing rigidity, halting hyperthermia
By promoting muscle relaxation, dantrolene prevents or reduces the rigidity that contributes to the life-threatening body temperatures of malignant hyperthermia.

Slow to a stop

It can take from hours to weeks before the patient notices any beneficial effects of baclofen. The elimination half-life of baclofen is 2½ to 4 hours. Abrupt withdrawal of the drug can cause hallucinations, seizures, and worsening of spasticity.

Pharmacodynamics

It isn't known exactly how baclofen works. Baclofen is chemically similar to the neurotransmitter gamma-aminobutyric acid and probably acts in the spinal cord.

Baclofen seems to lessen neuron activity, decreasing the number and severity of muscle spasms, and reduces the associated pain.

Elasticity vs. spasticity

Because baclofen produces less sedation than diazepam and less peripheral muscle weakness than dantrolene, it's the drug of choice to treat spasticity.

Pharmacotherapeutics

Baclofen's major clinical use is for paraplegic or quadriplegic patients with spinal cord lesions, most commonly caused by MS or trauma. For these patients, baclofen significantly reduces the number and severity of painful

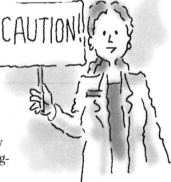

Stopping baclofen treatment abruptly could result in seizures!

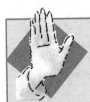

Before you give that drug!

Diazepam as a skeletal muscle relaxant

Diazepam is a benzodiazepine drug that is used to treat acute muscle spasms as well as spasticity caused by chronic disorders. Other uses of diazepam include treating anxiety, alcohol withdrawal, and seizures. It seems to work by promoting the inhibitory effect of the neurotransmitter gamma-aminobutyric acid on muscle contraction.

The negatives: sedation and tolerance

Diazepam can be used alone or with other drugs to treat spasticity, especially in patients with spinal cord lesions and, occasionally, in patients with cerebral palsy. It's also helpful in patients with painful, continuous muscle spasms who aren't too susceptible to the drug's sedative effects. Unfortunately, diazepam's use is limited by its central nervous system effects and the tolerance that develops with prolonged use.

flexor spasms. Aside from these benefits, however, baclofen doesn't improve stiff gait, manual dexterity, or residual muscle function.

Drug interactions

Baclofen has few drug interactions:
• The most significant drug interaction is an increase in CNS depression when baclofen is administered with other CNS depressants, including alcohol.
• Analgesia can be prolonged when fentanyl and baclofen are administered together.
• Lithium carbonate and baclofen taken together can aggravate hyperkinesia (an abnormal increase in motor function or activity).
• Tricyclic antidepressants and baclofen together can increase muscle relaxation. (See *Adverse reactions to baclofen.*)

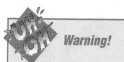

Warning!

Adverse reactions to baclofen

Most common
• Transient drowsiness

Less common
• Nausea
• Fatigue
• Vertigo
• Hypotonia
• Muscle weakness
• Depression
• Headache

Neuromuscular blocking drugs

Neuromuscular blocking drugs relax skeletal muscles by disrupting the transmission of nerve impulses at the motor end plate (the branching terminals of a motor nerve axon). (See *Motor end plate*, page 58.)

Neuromuscular blockers have three major clinical indications:
• to relax skeletal muscles during surgery
• to reduce the intensity of muscle spasms in drug or electrically induced seizures
• to manage patients who are fighting the use of a ventilator to help with breathing.

Two main classifications

There are two main classes of natural and synthetic drugs used as neuromuscular blockers — nondepolarizing and depolarizing.

Nondepolarizing blocking drugs

Nondepolarizing blocking drugs, also called competitive or stabilizing drugs, are derived from curare alkaloids and synthetically similar compounds. They include:
• atracurium

Now I get it!

Motor end plate

The motor nerve axon divides to form branching terminals called motor end plates. These are enfolded in muscle fibers, but separated from the fibers by the synaptic cleft.

Competing with contraction
A stimulus to the nerve causes the release of acetylcholine into the synaptic cleft. There, acetylcholine occupies receptor sites on the muscle cell membrane, depolarizing the membrane and causing muscle contraction. Neuromuscular blocking agents act at the motor end plate by competing with acetylcholine for the receptor sites or by blocking depolarization.

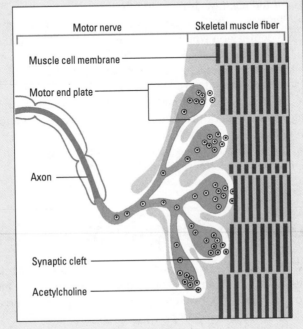

- cisatracurium
- doxacurium
- metocurine
- mivacurium
- pancuronium
- pipecuronium
- rocuronium
- tubocurarine (see *Tubocurarine tale*)
- vecuronium.

Pharmacokinetics

Because nondepolarizing blockers are absorbed poorly from the GI tract, they're administered parenterally. The I.V. route is preferred because the action is more predictable.

Distribution
These drugs are distributed rapidly throughout the body.

Metabolism and excretion
A variable but large proportion of the nondepolarizing drugs is excreted unchanged in the urine. Some drugs, such as atracurium, pancuronium, pipecuronium, and vecuronium, are partially metabolized in the liver.

Pharmacodynamics
Nondepolarizing blockers compete with acetylcholine at the cholinergic receptor sites of the skeletal muscle membrane. This blocks acetylcholine's neurotransmitter action, preventing the muscle from contracting.

The effect can be counteracted by anticholinesterase drugs, such as neostigmine or pyridostigmine, which inhibit the action of acetylcholinesterase, the enzyme that destroys acetylcholine.

From weakness to paralysis
The initial muscle weakness produced by these drugs quickly changes to a flaccid (loss of muscle tone) paralysis that affects the muscles in a specific sequence. The first muscles to exhibit flaccid paralysis are those of the eyes, face, and neck. Next, the limb, abdomen, and trunk muscles become flaccid. Finally, the intercostal muscles (between the ribs) and diaphragm (the breathing muscle) are paralyzed. Recovery from the paralysis usually occurs in the reverse order.

Conscious and aware
Because these drugs don't cross the blood-brain barrier, the patient remains conscious and able to feel pain. Even though the patient is paralyzed, he is aware of what is happening to him and can experience extreme anxiety but can't communicate his feelings. For this reason, an analgesic or antianxiety drug should be administered along with a neuromuscular blocker.

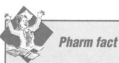

Pharm fact

Tubocurarine tale

Hundreds of years ago, the South American Indians used the neuromuscular blocker tubocurarine to paralyze the skeletal muscles of their enemies. They discovered this drug in the curare plant. The drug was placed on the tip of an arrow and shot at the unfortunate enemy, who quickly became paralyzed. The enemy finally died as his intercostal muscles and diaphragm became paralyzed and he could no longer breathe.

Remember, the effect of these drugs can be frightening for the patient. The patient can't move but is conscious. He can hear conversations and feel pain.

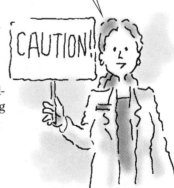

Pharmacotherapeutics

Nondepolarizing blockers are used for intermediate or prolonged muscle relaxation in the following situations to:

• ease the passage of an endotracheal (ET) tube (a tube placed in the trachea)
• decrease the amount of anesthetic required during surgery
• facilitate realigning broken bones and dislocated joints
• paralyze patients who need ventilatory support but who fight the ET tube and ventilation
• prevent muscle injury during electroconvulsive therapy (ECT) (passing an electric current through the brain to treat depression) by reducing the intensity of muscle spasms.

Drug interactions

Several drugs alter the effects of nondepolarizing neuromuscular blockers:

• Aminoglycoside antibiotics and anesthetics potentiate or exaggerate the neuromuscular blockade.
• Drugs that alter the serum levels of the electrolytes calcium, magnesium, or potassium also alter the effects of the nondepolarizing blockers.
• The anticholinesterases (neostigmine, pyridostigmine, and edrophonium) antagonize nondepolarizing blockers and are used as antidotes to them.
• Drugs that can increase the intensity and duration of paralysis when taken with a nondepolarizing blocking drug include inhalation anesthetics, aminoglycosides, carbamazepine, clindamycin, polymyxin, verapamil, quinine derivatives, ketamine, lithium, nitrates, piperacillin, thiazide diuretics, tetracyclines, and magnesium salts.
• Drugs that can cause decreased neuromuscular blockade when taken with a nondepolarizing blocking drug include corticosteroids, hydantoins, ranitidine, and theophylline. (See *Adverse reactions to nondepolarizing blockers.*)

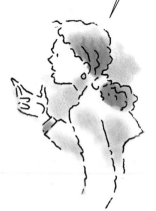

Paralysis from neuromuscular blocking drugs proceeds in a specific sequence. Recovery occurs in the reverse order.

Depolarizing blocking drugs

Succinylcholine is the only therapeutic depolarizing blocking drug. Although it's similar to the nondepolarizing blockers in its therapeutic effect, its mechanism of action differs. Succinylcholine acts like acetylcholine, but it isn't inactivated by cholinesterase. It's the drug of choice when short-term muscle relaxation is needed.

Pharmacokinetics

Because succinylcholine is absorbed poorly from the GI tract, the preferred administration route is I.V.; the I.M. route can be used if necessary.

Metabolism and excretion

Succinylcholine is hydrolyzed in the liver and plasma by the enzyme pseudocholinesterase, producing a metabolite with a nondepolarizing blocking action. Succinylcholine is excreted by the kidneys, with a small amount excreted unchanged.

Pharmacodynamics

After administration, succinylcholine is rapidly metabolized, but at a slower rate than acetylcholine is metabolized. As a result, succinylcholine remains attached to receptor sites on the skeletal muscle membrane for a longer period of time. This prevents repolarization of the motor end plate and results in muscle paralysis.

Pharmacotherapeutics

Succinylcholine is the drug of choice for short-term muscle relaxation, such as during intubation and ECT.

Drug interactions

The action of succinylcholine is potentiated by a number of anesthetics and antibiotics. In contrast to their interaction with nondepolarizing blockers, anticholinesterases increase succinylcholine blockade. (See *Adverse reactions to succinylcholine*, page 62.)

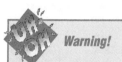

Warning!

Adverse reactions to nondepolarizing blockers

To all drugs
- Apnea
- Hypotension
- Skin reactions
- Bronchospasm
- Excessive bronchial and salivary secretions

To pancuronium
- Tachycardia
- Cardiac arrhythmias
- Hypertension

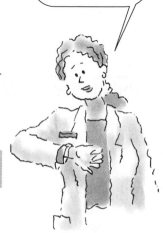

Because succinylcholine is administered I.V. or I.M., it has a very fast onset.

Antiparkinsonian drugs

Drug therapy is an important part of the treatment for Parkinson's disease, a progressive neurologic disorder characterized by four cardinal features:

- muscle rigidity (inflexibility)
- akinesia (loss of muscle movement)
- tremors at rest
- disturbances of posture and balance.

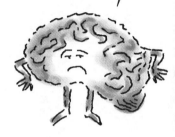

A deficiency of dopamine isn't good news...it prevents me from performing normally.

A defect in the dopamine pathway...

Parkinson's disease affects the extrapyramidal system, which influences movement. The extrapyramidal system includes the corpus striatum, globus pallidus, and substantia nigra of the brain.

In Parkinson's disease, a dopamine deficiency occurs in the basal ganglia, the dopamine-releasing pathway that connects the substantia nigra to the corpus striatum.

...causes an imbalance of neurotransmitters

Reduction of dopamine in the corpus striatum upsets the normal balance between two neurotransmitters, acetylcholine and dopamine. This results in increased cholinergic activity. The excessive excitation caused by cholinergic activity creates the movement disorders of Parkinson's disease.

Other causes

Parkinsonism can also result from drugs, encephalitis, neurotoxins, trauma, arteriosclerosis, or other neurologic disorders and environmental factors.

Two types of drugs

The goals of drug intervention are twofold:
- promoting the secretion of dopamine (with dopaminergic drugs)
- inhibiting cholinergic effects (with anticholinergic drugs).

Anticholinergic drugs

Anticholinergic drugs are sometimes called parasympatholytic drugs because they inhibit the action of acetylcholine at special receptors in the parasympathetic nervous system.

Two classes

Anticholinergics used to treat parkinsonism are classified in two chemical categories according to their chemical structure:

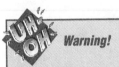

Warning!

Adverse reactions to succinylcholine

The primary adverse drug reactions to succinylcholine are:
- prolonged apnea
- hypotension.

Genetics increases the risk

The risk associated with succinylcholine is increased with certain genetic predispositions, such as a low pseudocholinesterase level and the tendency to develop malignant hyperthermia .

• synthetic tertiary amines, such as benztropine, biperiden hydrochloride, biperiden lactate, procyclidine, and trihexyphenidyl
• antihistamines, such as diphenhydramine and orphenadrine.

Pharmacokinetics

Typically, anticholinergic drugs are well absorbed from the GI tract and cross the blood-brain barrier to their action site in the brain. Most are metabolized in the liver, at least partially, and are excreted by the kidneys as metabolites and unchanged drug. The exact distribution of these drugs is unknown.

Up to 24 hours

Benztropine is a long-acting drug with a duration of action up to 24 hours in some patients. For most anticholinergics, half-life is undetermined. In addition to the oral route, some anticholinergics can also be given I.M. or I.V.

Pharmacodynamics

High acetylcholine levels produce an excitatory effect on the CNS, which can cause parkinsonian tremor. Patients with Parkinson's disease take anticholinergic drugs to inhibit the action of acetylcholine at receptor sites in the CNS and autonomic nervous system, thus reducing the tremor.

Pharmacotherapeutics

Anticholinergics are used to treat all forms of parkinsonism. They're used most commonly in the early stages of Parkinson's disease when symptoms are mild and don't have a major impact on the patient's lifestyle. These drugs effectively control sialorrhea (excessive flow of saliva) and are about 20% effective in reducing the incidence and severity of akinesia and rigidity.

During the early stages...

Anticholinergics can be used alone or with amantadine in the early stages of Parkinson's disease.

...and in the later stages

Anticholinergics can be given with levodopa during the later stages to further relieve symptoms.

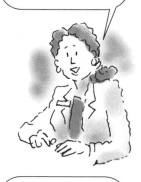

Anticholinergic drugs can be used alone to treat Parkinson's disease...

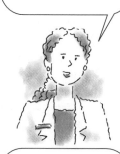

...or with the dopaminergic drug amantidine during the early stages...

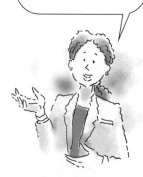

...adding levodopa when the disorder reaches more advanced stages.

Drug interactions

Interactions can occur when certain medications are taken with anticholinergics:
• Amantadine can cause increased anticholinergic adverse effects.
• Absorption of levodopa can be decreased, which could lead to worsening of parkinsonian signs and symptoms.
• Antipsychotics (such as phenothiazines, thiothixene, haloperidol, loxapine) decrease the effectiveness of both anticholinergics and antipsychotics. The incidence of anticholinergic adverse effects can also be increased.
• Over-the-counter cough or cold preparations, diet aids, or analeptics (drugs used to stay awake) increase anticholinergic effects.
• Alcohol increases CNS depression. (See *Adverse reactions to anticholinergics.*)

Dopaminergic drugs

Dopaminergics include drugs that are chemically unrelated:
• levodopa, the metabolic precursor to dopamine
• carbidopa-levodopa, a combination drug composed of carbidopa and levodopa
• amantadine, an antiviral drug
• bromocriptine, a semisynthetic ergot alkaloid
• pergolide and pramipexole, two dopamine agonists
• selegiline, a type B MAO inhibitor.

Pharmacokinetics

Like anticholinergic drugs, dopaminergic drugs are absorbed from the GI tract into the bloodstream and are delivered to their action site in the brain.

Absorption of levodopa is slowed and reduced when it's ingested with food. The body absorbs most levodopa, carbidopa-levodopa, pramipexole, or amantadine from the GI tract after oral administration, but only about 28% of bromocriptine is absorbed. The body can absorb a significant amount of pergolide, although how much is absorbed isn't fully known. About 73% of an oral dose of selegiline is absorbed.

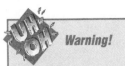

Warning!

Adverse reactions to anticholinergics

Mild, dose-related adverse reactions to anticholinergics are seen in 30% to 50% of patients. Dry mouth may be a dose-related reaction to trihexyphenidyl.

Common reactions
• Confusion
• Restlessness
• Agitation and excitement
• Drowsiness or insomnia
• Tachycardia and palpitations
• Constipation
• Nausea and vomiting
• Urinary retention
• Increased intraocular pressure, blurred vision, pupil dilation, and photophobia

Sensitivity-related reactions
• Hives
• Allergic rashes

Distribution

Levodopa is widely distributed in body tissues, including the GI tract, liver, pancreas, kidneys, salivary glands, and skin. Carbidopa-levodopa and pramipexole are also widely distributed. Amantadine is distributed in saliva, nasal secretions, and breast milk. Bromocriptine and pergolide are highly protein-bound. The distribution of selegiline is unknown.

Metabolism and excretion

Dopaminergic drugs are metabolized extensively in various areas of the body and eliminated by the liver, the kidneys, or both:

• Large amounts of levodopa are metabolized in the stomach and during the first pass through the liver. It's metabolized extensively to various compounds that are excreted by the kidneys.

• Carbidopa isn't metabolized extensively. The kidneys excrete approximately one-third of it as unchanged drug within 24 hours.

• Amantadine and pramipexole are excreted mostly unchanged by the kidneys.

• Almost all of a bromocriptine dose is metabolized by the liver to pharmacologically inactive compounds and primarily eliminated in the feces; only a small amount is excreted in the urine.

• After pergolide is metabolized, it's excreted by the kidneys.

• Selegiline is metabolized to amphetamine, methamphetamine, and N-desmethylselegiline (the major metabolite), which are eliminated in the urine.

Pharmacodynamics

Dopaminergic drugs act in the brain to improve motor function in one of two ways: by increasing the dopamine concentration or by enhancing neurotransmission of dopamine.

Getting the job done

Levodopa is inactive until it crosses the blood-brain barrier and is converted to dopamine by enzymes in the brain, increasing dopamine concentrations in the basal ganglia. Carbidopa enhances levodopa's effectiveness.

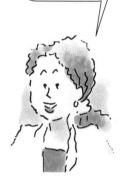

Levodopa, a dopaminergic drug, is the most effective drug used to treat Parkinson's disease.

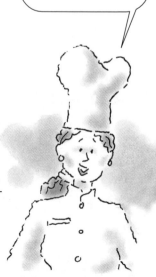

Absorption of levodopa is slowed and reduced when taken with food.

The other dopaminergic drugs have various mechanisms of action:
• Amantadine's mechanism of action isn't clear. It can increase the amount of dopamine in the brain by increasing dopamine release or by blocking dopamine reuptake from presynaptic neurons.
• Bromocriptine and pramipexole stimulate dopamine receptors in the brain, producing effects that are similar to dopamine's.
• Pergolide directly stimulates postsynaptic dopamine receptors in the CNS.
• Selegiline can increase dopaminergic activity by inhibiting type B MAO activity or by other mechanisms.

Pharmacotherapeutics

Usually, dopaminergic drugs are used to treat patients with severe parkinsonism or those who don't respond to anticholinergics alone. Levodopa is the most effective drug used to treat Parkinson's disease; however, it loses its effectiveness after 3 to 5 years. (See *Levodopa toxicity? Or worsening of Parkinson's disease?*)

Add carbidopa, reduce levodopa

When carbidopa is given with levodopa, the dosage of levodopa can be reduced, decreasing the risk of GI and cardiovascular adverse effects.

Tapered treatment

Some dopaminergic drugs, such as amantadine, pramipexole, and bromocriptine, must be gradually tapered to avoid precipitating parkinsonian crisis (sudden marked clinical deterioration) and possible life-threatening complications.

Food competition

In some patients, levodopa can produce a significant interaction with foods. Dietary amino acids can decrease levodopa's effectiveness by competing with it for absorption from the intestine and slowing its transport to the brain.

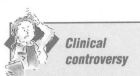

Clinical controversy

Levodopa toxicity? Or worsening of Parkinson's disease?

Levodopa is commonly used to treat Parkinson's disease; however, this use isn't without controversy. Initially, levodopa is very effective in controlling symptoms. But after several years, the effects of the drug sometimes don't last as long (the wearing-off effect) or lead to sharp fluctuations in symptoms (the on-off phenomenon).

Low doses? Or later?
Some doctors feel that levodopa should be used in low doses or started later in the course of the disease. Other doctors feel that these effects are from the progression of Parkinson's disease and not from the effects of levodopa. Some doctors are even concerned that levodopa accelerates the progression of Parkinson's disease by providing a source of free radicals that contribute to the degeneration of dopaminergic neurons.

Drug interactions

There are a number of drug interactions related to dopaminergic drugs, including some that are potentially fatal:

• The effectiveness of levodopa can be reduced when taking pyridoxine (vitamin B$_6$), phenytoin, benzodiazepines, reserpine, and papaverine.

• A type A MAO inhibitor increases the risk of hypertensive crisis.

• Antipsychotics, such as phenothiazines, thiothixene, haloperidol, and loxapine, can reduce the effectiveness of levodopa and pergolide.

• Anticholinergic drugs can increase the anticholinergic effects of amantadine and reduce the absorption of levodopa.

• Meperidine taken with selegiline can cause a fatal reaction. (See *Adverse reactions to dopaminergic drugs*.)

Anticonvulsant drugs

Anticonvulsants inhibit neuromuscular transmission, and are prescribed for:

• long-term management of chronic epilepsy (recurrent seizures)

• short-term management of acute isolated seizures not caused by epilepsy, such as after trauma or brain surgery.

In addition, some anticonvulsants are used in the emergency treatment of status epilepticus (a continuous seizure state).

Five types

Anticonvulsants fall into five major classes:

• hydantoins
• barbiturates
• iminostilbenes
• benzodiazepines
• valproic acid.

Hydantoins

The two most commonly prescribed anticonvulsant drugs—phenytoin and phenytoin sodium—belong to the *hydantoin* class.

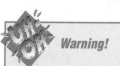

Warning!

Adverse reactions to dopaminergic drugs

Levodopa
• Nausea and vomiting
• Orthostatic hypotension
• Anorexia
• Neuroleptic malignant syndrome
• Arrhythmias
• Irritability
• Confusion

Amantadine
• Orthostatic hypotension
• Constipation

Bromocriptine
• Persistent orthostatic hypotension
• Ventricular tachycardia
• Bradycardia
• Worsening angina

Pergolide
• Confusion
• Dyskinesia
• Hallucinations
• Nausea

Pramipexole
• Orthostatic hypotension
• Dizziness
• Confusion
• Insomnia

Less commonly used hydantoins include fosphenytoin, mephenytoin, and ethotoin.

> The most commonly prescribed anticonvulsant drugs are phenytoin and phenytoin sodium. They share the trade name Dilantin.

Pharmacokinetics

The pharmacokinetics of hydantoins vary from drug to drug.

Phenytoin fits in slowly

Phenytoin is absorbed slowly after both oral and I.M. administration. It's distributed rapidly to all tissues and is highly (90%) protein-bound. Phenytoin is metabolized in the liver. Inactive metabolites are excreted in bile and then reabsorbed from the GI tract. Eventually, however, they're excreted in the urine.

Mephenytoin moves

Mephenytoin is absorbed rapidly after oral administration and is only moderately (60%) protein-bound. It's metabolized by the liver to an active metabolite believed to possess the therapeutic and toxic effects attributed to mephenytoin. Excretion occurs via the urine.

Ethotoin is metabolized by the liver. Extensively protein-bound, ethotoin is excreted in the urine, primarily as metabolites.

Fosphenytoin for the short-term

Fosphenytoin is indicated for short-term I.M. or I.V. administration. It's widely distributed throughout the body and is highly (90%) protein-bound. Fosphenytoin is metabolized by the liver and excreted in the urine.

> Hydantoins interact with many drugs — sometimes their action is increased and sometimes it's decreased.

Pharmacodynamics

In most cases, the hydantoin anticonvulsants stabilize nerve cells to keep them from getting overexcited. Phenytoin appears to work in the motor cortex of the brain, where it stops the spread of seizure activity. The pharmacodynamics of fosphenytoin, mephenytoin, and ethotoin are thought to mimic those of phenytoin. Phenytoin is also used as an antiarrhythmic drug to control irregular heart rhythms, with properties similar to those of quinidine or procainamide.

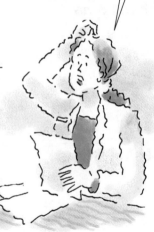

Pharmacotherapeutics

Because of its effectiveness and relatively low toxicity, phenytoin is the most commonly prescribed anticonvulsant. It's one of the drugs of choice to treat:
• complex partial seizures (also called psychomotor or temporal lobe seizures)
• tonic-clonic seizures.

Resistance is futile

Health care providers sometimes prescribe mephenytoin and ethotoin in combination with other anticonvulsants for partial and tonic-clonic seizures in patients who are resistant to or intolerant of other anticonvulsants.

Drug interactions

Hydantoins interact with a number of other drugs. Here are some drug interactions of major to moderate clinical significance:
• The effect of phenytoin is reduced when taken with phenobarbital, diazoxide, theophylline, carbamazepine, rifampin, antacids, and sucralfate.
• The effect of phenytoin is increased and the risk of toxicity increases when phenytoin is taken with allopurinol, cimetidine, disulfiram, fluconazole, isoniazid, omeprazole, sulfonamides, oral anticoagulants, chloramphenicol, and amiodarone.
• The effect of the following drugs is reduced when taken with an hydantoin anticonvulsant: oral anticoagulants, levodopa, amiodarone, corticosteroids, doxycycline, methadone, metyrapone, quinidine, theophylline, thyroid hormone, oral contraceptives, valproic acid, cyclosporine, and carbamazepine. (See *Adverse reactions to hydantoins.*)

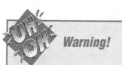

Warning!

Adverse reactions to hydantoins

Adverse reactions to hydantoins include:
• drowsiness
• ataxia
• irritability
• headache
• restlessness
• nystagmus
• dizziness and vertigo
• dysarthria
• nausea and vomiting
• abdominal pain
• anorexia
• depressed atrial and ventricular conduction
• ventricular fibrillation (in toxic states)
• bradycardia, hypotension, and cardiac arrest (with I.V. administration)
• hypersensitivity reactions.

Barbiturates

The long-acting *barbiturate* phenobarbital was formerly one of the most widely used anticonvulsants. It's now used less frequently because of its sedative effects. Phenobarbital is sometimes used for long-term treatment of epilepsy and is prescribed selectively for acute treatment of status epilepticus.

Other barbiturates

Mephobarbital, also a long-acting barbiturate, is some-times used as an anticonvulsant. Primidone, which is closely related chemically to the barbiturates, is also used in the chronic treatment of epilepsy.

Pharmacokinetics

Each barbiturate has a slightly different set of pharmaco-kinetic properties.

Phenobarbital for the long haul

Phenobarbital is absorbed slowly but well from the GI tract. Peak plasma concentration levels occur 8 to 12 hours after a single dose. The drug is 20% to 45% bound to serum proteins and to a similar extent to other tissues, including the brain. About 75% of a phenobarbital dose is metabolized by the liver and 25% is excreted un-changed in the urine.

Mephobarbital moves quickly

Almost half of a mephobarbital dose is absorbed from the GI tract and well distributed in body tissues. The drug is bound to tissue and plasma proteins. Mephobarbi-tal undergoes extensive metabolism by the liver; only 1% to 2% is excreted unchanged in the urine.

Primidone for new mothers?

Approximately 60% to 80% of a primidone dose is ab-sorbed from the GI tract and distributed evenly among body tissues. The drug is protein-bound to a small extent in the plasma. Primidone is metabolized by the liver to two active metabolites, phenobarbital and phenylethyl-malonamide (PEMA). From 15% to 25% of primidone is excreted unchanged in the urine, 15% to 25% is metabo-lized to phenobarbital, and 50% to 70% is excreted in the urine as PEMA. Primidone is also excreted in breast milk.

Pharmacodynamics

Barbiturates exhibit anticonvulsant action at doses below those that produce hypnotic effects. For this reason, the barbiturates usually don't produce addiction when used to treat epilepsy.

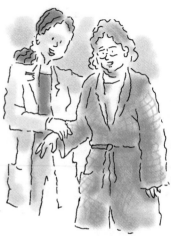

Barbiturates can have a paradoxical effect in elderly patients and in children.

Pharmacotherapeutics

The barbiturate anticonvulsants are effective in treating:
- partial seizures
- tonic-clonic seizures
- febrile seizures.

Barbiturates can be used alone or with other anticonvulsants. I.V. phenobarbital is also used to treat status epilepticus. The major disadvantage of using phenobarbital for status epilepticus is that it has a delayed onset of action when an immediate response is needed. Barbiturate anticonvulsants are ineffective in treating absence seizures.

Complex and partial? Try primidone

Mephobarbital has no advantage over phenobarbital and is used when the patient can't tolerate the adverse effects of phenobarbital. Primidone is used primarily with other anticonvulsants, although some consider it the drug of choice for complex partial seizures.

Drug interactions

The effects of barbiturates can be reduced when taken with rifampin. In addition, here are some other drug interactions:
- There is an increased risk of toxicity when phenobarbital is taken with CNS depressants, valproic acid, or chloramphenicol.
- The metabolism of methoxyflurane can be increased with long-term phenobarbital therapy, leading to the formation of metabolites toxic to the kidneys. (See *Adverse reactions to barbiturates.*)

Reduced rates

The effects of many drugs can be reduced when taken with a barbiturate, including beta blockers, chloramphenicol, doxycycline, oral anticoagulants, oral contraceptives, quinidine, phenothiazine, metronidazole, tricyclic antidepressants, theophylline, cyclosporine, carbamazepine, felodipine, and verapamil. Adverse effects of tricyclic antidepressants increase when they're taken with barbiturates.

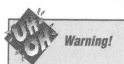

Warning!

Adverse reactions to barbiturates

Adverse reactions to phenobarbital and mephobarbital include:
- drowsiness, lethargy, and dizziness
- nystagmus, confusion, and ataxia (with large doses)
- laryngospasm, respiratory depression, and hypotension (when administered I.V.).

The same, plus psychoses
Primidone can cause the same CNS and GI adverse reactions as phenobarbital. Primidone can also cause acute psychoses, hair loss, impotence, and osteomalacia.

As a group
All three barbiturate anticonvulsants can produce a hypersensitivity rash, other rashes, lupus erythematosus–like syndrome (an inflammatory disorder), and enlarged lymph nodes.

Iminostilbenes

Carbamazepine is the most commonly used iminostilbene anticonvulsant. It effectively treats:
- partial and generalized tonic-clonic seizures
- mixed seizure types.

Pharmacokinetics

Carbamazepine is absorbed slowly and erratically from the GI tract. It's distributed rapidly to all tissues; 75% to 90% is bound to plasma proteins. Metabolism occurs in the liver, and carbamazepine is excreted in the urine. A small amount crosses the placenta, and some is secreted in breast milk. The half-life varies greatly.

Pharmacodynamics

Carbamazepine's anticonvulsant effect is similar to that of phenytoin. The drug's anticonvulsant action can occur because of its ability to inhibit the spread of seizure activity or neuromuscular transmission in general.

Pharmacotherapeutics

Carbamazepine is the drug of choice, in adults and children, for treating:
- generalized tonic-clonic seizures
- simple and complex partial seizures.

Carbamazepine also relieves pain when used to treat trigeminal neuralgia (tic douloureux, characterized by excruciating facial pain along the trigeminal nerve).

Drug interactions

Carbamazepine can reduce the effects of several drugs, including oral anticoagulants, oral contraceptives, doxycycline, felbamate, theophylline, and valproic acid. Other drug interactions can also occur:
- Increased carbamazepine levels and toxicity can occur with cimetidine, danazol, diltiazem, erythromycin, isoniazid, selective serotonin reuptake inhibitors, propoxyphene, troleandomycin, nonsedating antihistamines, valproic acid, and verapamil.
- Lithium and carbamazepine taken together increase the risk of toxic neurological effects.

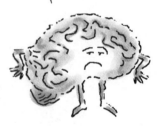

Be aware that, even when used as an anticonvulsant, carbamazepine will affect mood and behavior.

- Carbamazepine levels can be decreased when taken with warfarin, barbiturates, or felbamate. (See *Adverse reactions to carbamazepine*.)

Benzodiazepines

The three *benzodiazepine drugs* that provide anticonvulsant effects are:
- diazepam (in the parenteral form)
- clonazepam
- clorazepate.

Only one for ongoing treatment

Only clonazepam is recommended for long-term treatment of epilepsy. Diazepam is restricted to acute treatment of status epilepticus. Clorazepate is prescribed as an adjunct in treating partial seizures.

Pharmacokinetics

The patient can receive benzodiazepines orally or parenterally.

Absorption and distribution

Benzodiazepines are absorbed rapidly and almost completely from the GI tract but are distributed at different rates. Protein-binding of benzodiazepines ranges from 85% to 90%.

Metabolism and excretion

Benzodiazepines are metabolized in the liver to multiple metabolites and are then excreted in the urine. The benzodiazepines readily cross the placenta and are excreted in breast milk.

Pharmacodynamics

Benzodiazepines act as:
- anticonvulsants
- antianxiety agents
- sedative-hypnotics
- muscle-relaxants.
    Their mechanism of action is poorly understood.

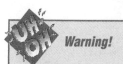
Warning!

Adverse reactions to carbamazepine

Occasionally, serious hematologic toxicity occurs. Because carbamazepine is related structurally to the tricyclic antidepressants, it can cause similar toxicities and affect behaviors and emotions.

When you're young
Hives and Stevens-Johnson syndrome (a potentially fatal inflammatory disease in children and young adults) can occur.

Pharmacotherapeutics

Each of the benzodiazepines can be used in slightly different ways.

Absence, atypical, atonic

Clonazepam is used to treat the following types of seizures:
- absence (petit mal)
- atypical absence (Lennox-Gastaut syndrome)
- atonic
- myoclonic.

I.V. or with others

Diazepam isn't recommended for long-term treatment because of its potential for addiction and the high serum concentrations required to control seizures.

I.V. diazepam is used to control status epilepticus. Because diazepam provides only short-term effects of less than 1 hour, the patient must also be given a long-acting anticonvulsant, such as phenytoin or phenobarbital, during diazepam therapy.

Clorazepate is used with other drugs to treat partial seizures.

Drug interactions

When benzodiazepines are taken with CNS depressants, sedative and other depressant effects become enhanced. This can cause motor skill impairment, respiratory depression, and even death at high doses.

Cimetidine and oral contraceptives, taken with a benzodiazepine drug, can cause excessive sedation and CNS depression. (See *Adverse reactions to benzodiazepines*.)

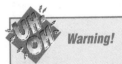 *Warning!*

Adverse reactions to benzodiazepines

Most common
- Drowsiness
- Confusion
- Ataxia
- Weakness
- Dizziness
- Nystagmus
- Vertigo
- Fainting
- Dysarthria
- Headache
- Tremor
- Glassy-eyed appearance

Less common
- Depression of the heart and breathing (with high doses and with I.V. diazepam)
- Rash and acute hypersensitivity reactions

Valproic acid

Valproic acid is unrelated structurally to the other anticonvulsants. The two major drugs in the valproic acid class are:
- valproate
- divalproex.

Pharm fact

Happy accident

The anticonvulsant properties of valproic acid were actually discovered when it was being used as a vehicle for *other* compounds being tested for anticonvulsant properties. Structurally, valproic acid is unlike other anticonvulsants. It's mechanism of action isn't completely understood.

Pharmacokinetics

Valproate is converted rapidly to valproic acid in the stomach. Divalproex is a precursor of valproic acid and separates into valproic acid in the GI tract. Valproic acid is absorbed well, strongly protein-bound, and is metabolized in the liver. Metabolites and unchanged drug are excreted in urine.

Valproic acid readily crosses the placental barrier and also appears in breast milk.

Pharmacodynamics

The mechanism of action for valproic acid remains unknown. It's thought to increase levels of gamma-aminobutyric acid (GABA), an inhibitory neurotransmitter. (See *Happy accident.*)

Pharmacotherapeutics

Valproic acid is prescribed for long-term treatment of:
• absence seizures
• myoclonic seizures
• tonic-clonic seizures.

It's also administered rectally for status epilepticus that doesn't respond to other anticonvulsants.

Liver risk

Valproic acid must be used cautiously in a young child or in a patient receiving multiple anticonvulsants. With these patients, valproic acid carries a risk of potentially fatal liver toxicity. This risk limits the use of valproic acid as a drug of choice for seizure disorders.

Drug interactions

The most significant drug interactions associated with valproic acid are:

• inhibition of platelet aggregation, which can cause prolonged bleeding times in patients who are also receiving anticoagulants

• inhibition of phenobarbital metabolism in the liver, causing increased levels of phenobarbital. (See *Adverse reactions to valproic acid*.)

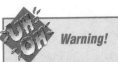

Warning!

Adverse reactions to valproic acid

Rare, but deadly, liver toxicity has occurred with this drug. For this reason, the drug isn't routinely prescribed. Most other adverse reactions to valproic acid are tolerable and dose-related. These include:
• nausea and vomiting
• diarrhea
• constipation
• sedation
• dizziness
• ataxia
• headache
• muscle weakness.

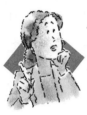

Quick quiz

1. A 15-year-old patient has a tonic-clonic seizure disorder and is prescribed phenytoin. Which term best describes the absorption rate of oral phenytoin?

    A. Rapid
    B. Slow
    C. Erratic

Answer: B. Phenytoin is absorbed slowly through the GI tract. It's absorbed much more rapidly when administered I.V.

2. An 11-year-old patient develops myoclonic seizures. Which potential adverse reaction makes it unlikely that valproate will be prescribed for this patient?

    A. Liver toxicity
    B. Central nervous system sedation
    C. Respiratory depression

Answer: A. When administered to children and patients taking other anticonvulsants, valproate carries a risk of potentially fatal liver toxicity.

3. Anticonvulsants fall into five major classes, including:

    A. sulfonamides.
    B. fluoroquinolones.
    C. iminostilbines.

Answer: C. The five major classes of anticonvulsants are iminostilbenes, hydantoins, barbiturates, benzodiazepines, and valproic acid.

4. A 48-year-old patient has been prescribed trihexyphenidyl for her Parkinson's disease. Which adverse reaction can be dose-related?
    A.   Excessive salivation
    B.   Dryness of mouth
    C.   Bradycardia
Answer: B. Dry mouth may be a dose-related adverse effect of trihexyphenidyl therapy.

5. Which antiparkinsonian drug is associated with the on-off phenomenon and end-of-dose deterioration?
    A.   Amantadine
    B.   Benztropine
    C.   Levodopa
Answer: C. Levodopa is associated with the on-off phenomenon and end-of-dose deterioration in patients taking the drug for many years. For that reason, some doctors believe the drug should be given in lower doses or started later in the course of the disorder.

6. The effectiveness of levodopa can be reduced when taking:
    A.   pyridoxine.
    B.   amantadine.
    C.   bromocriptine.
Answer: A. Levodopa effectiveness can be reduced when taking pyridoxine (vitamin B_{12}), phenytoin, benzodiazepines, reserpine, and papaverine.

7. Barbiturate anticonvulsants are effective in treating all of the following except:

    A.   absence seizures.

    B.   tonic-clonic seizures.

    C.   febrile seizures.

Answer: A. Barbiturate anticonvulsants are effective in treating partial, tonic-clonic, and febrile seizures. They're an ineffective treatment for absence seizures.

Scoring

☆☆☆   If you answered all seven questions correctly, marvelous! You're mighty fine with neuromusculars.

☆☆   If you answered five or six questions correctly, congrats! Your knowledge has a rapid onset and long duration.

☆   If you answered fewer than five questions correctly, don't worry. Just give yourself another dose of this chapter and recheck the results.

4

Pain medications

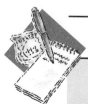

Just the facts

In this chapter, you'll review:

♦ classes of drugs used to control pain

♦ uses and varying actions of these drugs

♦ how these drugs are absorbed, distributed, metabolized, and excreted

♦ drug interactions and adverse reactions to these drugs.

Drugs and pain control

Drugs used to control pain range from mild, over-the-counter (OTC) preparations, such as acetaminophen, to potent general anesthetics. They include:
• nonnarcotic analgesics, antipyretics, and nonsteroidal anti-inflammatory drugs (NSAIDs)
• narcotic agonist and antagonist drugs
• anesthetic drugs.

Nonnarcotic analgesics, antipyretics, and NSAIDs

Nonnarcotic analgesics, antipyretics, and NSAIDs are a broad group of pain medications. They're discussed together because, in addition to pain control, they also produce antipyretic (fever control) and anti-inflammatory effects. The drug classes included in this group are:
• salicylates (especially aspirin), which are widely used

- the para-aminophenol derivative acetaminophen
- NSAIDs
- the urinary tract analgesic phenazopyridine hydrochloride.

Salicylates

Salicylates are among the most commonly used pain medications. They're used regularly to control pain and reduce fever and inflammation.

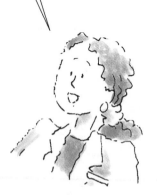

Salicylates are found in many OTC pain and cold preparations.

Cheap, easy, and reliable

Salicylates usually cost less than other analgesics and are readily available without a prescription. Aspirin, the most commonly used salicylate, remains the cornerstone of anti-inflammatory drug therapy. Other common salicylates include:

- choline magnesium trisalicylate
- choline salicylate
- diflunisal
- salsalate
- sodium salicylate.

Pharmacokinetics (how drugs circulate)

Taken orally, salicylates are absorbed partly in the stomach, but primarily in the upper part of the small intestine. The pure and buffered forms of aspirin are absorbed readily, but sustained-release and enteric-coated salicylate preparations or food or antacids in the stomach delay absorption. Salicylates given rectally have a slower, more erratic absorption.

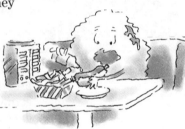

Taking a salicylate with an antacid or food slows absorption.

Distribution, metabolism, and excretion

Salicylates are distributed widely throughout body tissues and fluids, including breast milk. In addition, they easily cross the placenta.

The liver metabolizes salicylates extensively into several metabolites. The kidneys excrete the metabolites and some unchanged drug.

Pharmacodynamics (how drugs act)

The different effects of salicylates stem from their separate mechanisms of action. They relieve pain primarily by inhibiting the synthesis of prostaglandin. (Recall that prostaglandin is a chemical mediator that sensitizes nerve cells to pain.) In addition, they may also reduce inflammation by inhibiting the prostaglandin synthesis and release that occurs during inflammation.

Increase sweating, reduce temperature

Salicylates reduce fever by stimulating the hypothalamus, producing dilation of the peripheral blood vessels and increased sweating. This promotes heat loss through the skin and cooling by evaporation. Also, because prostaglandin E increases body temperature, inhibiting its production lowers a fever.

Bonus effect

One salicylate, aspirin, inhibits platelet aggregation (the clumping of platelets to form a clot) by interfering with the production of a substance called thromboxane A_2, necessary for platelet aggregation. As a result, aspirin can be used to enhance blood flow during myocardial infarction.

Pharmacotherapeutics (how drugs are used)

Salicylates are used primarily to relieve pain and reduce fever. However, they don't effectively relieve visceral pain (pain from the organs and smooth muscle) or severe pain from trauma.

You give me fever...

Salicylates won't reduce a normal body temperature. They can reduce an elevated body temperature, and will relieve headache and muscle ache at the same time.

Effective against arthritis

Salicylates can provide considerable relief in 24 hours when they're used to reduce inflammation in rheumatic fever and rheumatoid arthritis.

How low can you go?

No matter what the clinical indication, the main guideline of salicylate therapy is to use the lowest dose that provides relief. This reduces the likelihood of adverse reactions. (See *Adverse reactions to salicylates*, page 82.)

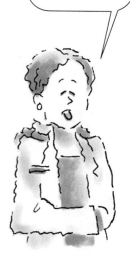

Because they relieve headache and muscle ache as well, salicylates are commonly used for fevers associated with colds and influenza.

Drug interactions

Because salicylates are highly protein bound, they can interact with many other protein-bound drugs by displacing those drugs from sites to which they normally bind. This increases the serum concentration of the unbound active drug, causing increased pharmacologic effects (the unbound drug is said to be *potentiated*). The following drug interactions may occur:

• Oral anticoagulants, heparin, methotrexate, oral antidiabetic agents, and insulin are among the drugs that have an increased effect or risk of toxicity when taken with salicylates.

• Probenecid, sulfinpyrazone, and spironolactone may have a decreased effect when taken with salicylates.

• Corticosteroids may decrease plasma salicylate levels and increase the risk of ulcers.

• Alkalinizing drugs and antacids may reduce salicylate levels.

• The antihypertensive effect of angiotensin-converting enzyme inhibitors and beta blockers may be reduced when these drugs are combined with salicylates.

• NSAIDs may have a reduced therapeutic effect and increased risk of GI effects when taken with salicylates.

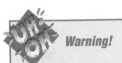

Warning!

Adverse reactions to salicylates

The most common adverse reactions to salicylates include gastric distress, nausea, and vomiting. Other adverse reactions include:

• hearing loss (when taken for prolonged periods)

• diarrhea, thirst, sweating, tinnitus, confusion, dizziness, impaired vision, and hyperventilation (rapid breathing)

• Reye's syndrome (when given to children with chickenpox or with flulike symptoms).

Acetaminophen

Although the class of para-aminophenol derivatives includes two drugs — phenacetin and acetaminophen — only acetaminophen is available in the United States. *Acetaminophen* is an OTC drug that produces analgesic and antipyretic effects. It appears in many products designed to relieve pain and symptoms associated with colds and influenza.

Pharmacokinetics

Acetaminophen is absorbed rapidly and completely from the GI tract. It's also absorbed well from the mucous membranes of the rectum.

Distribution, metabolism, and excretion

Acetaminophen is distributed widely in body fluids and readily crosses the placenta. After acetaminophen is metabolized by the liver, it's excreted by the kidneys and, in small amounts, in breast milk.

Pharmacodynamics

Acetaminophen reduces pain and fever, but unlike salicylates, it doesn't affect inflammation or platelet function.

Mystery theater

The pain-control effects of acetaminophen aren't well understood. It may work in the central nervous system (CNS) by inhibiting prostaglandin synthesis and in the peripheral nervous system in some unknown way. It reduces fever by acting directly on the heat-regulating center in the hypothalamus.

Pharmacotherapeutics

Acetaminophen is used to reduce fever and relieve headache, muscle ache, and general pain.

Child's play

Acetaminophen is the drug of choice to treat fever and flulike symptoms in children. Recently, the American Arthritis Association has indicated that acetaminophen is an effective pain reliever for some types of arthritis.

Drug interactions

Acetaminophen can produce the following drug interactions:
• It may slightly increase the effects of oral anticoagulants and thrombolytic drugs.
• The risk of liver toxicity is increased when chronic alcohol use, phenytoin, barbiturates, carbamazepine, and isoniazid are combined with acetaminophen.
• The effects of lamotrigine, loop diuretics, and zidovudine may be reduced when taken with acetaminophen. (See *Adverse reactions to acetaminophen*.)

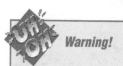

Warning!

Adverse reactions to acetaminophen

Most patients tolerate acetaminophen well. Unlike the salicylates, acetaminophen rarely causes gastric irritation or bleeding tendencies.

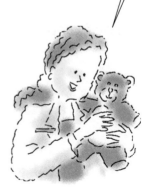

Acetaminophen is the drug of choice to treat fever and flulike symptoms in children.

Nonsteroidal anti-inflammatory drugs

As their name suggests, *NSAIDs* are often used to combat inflammation, and their anti-inflammatory action equals that of aspirin.

They also have analgesic and antipyretic effects, but are seldom prescribed for fever.

Drugs in this class include indomethacin, ibuprofen, mefenamic acid, phenylbutazone, celecoxib, piroxicam, and sulindac.

Pharmacokinetics

All NSAIDs are absorbed in the GI tract. They're mostly metabolized in the liver and excreted primarily by the kidneys.

Pharmacodynamics

Researchers believe that NSAIDs produce their effects by inhibiting prostaglandin synthesis. For example, a new class of NSAIDs, called cyclooxygenase-2 (Cox-2) inhibitors, inhibit Cox-2, an enzyme responsible for prostaglandin synthesis. Another type of NSAIDs, fenamates, may compete with prostaglandins at receptor-binding sites.

Pharmacotherapeutics

NSAIDs are used primarily to decrease inflammation. They're secondarily used to relieve pain, but are seldom prescribed to reduce fever.

Call and response

The following conditions respond favorably to treatment with NSAIDs:
- ankylosing spondylitis (an inflammatory joint disease that first affects the spine)
- moderate to severe rheumatoid arthritis (an inflammatory disease of peripheral joints)
- osteoarthritis (a degenerative joint disease) in the hip, shoulder, or other large joints
- osteoarthritis accompanied by inflammation
- acute gouty arthritis (urate deposits in the joints)
- dysmenorrhea (painful menstruation).

Drug interactions

A wide variety of drugs can interact with NSAIDs, especially with indomethacin, mefenamic acid, phenylbutazone, piroxicam, and sulindac. Because they're highly protein bound, NSAIDs are likely to interact with other protein-bound drugs such as oral anticoagulants. (See *Adverse reactions to NSAIDs.*)

Phenazopyridine hydrochloride

Phenazopyridine hydrochloride (Pyridium), an azo dye used in commercial coloring, produces a local analgesic effect on the urinary tract, usually within 24 to 48 hours after therapy begins. It relieves the pain, burning, urgency, and frequency that occur with urinary tract infections.

Dye job

When taken orally, phenazopyridine is 35% metabolized in the liver, with the remainder excreted unchanged in the urine, which may take on an orange or red color.

If the drug is accumulating, the skin and sclera of the eye may take on a yellow tinge and the phenazopyridine may need to be stopped.

Narcotic agonist and antagonist drugs

The word *narcotic* refers to any derivative of the opium plant or any synthetic drug that imitates natural narcotics. Narcotic agonists (also called narcotic analgesics) include opium derivatives and synthetic drugs with similar properties. They're used to relieve or decrease pain without causing the person to lose consciousness.

Some narcotic agonists may also have antitussive effects that suppress coughing and antidiarrheal actions that can control diarrhea.

Anta-dote

Narcotic antagonists aren't pain medications but block the effects of narcotic agonists and are used to reverse adverse drug reactions, such as respiratory and CNS depression produced by those drugs. Unfortunately, by reversing the analgesic effect, they also cause the patient's pain to recur.

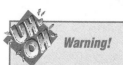

Warning!

Adverse reactions to NSAIDs

All nonsteroidal anti-inflammatory drugs (NSAIDs) produce similar adverse reactions which include:
• abdominal pain, bleeding, anorexia, diarrhea, nausea, ulcers, and liver toxicity
• drowsiness, headache, dizziness, confusion, tinnitus, vertigo, and depression
• bladder infection, blood in the urine, and kidney necrosis.

Risky business
Phenylbutazone has an unusually high incidence of adverse reactions, commonly causing nausea, vomiting, abdominal discomfort, dyspepsia (stomach discomfort after eating), diarrhea, and rashes.

Having it both ways

Some narcotic analgesics, called mixed narcotic agonist-antagonists, have both agonist and antagonist properties. The agonist component relieves pain, and the antagonist component decreases the risk of toxicity and drug dependence. These mixed narcotic agonist-antagonists reduce the risk of respiratory depression and drug abuse.

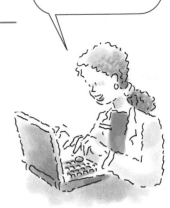

Narcotic refers to any derivative of the opium plant or to any synthetic drug that imitates the effects of natural narcotics.

Narcotic agonists

Narcotic agonists include:
- codeine
- fentanyl citrate
- hydromorphone hydrochloride
- levorphanol tartrate
- meperidine hydrochloride
- methadone hydrochloride
- morphine sulfate (including morphine sulfate sustained-release tablets and intensified oral solution).

Gold standard

Morphine sulfate is the standard against which the effectiveness and adverse reactions of other pain medications are measured.

Pharmacokinetics

A person may receive narcotic agonists by any administration route, although inhalation administration is uncommon. Oral doses are absorbed readily from the GI tract.

Instant help

Narcotic agonists administered I.V. provide the most rapid (almost immediate) and reliable pain relief. The S.C. and I.M. routes may result in delayed absorption, especially in patients with poor circulation.

Distribution

Narcotic agonists are distributed widely throughout body tissues. They have a relatively low plasma protein-binding capacity (30% to 35%).

Metabolism

Narcotic agonists are metabolized extensively in the liver. For example, meperidine is metabolized to normeperidine, a toxic metabolite with a longer half-life than meperidine.

Excretion

Metabolites are excreted by the kidneys. A small amount is excreted in stool through the biliary tract.

Pharmacodynamics

Narcotic agonists reduce pain by binding to opiate receptor sites in the peripheral nervous system and the CNS. When these drugs stimulate the opiate receptors, they mimic the effects of endorphins (naturally occurring opiates that are part of the body's own pain relief system). This receptor-site binding produces the therapeutic effects of analgesia and cough suppression as well as adverse reactions, such as respiratory depression and constipation. (See *How narcotic agonists control pain*, page 88.)

Smooth operator

Narcotic agonists, especially morphine, affect the smooth muscle of the GI and genitourinary tracts (the organs of the reproductive and urinary systems). This causes contraction of the bladder and ureters and slowed intestinal peristalsis (rhythmic contractions that move food along the digestive tract).

A fine line

These drugs also cause blood vessels to dilate, especially in the face, head, and neck. In addition, they suppress the cough center in the brain, producing antitussive effects and causing constriction of the bronchial muscles. Any of these effects can become adverse reactions if they're produced in excess. For example, if the blood vessels dilate too much, hypotension can occur.

Pharmacotherapeutics

Narcotic agonists are prescribed to relieve severe pain in acute, chronic, and terminal illnesses. They also reduce anxiety before a patient receives anesthesia and are sometimes prescribed to control diarrhea and suppress coughing.

Zoom in

How narcotic agonists control pain

Narcotic agonists, such as meperidine, inhibit pain transmission by mimicking the body's natural pain control mechanisms.

Where neurons meet

In the dorsal horn of the spinal cord, peripheral pain neurons meet central nervous system (CNS) neurons. At the synapse, the pain neuron releases substance P (a pain neurotransmitter). This agent helps transfer pain impulses to the CNS neurons that carry the impulses to the brain.

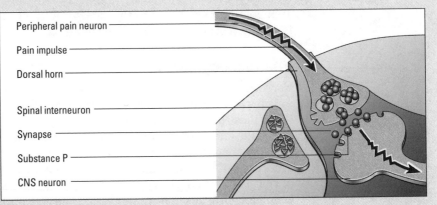

Peripheral pain neuron

Pain impulse

Dorsal horn

Spinal interneuron

Synapse

Substance P

CNS neuron

Taking up space

In theory, the spinal interneurons respond to stimulation from the descending neurons of the CNS by releasing endogenous opiates. These opiates bind to the peripheral pain neuron to inhibit release of substance P and to retard the transmission of pain impulses.

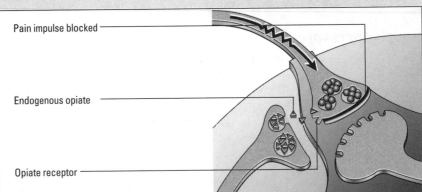

Pain impulse blocked

Endogenous opiate

Opiate receptor

Stopping substance P

Synthetic opiates supplement this pain-blocking effect by binding with free opiate receptors to inhibit the release of substance P. Opiates also alter consciousness of pain, but how this mechanism works remains unknown.

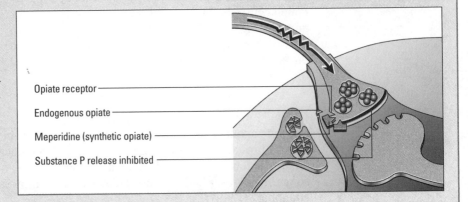

Opiate receptor

Endogenous opiate

Meperidine (synthetic opiate)

Substance P release inhibited

Cardio-assistance

Morphine relieves shortness of breath in patients with pulmonary edema (fluid in the lungs) and left-sided heart failure (inability of the heart to pump enough blood to meet the needs of the body).

Drug interactions

• The use of narcotic agonists with other drugs that also decrease respirations, such as alcohol, sedatives, hypnotics, and anesthetics, increases the patient's risk of severe respiratory depression.

• Taking tricyclic antidepressants, phenothiazines, or anticholinergics with narcotic agonists may cause severe constipation and urine retention. (See *Adverse reactions to narcotic agonists.*)

Mixed narcotic agonist-antagonists

Mixed narcotic agonist-antagonists attempt to relieve pain while reducing toxic effects and dependency. The mixed narcotic agonist-antagonists include:
• buprenorphine hydrochloride
• butorphanol tartrate
• dezocine
• nalbuphine hydrochloride
• pentazocine hydrochloride (combined with pentazocine lactate, naloxone hydrochloride, aspirin, or acetaminophen).

No free ride

Originally, mixed narcotic agonist-antagonists appeared to have less abuse potential than the pure narcotic agonists. However, butorphanol and pentazocine have reportedly caused dependence.

Pharmacokinetics

Absorption of mixed narcotic agonist-antagonists occurs rapidly from parenteral sites. These drugs are distributed to most body tissues and also cross the placenta. They're metabolized in the liver and excreted primarily by the kidneys, although more than 10% of a butorphanol dose and a small amount of dezocine and pentazocine doses are excreted in stool.

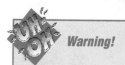
Warning!

Adverse reactions to narcotic agonists

One of the most common adverse reactions to narcotic agonists is decreased rate and depth of breathing that worsens as the dose of narcotic is increased. This may cause periodic, irregular breathing or trigger asthmatic attacks in susceptible patients.

Other adverse reactions include:
• flushing
• orthostatic hypotension
• pupil constriction.

Meperidine
• Tremors
• Palpitations
• Tachycardia
• Delirium

Pharmacodynamics

The exact mechanism of action of the mixed narcotic agonist-antagonists isn't known.

No rush to go

Buprenorphine binds with receptors in the CNS, altering both perception of and emotional response to pain through an unknown mechanism. It seems to release slowly from binding sites, producing a longer duration of action than the other drugs in this class.

It's believed that dezocine increases the amount of blood pumped by the heart and pulmonary vascular resistance.

Don't get emotional

The site of action of butorphanol may be opiate receptors in the limbic system (part of the brain involved in emotion).

Like pentazocine, butorphanol also acts on pulmonary circulation, increasing pulmonary vascular resistance (the resistance in the blood vessels of the lungs that the right ventricle must pump against). Both drugs also increase blood pressure and the workload of the heart.

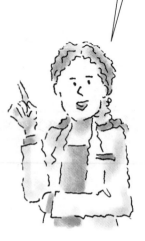

Mixed narcotic agonist-antagonists attempt to relieve pain while reducing toxic effects and dependency — but certain drugs may still cause dependence.

Pharmacotherapeutics

Mixed narcotic agonist-antagonists are prescribed primarily for relief of moderate to severe pain and as preoperative medication to reduce anxiety and pain. They're also used as analgesia during childbirth.

Independence day

Mixed narcotic agonist-antagonists are sometimes prescribed in place of narcotic agonists because they have a lower risk of drug dependence. Mixed narcotic agonist-antagonists also are less likely to cause respiratory depression, although they can produce some adverse reactions. (See *Adverse reactions to narcotic agonist-antagonists.*)

Drug interactions

Increased CNS depression and an additive decrease in respiratory rate and depth may result if mixed narcotic agonist-antagonists are administered to patients taking other CNS depressants, such as barbiturates and alcohol.

Clean and sober?

Patients with a history of narcotic abuse shouldn't receive any of the mixed narcotic agonist-antagonists because they can cause symptoms of withdrawal.

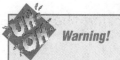

Narcotic antagonists

Narcotic antagonists attach to opiate receptors but don't stimulate them and have a greater attraction for opiate receptors than narcotics do. As a result, they prevent narcotic drugs, enkephalins, and endorphins from producing their effects.

Narcotic antagonists include:
- naloxone hydrochloride
- naltrexone hydrochloride.

Pharmacokinetics

Naloxone is administered I.M., S.C., or I.V. Naltrexone is administered orally in tablet or liquid form. Both drugs are metabolized by the liver and excreted by the kidneys.

Pharmacodynamics

Narcotic antagonists block the effects of narcotics by occupying the opiate receptor sites, displacing any narcotics attached to opiate receptors and blocking further narcotic binding at these sites. The process by which they work is known as competitive inhibition.

Pharmacotherapeutics

Naloxone is the drug of choice for managing a narcotic overdose. It reverses respiratory depression and sedation and helps stabilize the patient's vital signs within seconds after administration.

Because naloxone also reverses the analgesic effects of narcotic drugs, a patient who was given a narcotic drug for pain relief may complain of pain or even experience withdrawal symptoms.

> **Warning!**
>
> ## Adverse reactions to narcotic agonist-antagonists
>
> The most common adverse reactions to narcotic agonist-antagonists include nausea, vomiting, lightheadedness, sedation, and euphoria.

> Patients with a history of narcotic abuse shouldn't receive mixed narcotic agonist-antagonists — because withdrawal symptoms may result.

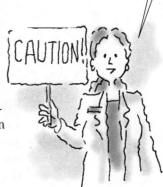

CAUTION!

Kicking the habit

Naltrexone is used along with psychotherapy or counseling to treat drug abuse. It's only given, however, to patients who have gone through a detoxification program to remove all narcotics from the body. That is because a patient who still has narcotics in the body may experience acute withdrawal symptoms if he receives naltrexone.

Drug interactions

Naloxone produces no significant drug interactions. Naltrexone will cause withdrawal symptoms if given to a patient receiving a narcotic agonist or to a narcotic addict. (See *Adverse reactions to naloxone and naltrexone.*)

Anesthetic drugs

Anesthetic drugs can be divided into three groups—general anesthetics, local anesthetics, and topical anesthetics.

Inhale or inject?

General anesthetic drugs are further subdivided into two main types, those given by inhalation and those given by injection.

Inhalation anesthetics

Commonly used general anesthetics given by inhalation include:
- desflurane
- sevoflurane
- enflurane
- halothane
- isoflurane
- nitrous oxide.

Pharmacokinetics

The absorption and elimination rates of an anesthetic are governed by its solubility in blood. *Inhalation anesthetics* enter the blood from the lungs and are distributed to other tissues. Distribution is most rapid to organs with high blood flow, such as the brain, liver, kidneys, and heart. In-

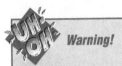

Warning!

Adverse reactions to naloxone and naltrexone

Naloxone and naltrexone produce different adverse reactions.

Watch the wake-up
Naloxone may cause nausea, vomiting and, occasionally, hypertension and tachycardia. An unconscious patient returned to consciousness abruptly after naloxone administration may hyperventilate and experience tremors.

Ear, nose, and throat
Naltrexone can cause a variety of adverse reactions, including:
- edema, hypertension, palpitations, phlebitis, and shortness of breath
- anxiety, depression, disorientation, dizziness, headache, and nervousness
- anorexia, diarrhea or constipation, nausea, thirst, and vomiting
- urinary frequency
- liver toxicity.

halation anesthetics are eliminated primarily by the lungs; enflurane, halothane, and sevoflurane are also eliminated by the liver. Metabolites are excreted in the urine.

Pharmacodynamics

Inhalation anesthetics work primarily by depressing the CNS, producing loss of consciousness, loss of responsiveness to sensory stimulation (including pain), and muscle relaxation. They also affect other organ systems.

Pharmacotherapeutics

Inhalation anesthetics are used for surgery because they offer more precise and rapid control of depth of anesthesia than injection anesthetics. These anesthetics, which are liquids at room temperature, require a vaporizer and special delivery system for safe use.

Of the inhalation anesthetics available, desflurane, isoflurane, and nitrous oxide are the most commonly used.

Stop signs

Inhalation anesthetics are contraindicated in a patient with known hypersensitivity to the drug, a liver disorder, or malignant hyperthermia (a potentially fatal complication of anesthesia characterized by skeletal muscle rigidity and high fever). They require cautious use in a pregnant or breast-feeding patient. (See *Adverse reactions to inhalation anesthetics* and *Unusual but serious*, page 94.)

Drug interactions

The most important drug interactions involving inhalation anesthetics are with other CNS, cardiac, or respiratory depressant drugs.

Injection anesthetics

Injection anesthetics are a type of general anesthesia usually used when anesthesia is needed for only a short period, such as with outpatient surgery. They're also used to promote rapid induction of anesthesia or to supplement inhalation anesthetics.

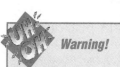
Warning!

Adverse reactions to inhalation anesthetics

The most common adverse reaction to inhalation anesthetics is an exaggerated patient response to a normal dose.

Waking up
After surgery, a patient may experience reactions similar to those seen with other central nervous system depressants, including depression of breathing and circulation, confusion, sedation, nausea, vomiting, ataxia, and hypothermia.

It happens with halothane
Rarely, liver necrosis develops several days after halothane use and occurs most commonly with multiple drug exposures. Symptoms include rash, fever, jaundice, nausea, vomiting, eosinophilia, and alterations in liver function.

Main options

The three drugs used solely as injected general anesthetics are:
- etomidate
- propofol
- ketamine hydrochloride.

In addition, various barbiturates, opiates, and opiate-like drugs may be used as injected general anesthetics.

Pharmacokinetics

All injection anesthetics bypass the mechanisms that reduce bioavailability, distributing rapidly into the CNS. Opiates given by I.M. injection have a more delayed absorption and reduced peak effect than when given I.V. Barbiturates depend on liver transformation for elimination, as do benzodiazepine and opiate drugs and the hypnotic etomidate.

Pharmacodynamics

Opiates work by occupying sites on specialized receptors scattered throughout the CNS and modifying the release of neurotransmitters from sensory nerves entering the CNS. Ketamine appears to induce a profound sense of dissociation from the environment by acting directly on the cortex and limbic system of the brain.

Getting sleepy

Barbiturates, benzodiazepines, and etomidate seem to enhance responses to the CNS neurotransmitter gamma-aminobutyric acid. This inhibits the brain's response to stimulation of the reticular activating system, the area of the brain stem that controls alertness. Barbiturates also depress the excitability of CNS neurons.

Pharmacotherapeutics

Because of the short duration of action of injection anesthetics, they're used in shorter surgical procedures, including outpatient surgery.

Alone or as a helper

Barbiturates are used alone in surgery that isn't expected to be painful and as adjuncts to other drugs in more ex-

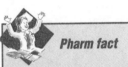

Pharm fact

Unusual but serious

Malignant hyperthermia, characterized by a sudden and often lethal increase in body temperature, is a serious and unexpected reaction to inhalation anesthetics. It occurs in genetically susceptible patients only and may result from a failure in calcium uptake by muscle cells. The skeletal muscle relaxant dantrolene is used to treat this condition.

tensive procedures. Benzodiazepines produce sedation and amnesia, but not pain relief.

Etomidate is used to induce anesthesia and to supplement low-potency inhalation anesthetics such as nitrous oxide. The opiates provide pain relief and supplement other anesthetic drugs.

Drug interactions

The injection anesthetics, particularly ketamine, can produce a variety of drug interactions:
• Verapamil enhances the anesthetic effects of etomidate, producing respiratory depression and apnea.
• Administering ketamine together with halothane increases the risk of hypotension and reduces cardiac output (the amount of blood pumped by the heart each minute).
• Giving ketamine and nondepolarizing drugs together increases neuromuscular effects, resulting in prolonged respiratory depression.
• Using barbiturates or narcotics with ketamine may prolong recovery time after anesthesia.
• Ketamine plus theophylline may promote seizures.
• Ketamine and thyroid hormones may cause hypertension and tachycardia (rapid heart rate). (See *Adverse reactions to injection anesthetics.*)

Local anesthetics

Local anesthetics are administered to prevent or relieve pain in a specific area of the body. In addition, these drugs are often used as an alternative to general anesthesia for elderly or debilitated patients.

Chain gang

Local anesthetics may be:
• "amide" drugs (with nitrogen in the molecular chain)
• "ester" drugs (with oxygen in the molecular chain). (See *Amides and esters*, page 96.)

Pharmacokinetics

Absorption of local anesthetics varies widely, but distribution occurs throughout the body. Esters and amides

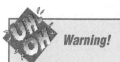

Warning!

Adverse reactions to injection anesthetics

Ketamine
• Prolonged recovery
• Irrational behavior
• Excitement
• Disorientation
• Delirium, hallucinations
• Increased heart rate
• Excess salivation
• Tearing, shivering, increased cerebrospinal fluid and eye pressure
• Seizures

Barbiturates
• Respiratory depression
• Anaphylaxis

Propofol
• Respiratory depression
• Hiccups, coughing, muscle twitching

Thiopental
• Hiccups, coughing, muscle twitching
• Depressed cardiac function and peripheral dilation

Etomidate
• Hiccups, coughing, muscle twitching

Fentanyl
• Seizures

undergo different types of metabolism, but both yield metabolites that are excreted in the urine.

Pharmacodynamics

Local anesthetics block nerve impulses at the point of contact in all kinds of nerves. They accumulate and cause the nerve cell membrane to expand. As the membrane expands, the cell loses its ability to depolarize, which is necessary for impulse transmission.

Pharmacotherapeutics

Local anesthetics are used to prevent and relieve pain from medical procedures, disease, or injury. Local anesthetics are used for severe pain that topical anesthetics or analgesics can't relieve.

When a general won't do

Local anesthetics are usually preferred to general anesthetics for surgery in an elderly or debilitated patient or a patient with a disorder that affects respiratory function, such as chronic obstructive pulmonary disease and myasthenia gravis.

Combining and coordinating

For some procedures, a local anesthetic is combined with a drug such as epinephrine that constricts blood vessels. Vasoconstriction helps control local bleeding and reduces absorption of the anesthetic. Reduced absorption prolongs the anesthetic's action at the site and limits its distribution and CNS effects.

Drug interactions

Local anesthetics produce few significant interactions with other drugs. Local anesthetics can produce adverse reactions. (See *Adverse reactions to local anesthetics.*)

Topical anesthetics

Topical anesthetics are applied directly to the skin or mucous membranes. All topical anesthetics are used to prevent or relieve minor pain.

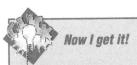
Now I get it!

Amides and esters

Amide anesthetics are local anesthetics that have nitrogen as part of their molecular makeup. They include:
• bupivacaine hydrochloride
• ropivacaine hydrochloride
• etidocaine hydrochloride
• lidocaine hydrochloride
• mepivacaine hydrochloride
• prilocaine hydrochloride.

Give them oxygen
Ester anesthetics have oxygen, not nitrogen, as part of their molecular makeup. They include:
• chloroprocaine hydrochloride
• procaine hydrochloride
• tetracaine hydrochloride.

All together now

Some injectable local anesthetics, such as lidocaine and tetracaine, also are effective topically. In addition, some topical anesthetics are combined in products.

Pharmacokinetics

Topical anesthetics produce little systemic absorption, except for the application of cocaine to mucous membranes. However, systemic absorption may occur if the patient receives frequent or high-dose applications to the eye or large areas of burned or injured skin.

Tetracaine and other esters are metabolized extensively in the blood and to a lesser extent in the liver. Dibucaine, lidocaine, and other amides are metabolized primarily in the liver. Both types of topical anesthetics are excreted in the urine.

Pharmacodynamics

Benzocaine, butacaine, butamben, cocaine, dyclonine, and pramoxine produce topical anesthesia by blocking nerve impulse transmission. They accumulate in the nerve cell membrane, causing it to expand and lose its ability to depolarize, thus blocking impulse transmission. Dibucaine, lidocaine, and tetracaine may block impulse transmission across the nerve cell membranes.

Drowning out input

The aromatic compounds, such as benzyl alcohol and clove oil, appear to stimulate nerve endings. This stimulation causes counterirritation that interferes with pain perception.

Freezing out nerve endings

Ethyl chloride superficially freezes the tissue, stimulating the cold sensation receptors and blocking the nerve endings in the frozen area. Menthol selectively stimulates the sensory nerve endings for cold, causing a cool sensation and some local pain relief.

Pharmacotherapeutics

Topical anesthetics are used to:
• relieve or prevent pain, especially minor burn pain
• relieve itching and irritation

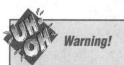

Warning!

Adverse reactions to local anesthetics

Dose-related central nervous system (CNS) reactions include anxiety, apprehension, restlessness, nervousness, disorientation, confusion, dizziness, blurred vision, tremors, twitching, shivering, and seizures. Dose-related cardiovascular reactions may include myocardial depression, bradycardia (slow heart rate), arrhythmias, hypotension, cardiovascular collapse, and cardiac arrest.

All the rest
Local anesthetic solutions that contain vasoconstrictors such as epinephrine also can produce CNS and cardiovascular reactions, including anxiety, dizziness, headache, restlessness, tremors, palpitations, tachycardia, angina, and hypertension.

• anesthetize an area before an injection is given
• numb mucosal surfaces before a tube, such as a urinary catheter, is inserted
• alleviate sore throat or mouth pain when used in a spray or solution.

Eyes and ears

Tetracaine also is used as a topical anesthetic for the eye. Benzocaine is used with other drugs in several ear preparations.

Drug interactions

Few interactions with other drugs occur with topical anesthetics because they aren't absorbed well into the systemic circulation. (See *Adverse reactions to topical anesthetics.*)

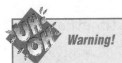

Warning!

Adverse reactions to topical anesthetics

Topical anesthetics can cause several different adverse reactions.
• Benzyl alcohol can cause topical reactions such as skin irritation.
• Refrigerants such as ethyl chloride may produce frostbite where it's been applied.
• Any topical anesthetic can cause a hypersensitivity reaction, including a rash, itching, hives, swelling of the mouth and throat, and breathing difficulty.

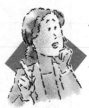

Quick quiz

1. How does the topical anesthetic benzocaine relieve sunburn pain?
   A. It numbs the skin surface, decreasing the perception of pain.
   B. It freezes the skin, which prevents nerve impulse transmission.
   C. It blocks nerve impulse transmission by preventing nerve cell depolarization.

Answer: C. Benzocaine prevents nerve cell depolarization, thus blocking nerve impulse transmission and relieving pain.

2. Which of the following adverse reactions is a patient most likely to experience postsurgery after receiving general anesthesia?
   A. Nausea and vomiting
   B. Seizures
   C. Cyanosis

Answer: A. After surgery involving general anesthesia, a patient is most likely to experience adverse reactions similar to those produced by other CNS depressant drugs, including nausea and vomiting.

3. Before administering dezocine, the nurse asks a patient if he has used narcotics. That is because administering a mixed narcotic agonist-antagonist to a patient dependent on narcotic agonists may cause which of the following reactions?

    A.   Hypersensitivity reaction

    B.   Withdrawal symptoms

    C.   Urinary incontinence

Answer: B. Because they can counteract the effects of narcotic agonists, mixed narcotic agonist-antagonists can cause withdrawal symptoms in patients dependent on narcotic agonists.

4. The drug commonly prescribed to treat a narcotic overdose is:

    A.   butorphanol.

    B.   naloxone.

    C.   pentazocine.

Answer: B. Naloxone is the drug of choice for managing narcotic overdose.

5. What are the most common adverse reactions to aspirin?

    A.   Increased rate and depth of respirations

    B.   Nausea, vomiting, and GI distress

    C.   Dizziness and vision changes

Answer: B. Aspirin most commonly produces adverse GI reactions, such as nausea, vomiting, and GI distress.

6. Desflurane is which type of anesthetic?

    A.   General

    B.   Local

    C.   Topical

Answer: A. Desflurane is a commonly used general anesthetic that is administered by inhalation.

7. Topical anesthetics are used:
   A. as an alternative to general anesthesia for elderly or debilitated patients.
   B. to numb mucosal surfaces before tube insertion.
   C. when anesthesia is needed for only a short period.

Answer: B. Topical anesthetics are used to numb mucosal surfaces as well as relieve or prevent pain, relieve itching and irritation, anesthetize an area for an injection, and alleviate sore throat or mouth pain.

Scoring

☆☆☆   If you answered all seven questions correctly, bravo! You're a pain medication powerhouse.

☆☆   If you answered five or six questions correctly, fabulous! For you, this chapter was painless.

☆   If you answered fewer than five questions correctly, hey, don't give up! Remember: No pain, no gain.

5

Cardiovascular drugs

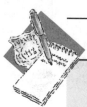

Just the facts

In this chapter, you'll review:

♦ classes of drugs used to treat cardiovascular disorders

♦ uses and varying actions of these drugs

♦ how these drugs are absorbed, distributed, metabolized, and excreted

♦ drug interactions and adverse reactions to these drugs.

Drugs and the cardiovascular system

The heart, arteries, veins, and lymphatics make up the cardiovascular system. These structures transport life-supporting oxygen and nutrients to cells, remove metabolic waste products, and carry hormones from one part of the body to another. Because this system performs such vital functions, any problem with the heart or blood vessels can seriously affect a person's health.

Types of drugs used to improve cardiovascular function include:
• digitalis glycosides and phosphodiesterase (PDE) inhibitors
• antiarrhythmic drugs
• antianginal drugs
• antihypertensive drugs
• diuretic drugs
• antilipemic drugs.

Digitalis glycosides and PDE inhibitors

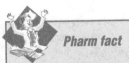

Digitalis glycosides and PDE inhibitors increase the force of the heart's contractions. Increasing the force of contractions is known as a positive inotropic effect, so these drugs are also called inotropic drugs. (Inotropic means effecting the force or energy of muscular contractions.)

Digitalis glycosides also slow the heart rate (called a negative chronotropic effect) and slow electrical impulse conduction through the atrioventricular (AV) node (called a negative dromotropic effect).

Load that dose

Because digoxin has a long half-life, a loading dose must be given to a patient who requires immediate drug effects, as in supraventricular arrhythmia.

By giving a larger initial dose, a minimum effective concentration of the drug in the blood may be reached faster.

Digitalis glycosides

Digitalis glycosides are a group of drugs derived from digitalis, a substance that occurs naturally in foxglove plants and certain toads. The most frequently used digitalis glycoside is *digoxin*. Another digitalis glycoside, digitoxin, is no longer available in the United States.

Pharmacokinetics (how drugs circulate)

The intestinal absorption of digoxin varies greatly; the capsules are absorbed most efficiently, followed by the elixir form, and then tablets. Digoxin is distributed widely throughout the body, is bound extensively to skeletal muscles, and doesn't penetrate body fat easily. Digoxin is poorly bound to plasma proteins.

In most patients, a small amount of digoxin is metabolized in the liver and gut by bacteria. This effect varies and may be substantial in some people. Most of the drug is excreted by the kidneys as unchanged drug.

Pharmacodynamics (how drugs act)

Digoxin is used to treat heart failure because it strengthens the contraction of the ventricles. It does this by boosting intracellular calcium at the cell membrane, enabling stronger heart contractions.

Digoxin also may enhance the movement of calcium into the myocardial cells and stimulate the release, or block the reuptake, of norepinephrine at the adrenergic nerve terminal.

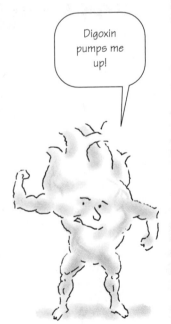

Digoxin pumps me up!

Stop that impulse

Digoxin acts on the central nervous system (CNS) to slow the heart rate, thus making it useful for treating supraventricular arrhythmias (an abnormal heart rhythm that originates above the bundle branches of the heart's conduction system), such as atrial fibrillation and atrial flutter. It also increases the refractory period (the period when the cells of the conduction system can't conduct an impulse).

Pharmacotherapeutics (how drugs are used)

In addition to treating heart failure and supraventricular arrhythmias, digoxin is used to treat paroxysmal atrial tachycardia (an arrhythmia marked by brief periods of tachycardia that alternate with brief periods of sinus rhythm). (See *Load that dose.*)

Drug interactions

Many drugs can interact with digoxin.
- Rifampin, phenytoin, barbiturates, cholestyramine resin, antacids, kaolin and pectin, sulfasalazine, neomycin, metoclopramide, and phenytoin reduce the therapeutic effects of digoxin.
- Calcium preparations, quinidine, verapamil, anticholinergics, amiodarone, spironolactone, hydroxychloroquine, erythromycin, itraconazole, and omeprazole increase the risk of digitalis toxicity.
- Amphotericin B, potassium-wasting diuretics, and steroids taken with digoxin may cause hypokalemia (low potassium levels) and increase the risk of digitalis toxicity.
- Beta blockers taken with digoxin may cause an excessively slow heart rate and arrhythmias.
- Succinylcholine and thyroid preparations increase the risk of arrhythmias when they're taken with digoxin.

Digoxin can also produce adverse reactions, mostly involving digitalis toxicity. (See *Adverse reactions to digitalis glycosides.*)

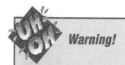 **Warning!**

Adverse reactions to digitalis glycosides

Because digitalis glycosides have a narrow therapeutic index (margin of safety), they may produce digitalis toxicity. To prevent digitalis toxicity, the dosage should be individualized based on the patient's serum digitalis concentration.

Signs and symptoms of digitalis toxicity include:
- nausea, abdominal pain
- headache, irritability, depression, insomnia, and vision changes
- arrhythmias, complete heart block.

PDE inhibitors

PDE inhibitors are typically used for short-term management of heart failure or long-term management in patients awaiting heart transplant surgery.

In the United States, two PDE inhibitors, inamrinone lactate and milrinone, have been approved for use.

Pharmacokinetics

Inamrinone is administered I.V., distributed rapidly, metabolized by the liver, and excreted by the kidneys.

Quick and short

Milrinone is also administered I.V. and is distributed rapidly and excreted by the kidneys, primarily as unchanged drug.

Pharmacodynamics

PDE inhibitors improve cardiac output by strengthening contractions. These drugs are thought to help move calcium into the cardiac cell or to increase calcium storage in the sarcoplasmic reticulum. By directly relaxing vascular smooth muscle, they also decrease peripheral vascular resistance (afterload) and the amount of blood returning to the heart (preload).

Pharmacotherapeutics

Inamrinone and milrinone are used for the management of heart failure in patients who haven't responded adequately to treatment with digitalis glycosides, diuretics, or vasodilators. Prolonged use of these drugs may increase the patient's risk of complications and death. (See *Adverse reactions to PDE inhibitors.*)

Drug interactions

• PDE inhibitors may interact with disopyramide, causing hypotension.
• Because PDE inhibitors reduce serum potassium levels, taking them with a potassium-wasting diuretic may lead to hypokalemia.

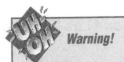

Warning!

Adverse reactions to PDE inhibitors

Adverse reactions to phosphodiesterase (PDE) inhibitors are uncommon, but the likelihood increases significantly when a patient is on prolonged therapy.

Adverse reactions may include:
• arrhythmias
• nausea and vomiting
• headache
• fever
• chest pain
• hypokalemia
• thrombocytopenia
• mild increase in heart rate.

Antiarrhythmic drugs

Antiarrhythmic drugs are used to treat arrhythmias, disturbances of the normal heart rhythm.

Benefits vs. risks

Unfortunately, many antiarrhythmic drugs are also capable of worsening or causing the very arrhythmias they're supposed to treat. The benefits need to be weighed against the risks of antiarrhythmic therapy.

Four classes plus...

Antiarrhythmics are categorized into four classes:
• I (which includes class IA, IB, and IC)
• II
• III
• IV.
　　Class I antiarrhythmics consist of sodium channel blockers. This is the largest group of antiarrhythmic drugs. Class I agents are frequently subdivided into Class IA, IB, and IC. One drug, adenosine, doesn't fall into any of these classes.
　　The mechanisms of action of antiarrhythmic drugs vary widely, and a few drugs exhibit properties common to more than one class.

Class IA antiarrhythmics

Class IA antiarrhythmics are used to treat a wide variety of atrial and ventricular arrhythmias. Class IA antiarrhythmics include:
• disopyramide phosphate
• procainamide hydrochloride
• quinidine sulfate
• quinidine gluconate
• quinidine polygalacturonate.

Pharmacokinetics

When administered orally, class IA drugs are rapidly absorbed and metabolized. Because they work so quickly, sustained-release forms of these drugs were developed to help maintain therapeutic levels.

One to the brain

These drugs are distributed through all body tissues. Quinidine, however, is the only one that crosses the blood-brain barrier.

All class IA antiarrhythmics are metabolized in the liver and are excreted unchanged by the kidneys. Acidic urine increases the excretion of quinidine.

> Because class IA antiarrhythmics work so quickly, sustained-release forms of the drugs were created to maintain therapeutic levels.

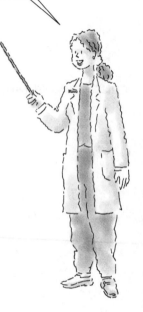

Pharmacodynamics

Class IA antiarrhythmics control arrhythmias by altering the myocardial cell membrane and interfering with autonomic nervous system control of pacemaker cells.

No (para)sympathy

Class IA antiarrhythmics also block parasympathetic stimulation of the sinoatrial (SA) and AV nodes. Because stimulation of the parasympathetic nervous system causes the heart rate to slow down, drugs that block the parasympathetic nervous system increase the conduction rate of the AV node.

Rhythmic risks

This increase in the conduction rate can produce dangerous increases in the ventricular heart rate if rapid atrial activity is present, as in a patient with atrial fibrillation. In turn, the increased ventricular heart rate can offset the ability of the antiarrhythmics to convert atrial arrhythmias to a regular rhythm.

Pharmacotherapeutics

Class IA antiarrhythmics are prescribed to treat such arrhythmias as premature ventricular contractions, ventricular tachycardia, atrial fibrillation, atrial flutter, and paroxysmal atrial tachycardia.

Drug interactions

Class IA antiarrhythmics can interact with other drugs in various ways:
• Disopyramide taken with anticholinergics may increase anticholinergic effects.

• Disopyramide plus verapamil may cause myocardial depression.
• Quinidine plus neuromuscular blockers causes increased skeletal muscle relaxation.
• Quinidine increases the risk of digitalis toxicity.
• Rifampin, phenytoin, and phenobarbital can reduce the effects of quinidine and disopyramide.

Abdominal problems are common adverse reactions to class IA antiarrhythmics. (See *Adverse reactions to class IA antiarrhythmics.*)

Class IB antiarrhythmics

Lidocaine hydrochloride, a *class IB antiarrhythmic*, is one of the antiarrhythmics most widely used for treating acute ventricular arrhythmias. Other class IB antiarrhythmics include mexiletine hydrochloride and tocainide hydrochloride.

Pharmacokinetics

With the exception of lidocaine, which is typically administered I.V., all class IB antiarrhythmics are absorbed well from the GI tract after oral administration.

All bound up?

Lidocaine is distributed widely throughout the body, including the brain. Lidocaine and mexiletine are moderately bound to plasma proteins. (Remember, only that portion of a drug that is unbound can produce a response.) Tocainide, on the other hand, is mostly unbound.

Class IB antiarrhythmics are metabolized in the liver and excreted in the urine. Mexiletine also is excreted in breast milk.

Pharmacodynamics

Class IB drugs work by blocking the rapid influx of sodium ions during the depolarization phase of the heart's depolarization-repolarization cycle, resulting in a decreased refractory period, which reduces the risk of arrhythmia.

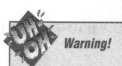

Warning!

Adverse reactions to class IA antiarrhythmics

Class IA antiarrhythmics, especially quinidine, may produce GI symptoms, such as diarrhea, cramping, nausea, vomiting, anorexia, and bitter taste.

Dramatic irony
Ironically, not only do class IA antiarrhythmics treat arrhythmias, but they can also induce arrhythmias, especially conduction delays that may worsen existing heart blocks.

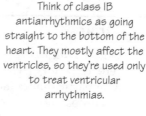

Think of class IB antiarrhythmics as going straight to the bottom of the heart. They mostly affect the ventricles, so they're used only to treat ventricular arrhythmias.

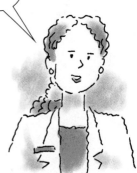

Make a IB-line for the ventricle

Because class IB antiarrhythmics especially affect the Purkinje fibers (fibers in the conducting system of the heart) and myocardial cells in the ventricles, they're used only to treat ventricular arrhythmias.

Pharmacotherapeutics

Class IB antiarrhythmics are used to treat ventricular ectopic beats, ventricular tachycardia, and ventricular fibrillation.

Because class IB antiarrhythmics usually don't produce serious adverse reactions, they're the drugs of choice in acute care.

Drug interactions

Class IB antiarrhythmics may exhibit additive or antagonistic effects when administered with other antiarrhythmics, such as phenytoin, propranolol, procainamide, and quinidine. Other drug interactions include the following:
• Rifampin may reduce the effects of mexiletine or tocainide.
• Theophylline plasma levels are increased when theophylline is given with mexiletine.
• Use of a beta blocker or disopyramide with mexiletine may reduce the contractility of the heart. (See *Adverse reactions to class IB antiarrhythmics.*)

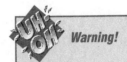
Warning!

Adverse reactions to class IB antiarrhythmics

Adverse reactions to class IB antiarrhythmics include drowsiness, light-headedness, paresthesia, sensory disturbances, hypotension, and bradycardia.

Lidocaine toxicity can cause seizures and respiratory arrest.

Adverse reactions to mexiletine include hypotension, atrioventricular block, bradycardia, confusion, ataxia, and double vision. Mexiletine or tocainide may produce nausea and vomiting.

Class IC antiarrhythmics

Class IC antiarrhythmics are used to treat certain severe, refractory (resistant) ventricular arrhythmias. Class IC antiarrhythmics include flecainide acetate, moricizine, and propafenone hydrochloride.

Pharmacokinetics

After oral administration, class IC antiarrhythmics are absorbed well, distributed in varying degrees, and probably metabolized by the liver. They're excreted primarily by the kidneys, except for propafenone, which is excreted primarily in stool.

After oral administration, about 38% of moricizine is absorbed. It undergoes extensive metabolism, with less than 1% of a dose excreted unchanged in the urine. Moricizine is highly protein bound, leaving only a small portion of the drug free to produce its antiarrhythmic effect.

Pharmacodynamics

Class IC antiarrhythmics primarily slow conduction along the heart's conduction system. Moricizine decreases the fast inward current of sodium ions of the action potential, depressing the depolarization rate and effective refractory period.

Pharmacotherapeutics

Like class IB antiarrhythmics, class IC antiarrhythmic drugs are used to treat life-threatening ventricular arrhythmias. They're also used to treat supraventricular arrhythmias (abnormal heart rhythms that originate above the bundle branches of the heart's conduction system).

Flecainide also may be used to prevent paroxysmal supraventricular tachycardia (PSVT) in patients without structural heart disease. Moricizine is used to manage life-threatening ventricular arrhythmias such as sustained ventricular tachycardia.

Drug interactions

Class IC antiarrhythmics may exhibit additive effects with other antiarrhythmics. Other interactions include the following:
• When used with digoxin, flecainide and propafenone increase the risk of digitalis toxicity.
• Quinidine increases the effects of propafenone.
• Cimetidine may increase the plasma level and the risk of toxicity of moricizine.
• Propanolol or digoxin given with moricizine may increase the PR interval on the electrocardiogram.
• Theophylline levels may be reduced in the patient receiving moricizine.
• Propafenone increases the serum concentration and effects of metoprolol and propranolol. (See *Adverse reactions to class IC arrhythmics.*)

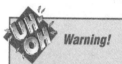

Class II antiarrhythmics

Class II antiarrhythmics are composed of beta-adrenergic antagonists, or beta blockers. Beta blockers used as antiarrhythmics include acebutolol hydrochloride, esmolol hydrochloride, and propranolol hydrochloride.

Pharmacokinetics

Acebutolol and propranolol are absorbed almost entirely from the GI tract after an oral dose. Esmolol, which can only be given I.V., is immediately available throughout the body.

Fat keeps out

Acebutolol has low lipid solubility. That means that it can't penetrate the highly fatty cells that act as barriers between the blood and brain, called the blood-brain barrier.

Propranolol has high lipid solubility and readily crosses the blood-brain barrier. Esmolol is distributed rapidly throughout all body tissues.

Acebutolol is poorly protein bound in plasma, esmolol is moderately protein bound, and propranolol is highly protein bound.

First-pass leaves little

Acebutolol and propranolol undergo significant first-pass effect, leaving only a small portion of these drugs available to reach the circulation to be distributed to the body.

About 35% of an acebutolol dose is excreted in the urine and 55% in stool. Most of an esmolol dose is metabolized to an inactive metabolite, which is excreted in the urine. Propranolol's metabolites are excreted in the urine as well.

Pharmacodynamics

Class II antiarrhythmics block beta-adrenergic receptor sites in the conduction system of the heart. As a result, the ability of the SA node to fire spontaneously (automaticity) is slowed. The ability of the AV node and other cells to receive and conduct an electrical impulse to nearby cells (conductivity) is also reduced.

Class II antiarrhythmics also reduce the strength of the heart's contractions. When the heart beats less forcefully, it doesn't require as much oxygen to do its work.

Class II antiarrhythmics also serve as antihypertensives — when these drugs are taken with phenothiazines or other antihypertensives, the patient can experience hypotension.

CAUTION!

Pharmacotherapeutics

Class II antiarrhythmics slow ventricular rates in patients with atrial flutter, atrial fibrillation, and paroxysmal atrial tachycardia. (See *Adverse reactions to class II antiarrhythmics.*)

Drug interactions

Class II antiarrhythmics can cause a variety of drug interactions:
• Administering them with phenothiazines and antihypertensive drugs increases the antihypertensive effect.
• The effects of sympathomimetics may be reduced when taken with class II antiarrhythmics.
• Beta blockers given with verapamil can depress the heart, causing hypotension, bradycardia, AV block, and asystole.
• Beta blockers reduce the effects of sulfonylureas.
• The risk of digitalis toxicity increases when digoxin is taken with esmolol.

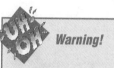

Warning!

Adverse reactions to class II antiarrhythmics

Common adverse reactions include:
• arrhythmias
• bradycardia
• heart failure
• hypotension
• GI reactions, such as nausea, vomiting, and diarrhea
• bronchoconstriction.

Class III antiarrhythmics

Class III antiarrhythmics are used to treat ventricular arrhythmias. The two drugs in this class are amiodarone hydrochloride and bretylium tosylate.

Pharmacokinetics

The absorption of these two antiarrhythmics varies widely.

Slow going

After oral administration, amiodarone is absorbed slowly at widely varying rates. The drug is distributed extensively and accumulates in many sites, especially in organs with a rich blood supply and fatty tissue. It's highly protein bound in plasma, mainly to albumin.

Erratic antics

Because GI absorption is so erratic, bretylium is given I.V. Bretylium is distributed widely throughout the body and is poorly protein bound, and is excreted unchanged by the kidneys.

Bretylium (a class III antiarrhythmic) is absorbed erratically in the GI tract, so it's only given I.V.

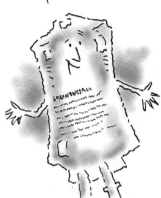

Pharmacodynamics

Although the exact mechanism of action isn't known, class III antiarrhythmics are thought to suppress arrhythmias by converting a unidirectional block to a bidirectional block. They have little or no effect on depolarization.

Pharmacotherapeutics

Because of their adverse effects, class III antiarrhythmics aren't the drugs of choice for antiarrhythmic therapy. They're used for life-threatening arrhythmias that are resistant to other antiarrhythmic treatment.

Drug interactions

- Amiodarone increases quinidine, procainamide, and phenytoin levels and may cause bleeding in patients receiving coumadin.
- Amiodarone also increases the risk of digitalis toxicity.

Pressure plunge

- Because of the risk of severe hypotension, bretylium can't be given with epinephrine, norepinephrine, or other sympathomimetics. Bretylium may potentiate the effects of the drugs given to correct hypotension.
- Severe hypotension may develop when amiodarone is given with antihypertensive drugs. (See *Adverse reactions to class III antiarrhythmics.*)

Class IV antiarrhythmics

Class IV antiarrhythmics are composed of calcium channel blockers. Calcium channel blockers used to treat arrhythmias include verapamil and diltiazem.

One main use

Verapamil and diltiazem are used to treat supraventricular arrhythmias with rapid ventricular response rates (rapid heart rate in which the rhythm originates above the ventricles).

For a thorough discussion of calcium channel blockers and how they work, see "Calcium channel blockers," page 118.

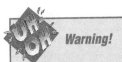

Warning!

Adverse reactions to class III antiarrhythmics

Adverse reactions to class III antiarrhythmics, especially amiodarone, vary widely and commonly lead to drug discontinuation. A common adverse effect is aggravation of arrhythmias.

Adverse reactions to amiodarone...
Amiodarone may produce hypotension, nausea, and anorexia. Severe pulmonary toxicity occurs in 15% of patients and can be fatal.

...and bretylium
After I.V. administration, orthostatic (on standing) and supine (while lying down) hypotension commonly occur, producing dizziness.

Adenosine

Adenosine is an injectable antiarrhythmic drug indicated for acute treatment of PSVT.

Pharmacokinetics

After I.V. administration, adenosine probably is distributed rapidly throughout the body and metabolized inside red blood cells as well as in vascular endothelial cells.

Pharmacodynamics

Adenosine depresses the pacemaker activity of the SA node, reducing the heart rate and the ability of the AV node to conduct impulses from the atria to the ventricles.

Pharmacotherapeutics

Adenosine is especially effective against reentry tachycardias (when an impulse depolarizes an area of heart muscle and returns and repolarizes it) that involve the AV node.

No slouch

Adenosine is also effective with more than 90% of PSVT cases. It's particularly used to treat arrhythmias associated with accessory bypass tracts, as in Wolff-Parkinson-White syndrome (brief periods of rapid heart rate in which the rhythm's origin is above the ventricle), a condition in which strands of heart tissue formed during fetal development abnormally connect structures, such as the atria and ventricles, bypassing normal conduction, also called a preexcitation syndrome.

Drug interactions

• Methylxanthines antagonize the effects of adenosine so that larger doses of adenosine may be necessary.
• Dipyridamole potentiates the effects of adenosine; therefore, smaller doses of adenosine may be necessary.
• When adenosine is administered with carbamazepine, there is an increased risk of heart block. (See *Adverse reactions to adenosine.*)

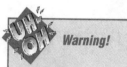

Warning!

Adverse reactions to adenosine

• Facial flushing
• Shortness of breath
• Dyspnea
• Chest discomfort

Remember, caffeine antagonizes the effect of adenosine, so larger doses of the drug may become necessary.

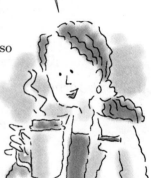

Antianginal drugs

Although angina's cardinal symptom is chest pain, the drugs used to treat angina aren't typically analgesics.

Instead, *antianginal drugs* treat angina by reducing myocardial oxygen demand (reducing the amount of oxygen the heart needs to do its work), by increasing the supply of oxygen to the heart, or both. (See *How antianginal drugs work.*)

The three classes of antianginal drugs discussed in this section include:
- nitrates (for treating acute angina)
- beta blockers (for long-term prevention of angina)
- calcium channel blockers (used when other drugs fail to prevent angina).

Nitrates

Nitrates are the drugs of choice for relieving acute angina. Nitrates commonly prescribed to treat angina include:
- erythrityl tetranitrate
- isosorbide dinitrate
- isosorbide mononitrate
- nitroglycerin
- pentaerythritol tetranitrate.

Pharmacokinetics

Nitrates can be administered in a variety of ways.

All absorbed...

Nitrates given sublingually (under the tongue), buccally (in the pocket of the cheek), as chewable tablets, or as lingual aerosols (sprayed onto or under the tongue) are absorbed almost completely. That is because the mucous membranes of the mouth have a rich blood supply.

...half-absorbed...

Swallowed nitrate capsules are absorbed through the mucous membranes of the GI tract, and only about half the dose enters circulation.

Transdermal nitrates (a patch or ointment placed on the skin) are absorbed slowly and in varying amounts, depending on the quantity of drug applied, the location

Zoom in

How antianginal drugs work

Angina occurs when the coronary arteries, the heart's primary source of oxygen, supply insufficient oxygen to the myocardium. This increases the heart's workload, increasing heart rate, preload (blood volume in ventricle at end of diastole), afterload (pressure in arteries leading from ventricle), and force of myocardial contractility. The antianginal drugs (nitrates, beta blockers, and calcium channel blockers) relieve angina by *decreasing* one or more of these four factors. This diagram summarizes how antianginal drugs affect the cardiovascular system.

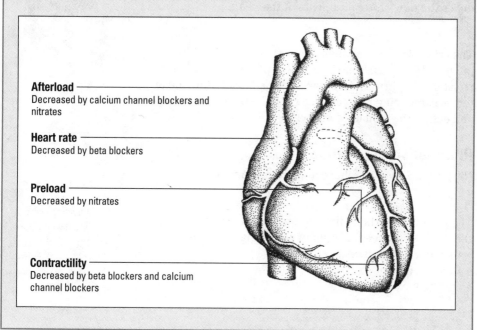

Afterload
Decreased by calcium channel blockers and nitrates

Heart rate
Decreased by beta blockers

Preload
Decreased by nitrates

Contractility
Decreased by beta blockers and calcium channel blockers

where the patch is applied, the surface area of skin used, and the circulation to the skin.

...or no absorption required

I.V. nitroglycerin, which doesn't need to be absorbed, goes directly into circulation.

Pharmacodynamics

Nitrates cause the smooth muscle of the veins and, to a lesser extent, the arteries to relax and dilate. This is what happens:

• When the veins dilate, less blood returns to the heart.
• This, in turn, reduces the amount of blood in the ventricles at the end of diastole, when the ventricles are full. (This blood volume in the ventricles just before contraction is called preload.)
• By reducing preload, nitrates reduce ventricular size and ventricular wall tension (the left ventricle doesn't have to stretch as much to pump blood). This, in turn, reduces the oxygen requirements of the heart.

Reducing resistance

The arterioles provide the most resistance to the blood pumped by the left ventricle (called peripheral vascular resistance). Nitrates decrease afterload by dilating the arterioles, reducing resistance, easing the heart's workload, and easing the demand for oxygen.

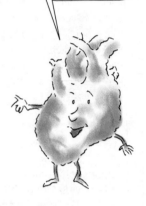

The more blood that fills my ventricles, the harder I have to work...

Pharmacotherapeutics

Nitrates are used to relieve and prevent angina.

For speedy relief...

The rapidly absorbed nitrates, such as nitroglycerin, are the drugs of choice for relief of acute angina because:
• they have a rapid onset of action
• they're easy to take
• they're inexpensive.

...or prevention

Longer-acting nitrates, such as the daily nitroglycerin transdermal patch, are convenient and can be used to prevent chronic angina. Oral nitrates are also used because they seldom produce serious adverse reactions.

...and the harder I work, the more oxygen I need. By dilating veins, nitrates reduce the blood in my ventricles — so I can get some rest.

Drug interactions

• Severe hypotension can result when nitrates interact with alcohol.

- Absorption of sublingual nitrates may be delayed when taken with an anticholinergic drug.
- Marked orthostatic hypotension (a drop in blood pressure when a person stands up) with light-headedness, fainting, or blurred vision may occur when calcium channel blockers and nitrates are used together. (See *Adverse reactions to nitrates.*)

Beta-adrenergic antagonists

Beta-adrenergic antagonists (also called *beta blockers*) are used for long-term prevention of angina and are one of the main types of drugs used to treat hypertension. Beta blockers include:
- atenolol
- metoprolol tartrate
- nadolol
- propranolol hydrochloride.

Pharmacokinetics

Metoprolol and propranolol are absorbed almost entirely from the GI tract, whereas less than half the dose of atenolol or nadolol is absorbed. These beta blockers are distributed widely. Propranolol is highly protein bound; the other beta blockers are poorly protein bound.

Excreted unchanged

Propranolol and metoprolol are metabolized in the liver, and their metabolites are excreted in the urine. Atenolol and nadolol aren't metabolized and are excreted unchanged in the urine and stool.

Pharmacodynamics

Beta blockers decrease blood pressure and block beta-adrenergic receptor sites in the heart muscle and conduction system, decreasing heart rate and reducing the force of the heart's contractions, resulting in lower demand for oxygen.

Pharmacotherapeutics

Beta blockers are indicated for long-term prevention of angina. Because of their longer onset, they aren't used to

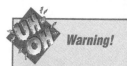
Warning!

Adverse reactions to nitrates

Most adverse reactions to nitrates are caused by changes in the cardiovascular system. The reactions usually disappear when the dosage is reduced.

The 3 H's
Headache is the most common adverse reaction. Hypotension may occur, accompanied by dizziness and increased heart rate.

provide immediate relief of an angina attack or to prevent an imminent one.

Because of their ability to reduce blood pressure, beta blockers are also first-line therapy for treating hypertension.

Drug interactions

A number of drugs interact with beta blockers.
- Antacids delay absorption of beta blockers.
- Nonsteroidal anti-inflammatory drugs (NSAIDs) can decrease the hypotensive effects of beta blockers.
- Lidocaine toxicity may occur when lidocaine is taken with beta blockers.
- The requirements for insulin and oral antidiabetic drugs can be altered by beta blockers.
- The ability of theophylline to produce bronchodilation is impaired by nonselective beta blockers. (See *Adverse reactions to beta blockers.*)

Calcium channel blockers

Calcium channel blockers are commonly used to prevent angina that doesn't respond to drugs in either of the other antianginal classes. As mentioned earlier, several of the calcium channel blockers are also used as antiarrhythmics. Calcium channel blockers include:
- amlodipine besylate
- diltiazem hydrochloride
- nicardipine hydrochloride
- nifedipine
- verapamil hydrochloride.

Pharmacokinetics

When administered orally, calcium channel blockers are absorbed quickly and almost completely. Because of the first-pass effect, however, the bioavailability of these drugs is much lower. The calcium channel blockers are highly bound to plasma proteins.

Look to the liver

All calcium channel blockers are metabolized rapidly and almost completely in the liver.

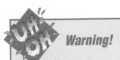

Warning!

Adverse reactions to beta blockers

Beta blockers may cause:
- bradycardia
- angina
- fainting
- fluid retention
- peripheral edema
- shock
- heart failure
- arrhythmias, especially atrioventricular block
- nausea and vomiting
- diarrhea
- significant constriction of the bronchioles.

Quick stop causes concern

Suddenly stopping a beta blocker may trigger:
- angina
- hypertension
- arrhythmias
- acute myocardial infarction.

Pharmacodynamics

Calcium channel blockers prevent the passage of calcium ions across the myocardial cell membrane and vascular smooth muscle cells. This causes dilation of the coronary and peripheral arteries, which decreases the force of the heart's contractions and reduces the workload of the heart. (See *How calcium channel blockers work*, page 120.)

Rate reductions

By preventing arterioles from constricting, calcium channel blockers also reduce afterload. Decreasing afterload also decreases the oxygen demands of the heart.

Calcium channel blockers also reduce the heart rate by slowing conduction through the SA and AV nodes. A slower heart rate reduces the heart's need for additional oxygen.

Pharmacotherapeutics

Calcium channel blockers are used only for long-term prevention of angina, not short-term relief of chest pain. Calcium channel blockers are particularly effective for preventing Prinzmetal's angina.

Drug interactions

• Calcium salts and vitamin D reduce the effectiveness of calcium channel blockers.
• Nondepolarizing blocking drugs may have an enhanced muscle relaxant effect when taken with calcium channel blockers.
• Verapamil and diltiazem increase the risk of digitalis toxicity, enhance the action of carbamazepine, and can produce myocardial depression. (See *Adverse reactions to calcium channel blockers.*)

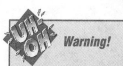

Warning!

Adverse reactions to calcium channel blockers

As with other antianginal drugs, cardiovascular reactions are the most common and serious adverse reactions to calcium channel blockers. These include orthostatic hypotension (a drop in blood pressure when a person stands up), heart failure, hypotension, and arrhythmias, such as bradycardia, sinus block, and atrioventricular block.

Others
Other possible adverse reactions include dizziness, headache, flushing, weakness, and persistent peripheral edema.

Antihypertensive drugs

Antihypertensive drugs, which act to reduce blood pressure, are used to treat hypertension, a disorder characterized by elevation in systolic blood pressure, diastolic blood pressure, or both.

Zoom in

How calcium channel blockers work

Calcium channel blockers increase the myocardial oxygen supply and slow the heart rate. Apparently, the drugs produce these effects by blocking the slow calcium channel. This action inhibits the influx of extracellular calcium ions across both myocardial and vascular smooth muscle cell membranes. Calcium channel blockers achieve this blockade without changing serum calcium concentrations.

No calcium = dilation

This calcium blockade causes the coronary arteries (and, to a lesser extent, the peripheral arteries and arterioles) to dilate, decreasing afterload and increasing myocardial oxygen supply. The blockade also slows sinoatrial and atrioventricular node conduction, slightly reducing heart rate.

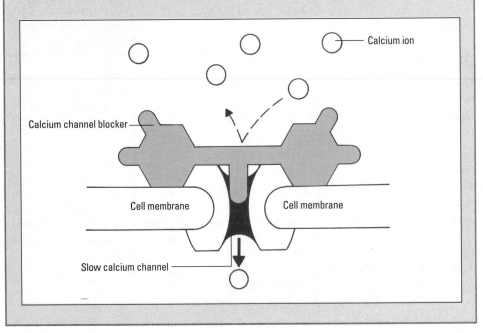

Calcium ion

Calcium channel blocker

Cell membrane

Cell membrane

Slow calcium channel

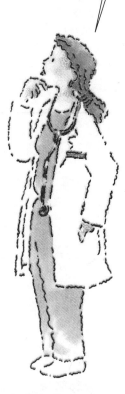

> Calcium channel blockers slow the heart rate but don't change the level of calcium in the blood.

Know the program

Treatment for hypertension begins with beta blockers and diuretics. (For more information, see "Beta-adrenergic antagonists," page 117, and "Thiazide and thiazide-like diuretics," page 125.) If those drugs don't prove effective, treatment continues with sympatholytic drugs (other than beta blockers), vasodilators, angiotensin-converting enzyme (ACE) inhibitors, or a combination of drugs.

Sympatholytic drugs

Sympatholytic drugs include several different types of drugs, but all reduce blood pressure by inhibiting or blocking the sympathetic nervous system. They are classified by their site or mechanism of action and include:
• central-acting sympathetic nervous system inhibitors (clonidine hydrochloride, guanabenz acetate, guanfacine, and methyldopa)
• alpha blockers (doxazosin mesylate, phentolamine, prazosin hydrochloride, and terazosin)
• mixed alpha and beta blockers (labetalol)
• norepinephrine depletors (guanadrel sulfate, guanethidine monosulfate, and reserpine).

Pharmacokinetics

Most sympatholytic drugs are absorbed well from the GI tract, distributed widely, metabolized in the liver, and excreted primarily in the urine.

Pharmacodynamics

All sympatholytic drugs inhibit stimulation of the sympathetic nervous system. This causes dilation of the peripheral blood vessels or decreased cardiac output, thereby reducing blood pressure.

Pharmacotherapeutics

Beta blockers (along with diuretics) are the initial drugs for treating hypertension. If blood pressure fails to come under control, an alpha blocker such as prazosin or an alpha-beta blocker such as labetalol may be used. If the patient fails to respond (achieves the desired blood pressure), the doctor may add a drug from a different class, substitute a drug in the same class, or increase the drug dosage.

Drug interactions

Sympatholytic drugs can create the following drug interactions:
• Clonidine plus tricyclic antidepressants may increase blood pressure.
• Clonidine taken with CNS depressants may worsen CNS depression.

Sympatholytic drugs can also produce significant adverse reactions. (See *Adverse reactions to sympatholytics*.)

Vasodilating drugs

There are two types of *vasodilating drugs*—direct vasodilators and calcium channel blockers. Both types decrease systolic and diastolic blood pressure.

Resistance is futile

Direct vasodilators act on arteries, veins, or both. They include:
- diazoxide
- hydralazine hydrochloride
- minoxidil
- nitroprusside sodium.

Hydralazine and minoxidil are usually used to treat resistant or refractory hypertension. Diazoxide and nitroprusside are reserved for use in hypertensive crisis.

Keep out calcium

Calcium channel blockers produce arteriolar relaxation by preventing the entry of calcium into the cells. This prevents the contraction of vascular smooth muscle. (See "Calcium channel blockers," page 118.)

Pharmacokinetics

Most of the drugs are absorbed rapidly and distributed well. They all are metabolized in the liver, and most are excreted by the kidneys.

Pharmacodynamics

The direct vasodilators relax peripheral vascular smooth muscles, causing the blood vessels to dilate. This lowers blood pressure by increasing the diameter of the blood vessels, reducing total peripheral resistance.

Pharmacotherapeutics

Vasodilating drugs are rarely used alone to treat hypertension. Instead they're usually used in combination with other drugs to treat the patient with moderate to severe hypertension (hypertensive crisis).

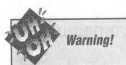
Warning!

Adverse reactions to sympatholytics

Alpha blockers
- Hypotension

Central-acting drugs
- Depression
- Drowsiness
- Edema
- Liver dysfunction
- Numbness, tingling
- Vertigo

Guanadrel
- Difficulty breathing
- Excessive urination
- Fainting
- Orthostatic hypotension

Guanethidine
- Decreased heart contractility
- Diarrhea
- Fluid retention
- Orthostatic hypotension

Reserpine
- Abdominal cramps, diarrhea
- Angina
- Blurred vision
- Bradycardia
- Bronchoconstriction
- Decreased libido
- Depression
- Drowsiness
- Weight gain

Calcium channel blockers are occasionally used alone to treat mild to moderate hypertension.

Drug interactions

- The antihypertensive effects of hydralazine and minoxidil are increased when they're given with other antihypertensive drugs, such as methyldopa or reserpine.
- Vasodilating drugs may produce additive effects when given with nitrates, such as isosorbide dinitrate or nitroglycerin.
- Few other drug interactions occur with vasodilating drugs. (See *Adverse reactions to direct vasodilators.*)

ACE inhibitors

ACE inhibitors reduce blood pressure by interrupting the renin-angiotensin-aldosterone system. Commonly prescribed ACE inhibitors include:
- benazepril hydrochloride
- captopril
- enalapril
- fosinopril sodium
- lisinopril
- quinapril hydrochloride
- ramipril.

Pharmacokinetics

ACE inhibitors are absorbed from the GI tract, distributed to most body tissues, metabolized somewhat in the liver, and excreted by the kidneys. Ramipril also is excreted in stool.

Pharmacodynamics

ACE inhibitors act by interfering with the renin-angiotensin-aldosterone system. Here is how they work.

Normally, the kidneys maintain blood pressure by releasing the hormone renin. Renin acts on the plasma protein angiotensinogen to form angiotensin I. Angiotensin I is then converted to angiotensin II. Angiotensin II, a potent vasoconstrictor, increases peripheral resistance and promotes the excretion of aldosterone. Aldosterone, in turn, promotes the retention of sodium and water, increasing the volume of blood the heart needs to pump.

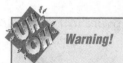

Warning!

Adverse reactions to direct vasodilators

Direct vasodilators commonly produce adverse reactions related to reflex activation of the sympathetic nervous system. As blood pressure falls, the sympathetic nervous system is stimulated, producing compensatory measures, such as vasoconstriction and tachycardia.

Other reactions to sympathetic stimulation include:
- palpitations
- angina
- edema
- breast tenderness
- fatigue
- headache
- rash
- severe pericardial effusion.

Conversion diversion

ACE inhibitors work by preventing the conversion of angiotensin I to angiotensin II. As angiotensin II is reduced, arterioles dilate, reducing peripheral vascular resistance.

Less water, less work

By reducing aldosterone secretion, ACE inhibitors promote the excretion of sodium and water, reducing the amount of blood the heart needs to pump and resulting in decreased blood pressure.

Pharmacotherapeutics

ACE inhibitors may be used alone or in combination with another drug, such as a thiazide diuretic, to treat hypertension. They're commonly used when beta blockers or diuretics are ineffective. They're also used to manage heart failure.

Drug interactions

ACE inhibitors can cause several different types of interactions with other cardiovascular drugs. All ACE inhibitors enhance the hypotensive effects of diuretics and other antihypertensives, such as beta blockers. They also can increase serum lithium levels, possibly resulting in lithium toxicity.

When ACE inhibitors are used with potassium-sparing diuretics, potassium supplements, or potassium-containing salt substitutes, hyperkalemia may occur.

Individual items

Captopril, enalapril, and lisinopril may become less effective when administered with NSAIDs. Antacids may impair the absorption of fosinopril, and quinapril may reduce the absorption of tetracycline. (See *Adverse reactions to ACE inhibitors.*)

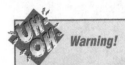

Warning!

Adverse reactions to ACE inhibitors

Angiotensin-converting enzyme (ACE) inhibitors can produce the following adverse reactions:
- headache and fatigue
- a dry, nonproductive, persistent cough
- angioedema
- GI reactions
- increased serum potassium concentrations
- tickling in the throat
- transient elevations of blood urea nitrogen and serum creatinine levels (indicators of kidney function).

Caused by captopril
Captopril may cause protein in the urine, reduced neutrophils and granulocytes (types of white blood cells), rash, loss of taste, hypotension, or a severe allergic reaction.

Diuretic drugs

Diuretics are used to promote the excretion of water and electrolytes by the kidneys. By doing so, diuretics play a major role in the treatment of hypertension as well as other cardiovascular conditions.

The major diuretics used as cardiovascular drugs include thiazide and thiazide-like diuretics, loop diuretics, and potassium-sparing diuretics.

Thiazide and thiazide-like diuretics

Thiazide and *thiazide-like diuretics* are sulfonamide derivatives.

Thiazide diuretics include:
- bendroflumethiazide
- benzthiazide
- chlorothiazide
- hydrochlorothiazide
- hydroflumethiazide
- methyclothiazide
- polythiazide
- trichlormethiazide.

Thiazide-like diuretics include:
- chlorthalidone
- indapamide.

Pharmacokinetics

Thiazide diuretics are absorbed rapidly but incompletely from the GI tract after oral administration. Thiazide diuretics cross the placenta and are secreted in breast milk. These drugs differ in how well they're metabolized; they're excreted primarily in the urine.

How the others move

Thiazide-like diuretics are absorbed from the GI tract. Indapamide is distributed widely into body tissues and metabolized in the liver. Chlorthalidone is 90% bound to erythrocytes. Little is known about chlorthalidone metabolism. These drugs are excreted primarily in the urine.

Pharmacodynamics

Thiazide and thiazide-like diuretics work by preventing sodium from being reabsorbed in the kidney. As sodium is excreted, it pulls water along with it. Thiazide and thiazide-like diuretics also increase the excretion of chloride, potassium, and bicarbonate, which can result in electrolyte imbalances.

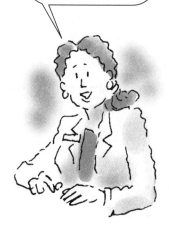

Thiazide diuretics promote the excretion of sodium from the kidneys, which in turn causes a loss of water...

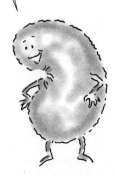

...but the process also causes me to excrete chloride, bicarbonate, and potassium. This increases the risk of electrolyte imbalances and hypokalemia.

Stability with time

Initially, these drugs decrease circulating blood volume, leading to a reduced cardiac output. However, if the therapy is maintained, cardiac output stabilizes, but plasma fluid volume decreases.

Pharmacotherapeutics

Thiazides are used as long-term treatment of hypertension and are also used to treat edema caused by mild or moderate heart failure, liver disease, kidney disease, and corticosteroid and estrogen therapy.

Preventing rolling stones

Because these drugs decrease the level of calcium in the urine, they're also used alone or with other drugs to prevent the development and recurrence of calcium kidney stones.

A paradoxical effect

In patients with diabetes insipidus (a disorder characterized by excessively large amounts of urine production and excessive thirst, caused by reduced secretion of antidiuretic hormone), thiazides paradoxically decrease urine volume, possibly through sodium depletion and plasma volume reduction.

Drug interactions

Drug interactions related to thiazide and thiazide-like diuretics result in altered fluid volume, blood pressure, and serum electrolyte levels.
• Thiazide and thiazide-like diuretics may increase blood glucose levels, requiring higher doses of insulin and oral antidiabetic drugs. Hyponatremia (low levels of sodium in the blood) and thiazide resistance may also occur.
• Taking corticosteroids, corticotropin, and amphotericin with these diuretics may cause hypokalemia.
• Lithium levels may be increased by thiazide and thiazide-like diuretics.
• These diuretics may increase the response to skeletal muscle relaxants.
• NSAIDs may reduce the antihypertensive effect of these diuretics. (See *Adverse reactions to thiazide and thiazide-like diuretics.*)

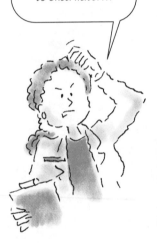

That's strange. Thiazide diuretics help treat edema and hypertension by causing the body to shed water…

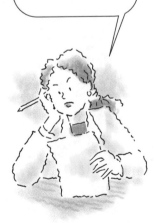

… but with diabetes insipidus, these drugs actually *reduce* urine volume — a beneficial effect.

Loop diuretics

Loop (high-ceiling) *diuretics* are highly potent drugs. They include bumetanide, ethacrynate sodium, ethacrynic acid, and furosemide.

Pharmacokinetics

Loop diuretics usually are absorbed well and distributed rapidly. These diuretics are highly protein bound. Loop diuretics, for the most part, undergo partial or complete metabolism in the liver, except for furosemide, which is excreted primarily unchanged. Loop diuretics are excreted primarily by the kidneys.

Pharmacodynamics

Loop diuretics are the most potent diuretics available, producing the greatest volume of diuresis (urine production). They also have a high potential for causing severe adverse reactions.

Bumetanide is the shortest-acting diuretic. It's even 40 times more potent than another loop diuretic, furosemide.

Locating the loop

Loop diuretics receive their name because they act primarily on the thick ascending loop of Henle (the part of the nephron responsible for concentrating urine) to increase the secretion of sodium, chloride, and water. These drugs also may inhibit sodium, chloride, and water reabsorption.

Pharmacotherapeutics

Loop diuretics are used to treat edema associated with heart failure, as well as hypertension (usually with a potassium-sparing diuretic or a potassium supplement to prevent hypokalemia).

Loop diuretics are also used to treat edema associated with liver disease or nephrotic syndrome (kidney disease).

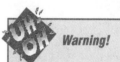

Warning!

Adverse reactions to thiazide and thiazide-like diuretics

The most common adverse reactions to thiazide and thiazide-like diuretics are reduced blood volume, orthostatic hypotension (a drop in blood pressure when a person stands up), hyponatremia (low blood sodium levels), and hypokalemia.

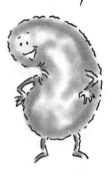

It's a logical label. Loop diuretics act primarily on the loop of Henle, the part of each nephron that concentrates urine.

Drug interactions

Loop diuretics produce a variety of drug interactions, as well as a significant number of adverse reactions. (See *Adverse reactions to loop diuretics.*)
• The risk of ototoxicity (damage to the organs of hearing) is increased when aminoglycosides and cisplatin are taken with loop diuretics.
• Loop diuretics reduce the hypoglycemic effect of oral antidiabetic drugs, possibly resulting in hyperglycemia.
• Loop diuretics may increase the risk of lithium toxicity.
• An increased risk of electrolyte imbalances that can trigger arrhythmias is present when digitalis glycosides and loop diuretics are taken together.

Potassium-sparing diuretics

Potassium-sparing diuretics have weaker diuretic and antihypertensive effects than other diuretics, but they have the advantage of conserving potassium.

Potassium-sparing diuretics include amiloride, spironolactone, and triamterene.

Pharmacokinetics

Potassium-sparing diuretics are only available orally and are absorbed in the GI tract. They're metabolized in the liver (except for amiloride, which isn't metabolized) and excreted primarily in the urine and bile.

Pharmacodynamics

The direct action of potassium-sparing diuretics on the distal tubule of the kidneys produces the following effects:
• Urinary excretion of sodium and water increases, as does excretion of chloride and calcium ions.
• The excretion of potassium and hydrogen ions decreases.

These effects lead to reduced blood pressure and increased serum potassium levels.

Aping aldosterone

Spironolactone, one of the main potassium-sparing diuretics, is structurally similar to aldosterone and acts as an aldosterone antagonist. Recall that aldosterone pro-

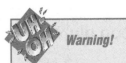

Warning!

Adverse reactions to loop diuretics

Because of the potent effects of these drugs, adverse reactions to loop diuretics may be severe. The most severe reactions involve fluid and electrolyte imbalances.

Levels go low

Common adverse reactions include:
• too great a loss of fluid volume (especially in elderly patients
• orthostatic hypotension
• hyperuricemia
• hypokalemia
• hypochloremia
• hyponatremia
• hypocalcemia
• hypomagnesemia.

motes the retention of sodium and water and loss of potassium. Spironolactone counteracts these effects by competing with aldosterone for receptor sites. As a result, sodium, chloride, and water are excreted and potassium is retained.

Pharmacotherapeutics

Potassium-sparing diuretics are used to treat:
• edema
• diuretic-induced hypokalemia in patients with heart failure
• cirrhosis
• nephrotic syndrome (abnormal condition of the kidneys)
• hypertension.

Spironolactone, in particular, is also used to treat hyperaldosteronism (excessive secretion of aldosterone) and hirsutism (excessive hair growth), including hirsutism associated with Stein-Leventhal (polycystic ovary) syndrome.

Potentiate or counteract

Potassium-sparing diuretics are commonly used with other diuretics to potentiate their action or counteract their potassium-wasting effects.

Drug interactions

Few drug interactions are associated with the use of amiloride, spironolactone, and triamterene. Those that do occur aren't directly related to the drug but to its potassium-sparing effects. (See *Adverse reactions to potassium-sparing diuretics.*)

Antilipemic drugs

Antilipemic drugs are used to lower abnormally high blood levels of lipids, such as cholesterol, triglycerides, and phospholipids. The risk of developing coronary artery disease increases when serum lipid levels are elevated. Drugs are used when lifestyle changes, such as proper diet, weight loss, exercise, and treatment of an un-

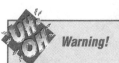

Warning!

Adverse reactions to potassium-sparing diuretics

Few adverse drug reactions occur with potassium-sparing diuretics. However, their potassium-sparing effects can lead to hyperkalemia, especially if a potassium-sparing diuretic is given with a potassium supplement or a high-potassium diet.

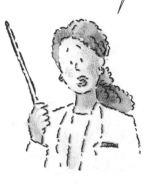

Be aware! Potassium-sparing diuretics can result in dangerously high potassium levels.

derlying disorder causing the lipid abnormality, fail to lower lipid levels.

Antilipemic drug classes include:
- bile-sequestering drugs (cholestyramine and colestipol hydrochloride)
- fibric acid derivatives (clofibrate and gemfibrozil)
- cholesterol synthesis inhibitors (lovastatin, pravastatin sodium, and simvastatin).

Bile-sequestering drugs

The two *bile-sequestering drugs* are cholestyramine and colestipol hydrochloride. These two drugs are resins that remove excess bile acids from the fat depots under the skin.

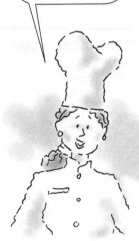

Bile-sequestering drugs are used to lower LDL levels that don't respond to changes in diet.

Pharmacokinetics

Bile-sequestering drugs aren't absorbed from the GI tract. Instead, they remain in the intestine, where they combine with bile acids for about 5 hours. Eventually, they're excreted in stool.

Pharmacodynamics

The bile-sequestering drugs lower blood levels of low-density lipoproteins (LDLs). These drugs combine with bile acids in the intestines to form an insoluble compound that is then excreted in stool. The decreasing level of bile acid in the gallbladder triggers the liver to synthesize more bile acids from their precursor, cholesterol.

Putting cholesterol to use

As cholesterol leaves the bloodstream and other storage areas to replace the lost bile acids, blood cholesterol levels decrease. Because the small intestine needs bile acids to emulsify lipids and form chylomicrons, absorption of all lipids and lipid-soluble drugs decreases until the bile acids are replaced.

Pharmacotherapeutics

Bile-sequestering drugs are the drugs of choice for treating type IIa hyperlipoproteinemia (familial hypercholesterolemia) in the patient who isn't able to lower LDL levels through dietary changes. A patient whose blood cholesterol levels indicate a severe risk of coronary artery disease is most likely to require one of these drugs to supplement his diet.

Drug interactions

Bile-sequestering drugs produce the following drug interactions:

• They may bind with acidic drugs in the GI tract, decreasing their absorption and effectiveness. Acidic drugs that are likely to be affected include barbiturates, phenytoin, penicillins, cephalosporins, thyroid hormones, thyroid derivatives, chenodiol, and digoxin.

• Bile-sequestering drugs also may reduce absorption of lipid-soluble vitamins, such as vitamins A, D, E, and K. Poor absorption of vitamin K can affect prothrombin times significantly, increasing the risk of bleeding.

• Absorption of many other drugs that normally are absorbed from the GI tract — including tetracyclines — also may be decreased. (See *Adverse reactions to bile-sequestering drugs.*)

Fibric acid derivatives

Fibric acid is produced by several fungi. Two derivatives of this acid are clofibrate and gemfibrozil. These drugs are used to reduce high triglyceride levels and, to a lesser extent, high LDL levels.

Pharmacokinetics

Clofibrate and gemfibrozil are absorbed readily from the GI tract and are highly protein bound. Clofibrate is hydrolyzed, and gemfibrozil undergoes extensive metabolism in the liver before both drugs are excreted in the urine.

Pharmacodynamics

Although the exact mechanism of action for these drugs isn't known, researchers believe that fibric acid derivatives may:

• reduce cholesterol production early in its formation
• mobilize cholesterol from the tissues
• increase cholesterol excretion
• decrease synthesis and secretion of lipoproteins
• decrease synthesis of triglycerides.

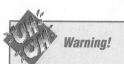
Warning!

Adverse reactions to bile-sequestering drugs

Short-term adverse reactions to these drugs are relatively mild. More severe reactions can result from long-term use. Adverse GI effects with long-term therapy include severe fecal impaction, vomiting, diarrhea, and hemorrhoid irritation.

Less likely
Rarely, peptic ulcers and bleeding, gallstones, and inflammation of the gallbladder may occur.

All to the "good..."

Gemfibrozil produces two other effects:
• It increases high-density lipoprotein levels in the blood (remember, this is "good" cholesterol).
• It increases the serum's capacity to dissolve additional cholesterol.

Pharmacotherapeutics

Fibric acid drugs are used primarily to reduce triglyceride levels, especially very-low-density triglycerides, and secondarily to reduce blood cholesterol levels.

Because of their ability to reduce triglyceride levels, fibric acid derivatives are useful in treating patients with types II, III, IV, and mild-type V hyperlipoproteinemia.

Drug interactions

• Fibric acid drugs may displace acidic drugs, such as barbiturates, phenytoin, thyroid derivatives, and digitalis glycosides.
• The risk of bleeding increases when fibric acid derivatives are taken with oral anticoagulants.
• Clofibrate may increase the hypoglycemic effect of oral antidiabetic drugs.
• Fibric acid derivatives can lead to adverse GI effects.

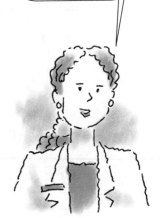

Gemfibrozil not only reduces triglycerides but also increases high-density lipoprotein levels and increases the blood's ability to dissolve cholesterol.

Cholesterol synthesis inhibitors

As their name implies, *cholesterol synthesis inhibitors* (also known as the "statins") lower lipid levels by interfering with cholesterol synthesis. These drugs include lovastatin, pravastatin sodium, and simvastatin.

Pharmacokinetics

These drugs each have slightly different pharmacokinetic properties.

Slow-movin' lovastatin

After oral administration, lovastatin is absorbed incompletely, and much of the drug dose is lost due to extensive first-pass metabolism in the liver. Food may increase the drug's systemic absorption.

Quick peaks of pravastatin

Pravastatin is absorbed rapidly but incompletely after being taken orally. Pravastatin also undergoes extensive first-pass metabolism in the liver.

Incomplete absorption of simvastatin

Simvastatin is absorbed incompletely and also undergoes extensive first-pass metabolism in the liver. Both simvastatin and its major metabolite are highly protein bound.

Pharmacodynamics

Cholesterol synthesis inhibitors reduce cholesterol levels by inhibiting enzyme activity. This interferes with an early step of cholesterol synthesis, thereby reducing the synthesis of LDL and enhancing LDL breakdown.

Pharmacotherapeutics

Cholesterol synthesis inhibitors are used to treat elevated total cholesterol and LDL levels in patients with primary hypercholesterolemia (types IIa and IIb). By lowering cholesterol levels, the cholesterol synthesis inhibitors reduce the risk of coronary artery disease.

Drug interactions

• When any of these drugs are administered with an immunosuppressant (especially cyclosporine), gemfibrozil, erythromycin, or niacin, the interaction may increase the risk of myopathy (muscle wasting and weakness) or rhabdomyolysis (potentially fatal breakdown of skeletal muscle, causing renal failure).

Just one or two

• Pravastatin and simvastatin may increase the risk of bleeding when administered with warfarin.
• Cholestyramine and colestipol may decrease the effectiveness of pravastatin. (See *Adverse reactions to cholesterol synthesis inhibitors.*)

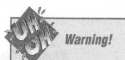

Warning!

Adverse reactions to cholesterol synthesis inhibitors

The most common adverse reactions to lovastatin include GI disturbances and headache. Increased liver enzyme levels may occur in the patient receiving long-term lovastatin therapy.

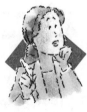

Quick quiz

1. Treatment with clofibrate, a type of fibric acid derivative, would have to proceed cautiously if the patient is also receiving which of the following drugs?

    A. Penicillin
    B. Thiazide diuretic
    C. Oral anticoagulant

Answer: C. Fibric acid derivatives cause an increased risk of bleeding when given with an oral anticoagulant.

2. A patient is taking lovastatin, a cholesterol synthesis inhibitor. Which of the following parameters should the patient monitor periodically?

    A. Liver function test results
    B. Electrolyte levels
    C. Vision testing

Answer: A. Because increased liver enzyme levels may occur in patients receiving long-term lovastatin therapy, liver function test results should be monitored.

3. A patient needs a diuretic drug but is allergic to sulfa-based drugs. Which of the following diuretics should he avoid?

    A. Thiazide and thiazide-like diuretics
    B. Loop diuretics
    C. Potassium-sparing diuretics

Answer: A. Thiazide and thiazide-like diuretics are sulfonamide derivatives, so they should be avoided in the patient allergic to sulfa-based drugs.

Scoring

✰✰✰   If you answered all three questions correctly, A+! You're aces with ACE inhibitors!

✰✰   If you answered two questions correctly, cool! Cardiovascular drugs aren't giving you any complications.

✰   If you answered fewer than two questions correctly, stay mellow. This is a complex chapter, and it might just take another go.

Hematologic drugs

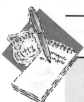

Just the facts

In this chapter, you'll review:

♦ classes of drugs used to treat hematologic disorders

♦ uses and varying actions of these drugs

♦ how these drugs are absorbed, distributed, metabolized, and excreted

♦ drug interactions and adverse reactions to these drugs.

Drugs and the hematologic system

The hematologic system includes plasma (the liquid component of blood) and blood cells, such as red blood cells (RBCs), white blood cells, and platelets. Types of drugs used to treat disorders of the hematologic system include:
- hematinic drugs
- anticoagulant drugs
- thrombolytic drugs.

Hematinic drugs

Hematinic drugs provide essential building blocks for RBC production. They do so by increasing hemoglobin, the necessary element for oxygen transportation.

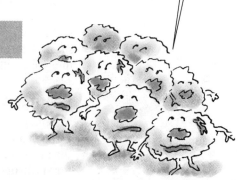

Need some RBCs built? Turn to hematinic drugs.

Iron, vitamin B$_{12}$, folic acid

This section discusses hematinic drugs used to treat microcytic and macrocytic anemia—iron, vitamin B$_{12}$, and folic acid.

It also describes the use of epoetin alfa to treat normocytic anemia.

Iron

Iron preparations are used to treat the most common form of anemia—iron deficiency anemia. Iron preparations discussed in this section include ferrous fumarate, ferrous gluconate, ferrous sulfate, and iron dextran.

Pharmacokinetics (how drugs circulate)

Iron is absorbed primarily from the duodenum and upper jejunum of the intestine.

Low iron increases absorption

The amount of iron absorbed depends partially on the body stores of iron. When body stores are low or RBC production is accelerated, iron absorption may increase by 20% to 30%. On the other hand, when total iron stores are large, only about 5% to 10% of iron is absorbed.

Enteric-coated preparations decrease iron absorption because in that form, iron isn't released until after it leaves the duodenum. The lymphatic system absorbs the parenteral form after I.M. injections.

> It takes about 6 months for iron therapy to correct iron deficiency anemia.

Hemoglobin has it

Iron is transported by the blood and bound to transferrin, its carrier plasma protein. About 30% of the iron is stored primarily as hemosiderin or ferritin in the reticuloendothelial cells of the liver, spleen, and bone marrow. About two-thirds of the total body iron is contained in hemoglobin. Iron is excreted in urine, stool, sweat, and through intestinal cell sloughing and is secreted in breast milk.

Pharmacodynamics (how drugs act)

Although iron has other roles, its most important role is the production of hemoglobin. About 80% of iron in the plasma goes to the bone marrow, where it's used for erythropoiesis (production of RBCs).

Pharmacotherapeutics (how drugs are used)

Oral iron therapy is used to prevent or treat iron deficiency anemia. It's also used to prevent anemias in children age 6 months to 2 years because this is a period of rapid growth and development.

Pregnant women may need iron supplements to replace the iron used by the developing fetus. Treatment for iron deficiency anemia usually lasts for 6 months.

Ironclad options

Parenteral iron therapy is used for patients who can't absorb oral preparations, aren't compliant with oral therapy, or have bowel disorders (such as ulcerative colitis). The only currently available parenteral form is iron dextran, which builds up iron stores more rapidly than the oral drugs but doesn't correct anemia any faster.

Drug interactions

Iron absorption is reduced by antacids as well as by such foods as coffee, tea, eggs, and milk. Other drug interactions involving iron include the following:
• Tetracycline, oxytetracycline, methacycline, doxycycline, methyldopa, ciprofloxacin, ofloxacin, chloramphenicol, and penicillamine absorption may be reduced when taken with oral iron preparations.
• Cholestyramine and colestipol may reduce serum levels of iron.
• Cimetidine and other histamine$_2$–receptor antagonists may decrease GI absorption of iron. (See *Adverse reactions to iron therapy.*)

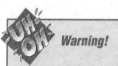

Warning!

Adverse reactions to iron therapy

The most common adverse reaction to iron therapy is gastric irritation. Iron preparations also darken the stool, and liquid ones can stain the teeth.

Some patients lack a crucial "intrinsic factor" that allows vitamin B$_{12}$ absorption...

...so they can't take the vitamin orally and must receive injections instead.

Vitamin B$_{12}$

Vitamin B$_{12}$ preparations are used to treat pernicious anemia. Common vitamin B$_{12}$ preparations include cyanocobalamin and hydroxocobalamin.

Pharmacokinetics

Vitamin B$_{12}$ is available in both oral and injectable forms. A substance called intrinsic factor, secreted by the gastric mucosa, is needed for vitamin B$_{12}$ absorption.

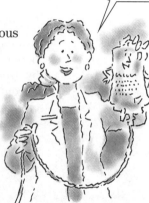

People who have a deficiency of intrinsic factor develop a special type of anemia known as vitamin B_{12}-deficiency pernicious anemia. Because people with this disorder can't absorb vitamin B_{12}, an injectable form of the drug is used to treat this type of anemia.

Parenteral possibilities

When cyanocobalamin is injected by the I.M. or S.C. route, it's absorbed and binds to transcobalamin II for transport to the tissues. It's then transported in the bloodstream to the liver, where 90% of the body's supply of vitamin B_{12} is stored.

Although hydroxocobalamin is absorbed more slowly from the injection site, its uptake in the liver may be greater than that of cyanocobalamin.

Most gets lost

With either drug, the liver slowly releases vitamin B_{12} as needed by the body. It's secreted in breast milk during lactation. About 3 to 8 mcg of vitamin B_{12} are excreted in bile each day and then reabsorbed in the ileum.

Within 48 hours after a vitamin B_{12} injection, 50% to 95% of the dose appears in urine, with the major portion excreted in the first 8 hours.

Pharmacodynamics

When vitamin B_{12} is administered, it replaces vitamin B_{12} that the body normally would absorb from the diet. This vitamin is essential for cell growth and replication and for the maintenance of myelin (nerve coverings) throughout the nervous system. Vitamin B_{12} also may be involved in lipid and carbohydrate metabolism.

Pharmacotherapeutics

Cyanocobalamin and hydroxocobalamin are used to treat pernicious anemia, a megaloblastic anemia characterized by decreased gastric production of hydrochloric acid and the deficiency of intrinsic factor, a substance normally secreted by the parietal cells of the gastric mucosa that is essential for vitamin B_{12} absorption.

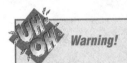
Warning!

Adverse reactions to vitamin B_{12} therapy

No dose-related adverse reactions occur with vitamin B_{12} therapy. However, some rare reactions may occur when vitamin B_{12} is administered parenterally.

Parenteral problems
Adverse reactions to parenteral administration can include hypersensitivity reactions that could result in anaphylaxis and death, pulmonary edema, heart failure, peripheral vascular thrombosis, polycythemia vera, hypokalemia, itching, transient rash, hives, and mild diarrhea.

Drug interactions

Alcohol, aminosalicylic acid, neomycin, chloramphenicol, and colchicine may decrease the absorption of oral cyanocobalamin. (See *Adverse reactions to vitamin B_{12} therapy.*)

Folic acid

Folic acid is given to treat folic acid deficiency. It's typically known simply as folic acid, although a preparation called leucovorin calcium is also used.

Pharmacokinetics

Folic acid is absorbed rapidly in the first third of the small intestine and distributed into all body tissues. Folic acid is metabolized in the liver. Excess folate is excreted unchanged in the urine, and small amounts of folic acid are excreted in stool. Folates are excreted in urine and stool and secreted in breast milk.

Pharmacodynamics

Folic acid is an essential component for normal RBC production and growth. A deficiency in folic acid results in pernicious anemia and low serum and RBC folate levels.

Pharmacotherapeutics

Folic acid is used to treat folic acid deficiency. Patients who are pregnant or undergoing treatment for liver disease, hemolytic anemia, alcohol abuse, skin disease, or renal failure typically need preventive folic acid therapy.

Drug interactions

• Methotrexate, antimalarial drugs, triamterene, pentamidine, and trimethoprim reduce the effectiveness of folic acid. Patients taking those drugs typically need to take leucovorin calcium to minimize interference.
• In large doses, folic acid may counteract the effects of anticonvulsants, such as phenytoin, phenobarbital, and primidone, potentially leading to seizures.

It takes a lot to make an RBC! Folic acid, iron, vitamin B_{12}, amino acids, copper, and cobalt are all necessary components...

...and hematinic drugs usually replace one of these missing parts.

• Folic acid may interfere with the antimicrobial action of pyrimethamine.
• Glutethimide, isoniazid, cycloserine, and oral contraceptives may interfere with folic acid absorption. (See *Adverse reactions to folic acid.*)

Epoetin alfa

Epoetin alfa stimulates RBC production.

Pharmacokinectics

Epoetin alfa may be given S.C. or I.V. After S.C. administration, peak serum levels occur with 5 to 24 hours. Distribution, metabolism, and excretion are still unknown.

Pharmacodynamics

Epoetin alfa boosts the production of erythropoietin, thus stimulating RBC production in the bone marrow. Normally, erythropoietin is formed in the kidneys in response to hypoxia (reduced oxygen) and anemia. Patients with conditions that decrease production of erythropoietin develop chronic normocytic anemia, necessitating epoetin alfa administration.

Pharmacotherapeutics

Epoetin alfa is used to:
• treat patients with normocytic anemia (characterized by a decrease in hemoglobin content, packed RBC volume, and the number of RBCs per cubic millimeter of blood) caused by chronic renal failure
• treat anemia associated with zidovudine therapy in patients with human immunodeficiency virus infection
• decrease the need for transfusions in patients with certain types of leukemia.

Drug interactions

No known drug interactions exist with epoetin alfa, although it can cause some adverse reactions. (See *Adverse reactions to epoetin alfa.*)

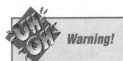

Warning!

Adverse reactions to folic acid

Adverse reactions to folic acid include:
• erythema
• itching
• rash.

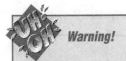

Warning!

Adverse reactions to epoetin alfa

Hypertension is the most common adverse reaction to epoetin alfa.

Other adverse reactions may include:
• headache
• joint pain
• nausea
• edema
• fatigue
• diarrhea
• vomiting
• chest pain
• skin reactions at the administration site
• weakness
• dizziness.

Anticoagulant drugs

Anticoagulant drugs are used to reduce the ability of the blood to clot. Major categories of anticoagulants include:
- heparin
- oral anticoagulants
- antiplatelet drugs.

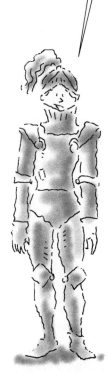

Heparin prevents clots from forming but doesn't dissolve blood clots.

Heparin

Heparin, prepared commercially from animal tissue, is used to prevent clot formation. Because it doesn't affect the synthesis of clotting factors, heparin can't dissolve already formed clots.

Breaking news

Low-molecular-weight heparins, such as dalteparin sodium and enoxaparin sodium, have been developed to prevent deep vein thrombosis (a blood clot in the deep veins, usually of the legs) in surgical patients.

Pharmacokinetics

Because heparin isn't absorbed well from the GI tract, it must be administered parenterally. Distribution is immediate after I.V. administration, but it isn't as predictable with S.C. injection.

I.M. is out

Heparin isn't given I.M. because of the risk of local bleeding. Heparin is metabolized in the liver, and its metabolites are excreted in urine.

Pharmacodynamics

Heparin prevents the formation of new thrombi. Here is how it works:
- Heparin inhibits the formation of thrombin and fibrin by activating antithrombin III.
- Antithrombin III then inactivates factors IXa, Xa, XIa, and XIIa in the intrinsic and common pathways. The end result is prevention of a stable fibrin clot.

- In low doses, heparin increases the activity of antithrombin III against factor Xa and thrombin and inhibits clot formation.
- Much larger doses are necessary to inhibit fibrin formation after a clot has been formed. This relationship between dose and effect is the rationale for using low-dose heparin to prevent clotting.
- Whole blood clotting time, thrombin time, and partial thromboplastin time are prolonged during heparin therapy. However, these times may be only slightly prolonged with low or ultra-low preventive doses.

Pharmacotherapeutics

Heparin may be used in a number of clinical situations to prevent the formation of new clots or the extension of existing clots. These situations include:
- preventing or treating venous thromboemboli, characterized by inappropriate or excessive intravascular activation of blood clotting
- treating disseminated intravascular coagulation, a complication of other diseases, resulting in accelerated clotting
- treating arterial clotting and preventing embolus formation in patients with atrial fibrillation, an arrhythmia in which ineffective atrial contractions cause blood to pool in the atria, increasing the risk of clot formation
- preventing thrombus formation and promoting cardiac circulation in an acute myocardial infarction (MI) by preventing further clot formation at the site of the already formed clot.

Circulate freely

Heparin can be used to prevent clotting whenever the patient's blood must circulate outside the body through a machine, such as the cardiopulmonary bypass machine and hemodialysis machine.

You're the one

Heparin is also useful for preventing clotting during orthopedic surgery. (This type of surgery, in many cases, activates the coagulation mechanisms excessively.) In fact, heparin is the drug of choice for orthopedic surgery.

Heparin increases the effects of oral anticoagulants... so if the patient is also taking warfarin or dicumarol, watch out for bleeding.

CAUTION!

Drug interactions

• Because heparin acts synergistically with all the oral anticoagulants, the risk of bleeding increases when the patient takes both drugs together. The prothrombin time and international normalized ratio, used to monitor the effects of oral anticoagulants, also may be prolonged.
• The risk of bleeding increases when the patient takes nonsteroidal anti-inflammatory drugs (NSAIDs), iron dextran, or an antiplatelet drug, such as aspirin, ticlopidine, and dipyridamole, while receiving heparin.

Another reason to quit

• Drugs that antagonize or inactivate heparin include antihistamines, digoxin, nicotine, phenothiazines, tetracycline hydrochloride, quinidine, neomycin sulfate, and I.V. penicillin.
• Nicotine may inactivate heparin; nitroglycerin may inhibit the effects of heparin. (See *Adverse reactions to heparin.*)

Oral anticoagulants

The major *oral anticoagulants* used in the United States are the coumarin compounds warfarin sodium and dicumarol.

Pharmacokinetics

Warfarin is absorbed rapidly and almost completely when it's taken orally. Dicumarol is absorbed more slowly and erratically. Warfarin and dicumarol are both bound extensively to plasma albumin, metabolized in the liver, and excreted in urine.

Because warfarin is highly protein bound, bleeding can occur if the patient takes other highly protein-bound drugs.

Pharmacodynamics

Oral anticoagulants alter the ability of the liver to synthesize vitamin K-dependent clotting factors, including prothrombin and factors VII, IX, and X. However, clotting

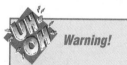

Warning!

Adverse reactions to heparin

One advantage of heparin is that it produces relatively few adverse reactions. These reactions can usually be prevented if the patient's partial thromboplastin time is maintained within the therapeutic range (1½ to 2½ times the control).

Bleeding, the most common adverse effect, can be reversed easily by administering protamine sulfate, which binds to heparin and forms a stable salt with it.

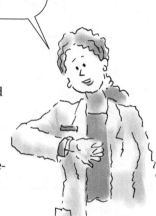

Although oral anticoagulants are absorbed quickly, it can take them a couple of days to take effect.

factors already in the bloodstream continue to coagulate blood until they become depleted, so anticoagulation doesn't begin immediately.

Pharmacotherapeutics

Oral anticoagulants are prescribed to treat thromboembolism and, in this situation, are started while the patient is still receiving heparin. Warfarin, however, may be started without heparin in outpatients at high risk for thromboembolism.

Deep in the veins

Oral anticoagulants also are the drugs of choice to prevent deep vein thrombosis and for patients with prosthetic heart valves or diseased mitral valves. They sometimes are combined with an antiplatelet drug, such as dipyridamole, to decrease the risk of arterial clotting. (See *Stretch that treatment?*)

Drug interactions

Many patients who take oral anticoagulants are also receiving other drugs. Serious interactions between oral anticoagulants and other drugs may occur.
• A diet high in vitamin K reduces the effectiveness of oral anticoagulants.

Clinical controversy

Stretch that treatment?

About 40,000 Americans each year develop potentially life-threatening deep vein thrombi (blood clots) in the leg. Approximately 15% suffer another clot within months. It's a well-known fact that prescribing oral anticoagulants for these patients helps prevent further clots from forming. The controversy is over how long the drugs should be taken.

Industry standard
Usually, deep vein thrombi are first treated with I.V. heparin for 1 week, followed by warfarin, an oral anticoagulant, for 3 months.

Lots more warfarin
Recent research, however, shows that patients who received warfarin for an average of 13 months—10 months longer than usual treatment—reduced their risk of another blood clot by 95% when compared to the typical 3-month treatment.

• The risk of phenytoin toxicity increases when phenytoin is taken with oral anticoagulants. Phenytoin may increase or decrease the effects of oral anticoagulants.
• The patient with chronic alcohol abuse has an increased risk of clotting when taking oral anticoagulants, and the patient with acute alcohol intoxication has an increased risk of bleeding.

Bleeding risk...

The risk of bleeding increases when the following drugs are taken with oral anticoagulants: salicylates, phenylbutazone, sulfinpyrazone, indomethacin, clofibrate, anabolic and androgenic steroids, chloral hydrate, chloramphenicol, disulfiram, heparin, gemfibrozil, meclofenamate, mefenamic acid, metronidazole, miconazole, nalidixic acid, piroxicam, allopurinol, cimetidine, dextrothyroxine, erythromycin, co-trimoxazole, sulindac, thyroid hormones, and influenza vaccine.

...and clotting risk

The risk of blood clotting increases when the following drugs are taken with oral anticoagulants: barbiturates, glutethimide, ethchlorvynol, griseofulvin, carbamazepine, rifampin, vitamin K, cholestyramine, colestipol, aminoglutethimide, propylthiouracil, methimazole, corticotropin, mercaptopurine, and spironolactone. (See *Adverse reactions to oral anticoagulants.*)

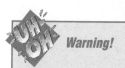

Warning!

Adverse reactions to oral anticoagulants

The primary adverse reaction to oral anticoagulant therapy is minor bleeding. Severe bleeding can occur, however, with the most common site being the GI tract. Bleeding into the brain may be fatal. Bruises and hematomas may form at arterial puncture sites (for example, after a blood gas sample is drawn).

Quick fix
The effects of oral anticoagulants can be reversed with phytonadione (vitamin K_1).

Antiplatelet drugs

Antiplatelet drugs are used to prevent arterial thromboembolism, particularly in patients at risk for MI, stroke, and arteriosclerosis (hardening of the arteries).

Aspirin, dipyridamole, sulfinpyrazone, and ticlopidine are examples of antiplatelet drugs.

Pharmacokinetics

All antiplatelet drugs are taken orally, absorbed very quickly, and reach peak concentration between 1 and 2 hours after administration. Aspirin maintains its antiplatelet effect approximately 10 days, or as long as platelets normally survive. Sulfinpyrazone may require several days of administration.

Pharmacodynamics

Antiplatelet drugs interfere with platelet activity in different drug-specific and dose-related ways.

Low dose

Low dosages of aspirin (325 mg/day) appear to inhibit clot formation by blocking the synthesis of prostaglandin, which in turn prevents formation of the platelet-aggregating substance thromboxane A_2.

Dipyridamole may inhibit platelet aggregation.

Single dose

Sulfinpyrazone appears to inhibit several platelet functions. At dosages of 400 to 800 mg/day, it lengthens platelet survival; dosages of more than 600 mg/day prolong the patency of arteriovenous shunts used for hemodialysis. A single dose rapidly inhibits platelet aggregation.

Broken bindings

Ticlopidine inhibits the binding of fibrinogen to platelets during the first stage of the clotting cascade.

Pharmacotherapeutics

Antiplatelet drugs have many different uses.

Managing MIs

Aspirin is used in patients with a previous MI or unstable angina to reduce the risk of death, and in men to reduce the risk of transient ischemic attacks (TIAs) (temporary reduction in circulation to the brain).

After an MI, sulfinpyrazone may be used to decrease the risk of sudden cardiac death. In patients with mitral stenosis (a narrowed mitral valve) caused by rheumatic fever, it may decrease the risk of systemic embolism.

Salve for surgery

Dipyridamole is used with a coumarin compound to prevent thrombus formation after cardiac valve replacement. Dipyridamole with aspirin has been used to prevent thromboembolic disorders in patients with aortocoronary bypass grafts (bypass surgery) or prosthetic (artificial) heart valves.

Circumventing stroke

Ticlopidine is used to reduce the risk of thrombotic stroke in high-risk patients (including those with a history of frequent TIAs) and in patients who have already had a thrombotic stroke.

Drug interactions

• Aspirin taken with heparin, oral anticoagulants, and dipyridamole increases the risk of bleeding.
• Sulfinpyrazone taken with aspirin and oral anticoagulants increases the risk of bleeding.

Tales of toxicity

• Aspirin increases the risk of toxicity of methotrexate and valproic acid.
• Aspirin and ticlopidine may reduce the effectiveness of sulfinpyrazone to relieve signs and symptoms of gout.
• Antacids may reduce the plasma levels of ticlopidine.
• Cimetidine increases the risk of ticlopidine toxicity and bleeding.

You just don't know

Because guidelines haven't been established for administrating of ticlopidine with heparin, oral anticoagulants, aspirin, or fibrinolytic drugs, these drugs should be discontinued before ticlopidine therapy begins. (See *Adverse reactions to antiplatelet drugs.*)

Thrombolytic drugs

Thrombolytic drugs are used to dissolve a preexisting clot or thrombus, often in an acute or emergency situation. Some of the thrombolytic drugs currently used include alteplase, anistreplase, and streptokinase.

Pharmacokinetics

After I.V. or intracoronary administration, thrombolytic drugs are distributed immediately throughout the circulation, quickly activating plasminogen (a precursor to plasmin, which dissolves fibrin clots).

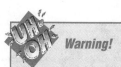
Warning!

Adverse reactions to antiplatelet drugs

Hypersensitivity reactions, particularly anaphylaxis, can occur.

Aspirin
• Stomach pain
• Heartburn, nausea
• Constipation
• Blood in the stool
• Slight gastric blood loss

Sulfinpyrazone
• Abdominal discomfort

Ticlopidine
• Diarrhea
• Nausea
• Dyspepsia
• Rash
• Elevated liver function test results
• Neutropenia

Dipyridamole
• Headache
• Dizziness
• Nausea
• Flushing
• Weakness
• Fainting
• Mild GI distress

How alteplase helps restore circulation

When a thrombus forms in an artery, it obstructs the blood supply, causing ischemia and necrosis. Alteplase can dissolve a thrombus in either the coronary or pulmonary artery, restoring the blood supply to the area beyond the blockage.

Obstructed artery
A thrombus blocks blood flow through the artery, causing distal ischemia.

Inside the thrombus
Alteplase enters the thrombus, which consists of plasminogen bound to fibrin. Alteplase binds to the fibrin-plasminogen complex, converting the inactive plasminogen into active plasmin. This active plasmin digests the fibrin, dissolving the thrombus. As the thrombus dissolves, blood flow resumes.

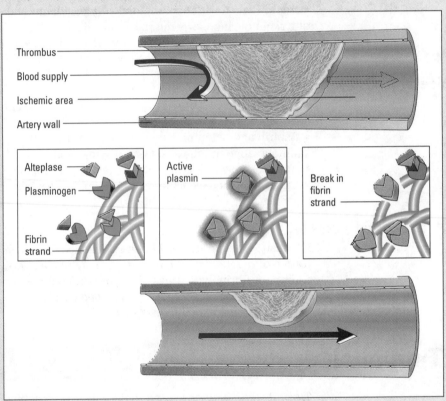

Blood work

Alteplase is cleared rapidly from circulating plasma, primarily by the liver; anistreplase is metabolized in the plasma. Streptokinase is removed rapidly from the circulation by antibodies and the reticuloendothelial system (a body system involved in defending against infection and disposing products of cell breakdown). It doesn't appear to cross the placental barrier.

Pharmacodynamics

Thrombolytic drugs convert plasminogen to plasmin, which lyses (dissolves) thrombi, fibrinogen, and other plasma proteins. (See *How alteplase helps restore circulation.*)

Pharmacotherapeutics

Thrombolytic drugs have a number of uses. They're used to treat certain thromboembolic disorders and have also been used to dissolve thrombi in arteriovenous cannulas (used in dialysis) and I.V. catheters to reestablish blood flow.

The sooner the better

Thrombolytic drugs are the drugs of choice to break down newly formed thrombi. They seem most effective when administered immediately after thrombosis, although they can be used for up to 6 hours after the onset of symptoms.

Acute MI and others

In addition, each drug has specific uses.
• Alteplase is used to treat acute MI, pulmonary embolism, and acute ischemic stroke.
• Anistreplase is also used in acute MI.
• Streptokinase is used to treat acute MI, pulmonary embolus, deep vein thrombosis, arterial thrombosis, and arterial embolism as well as to clear an occluded arteriovenous cannula.

Drug interactions

• Thrombolytic drugs interact with heparin, oral anticoagulants, antiplatelet drugs, and NSAIDs to increase the patient's risk of bleeding.
• Aminocaproic acid inhibits streptokinase and can be used to reverse its fibrinolytic effects. (See *Adverse reactions to thrombolytic drugs.*)

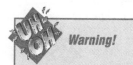

Warning!

Adverse reactions to thrombolytic drugs

The major reactions associated with the thrombolytic drugs are bleeding and allergic responses, especially with streptokinase and anistreplase.

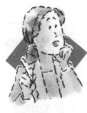

Quick quiz

1. A patient is given heparin to treat thrombophlebitis. If the patient starts to bleed excessively during heparin therapy, which of the following drugs is likely to be prescribed as an antidote?

    A.   vitamin K

    B.   factor VIII

    C.   protamine sulfate

Answer: C. Protamine sulfate reverses the effects of heparin.

2. Why is heparin administered concurrently with warfarin?

    A.   Warfarin's therapeutic effects don't occur until clotting factors are depleted.

    B.   Heparin activates warfarin.

    C.   Warfarin and heparin have a synergistic effect.

Answer: A. Heparin is administered concurrently with warfarin because warfarin is ineffective until clotting factors are depleted.

3. How soon after cyanocobalamin (vitamin B_{12}) therapy is begun can a patient expect to feel better?

    A.   24 hours

    B.   72 hours

    C.   1 week

Answer: A. The effects of cyanocobalamin can be felt 24 hours after initiation of treatment.

Scoring

  ☆☆☆   If you answered all three questions correctly, far out! You're hip to hematologic drugs.

    ☆☆   If you answered two questions correctly, that's great! You've caught the wave of anticoagulants.

      ☆   If you answered fewer than two questions correctly, play it cool. You just might need some time to get the blood flowing.

7

Respiratory drugs

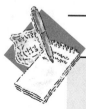

Just the facts

In this chapter, you'll review:

♦ classes of drugs used to improve respiratory function

♦ uses and varying actions of these drugs

♦ how these drugs are absorbed, distributed, metabolized, and excreted

♦ drug interactions and adverse reactions to these drugs.

Drugs and the respiratory system

The respiratory system, extending from the nose to the pulmonary capillaries, performs the essential function of gas exchange between the body and its environment. In other words, it takes in oxygen and expels carbon dioxide.

Breathe easy

Drugs used to improve respiratory function include:
- methylxanthines
- expectorants
- antitussives
- mucolytics
- decongestants.

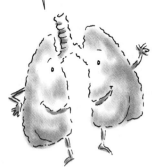

I've got an important job — gas exchange — and sometimes I need a little help from respiratory drugs to get it done.

Methylxanthines

Methylxanthines, also called *xanthines*, are used to treat breathing disorders.

Types of methylxanthines

Methylxanthines include *anhydrous theophylline* and its derivative salts:

- aminophylline
- oxtriphylline
- theophylline sodium glycinate.

Pharmacokinetics (how drugs circulate)

The pharmacokinetics of methylxanthines vary according to which drug the patient is receiving, the dosage form, and the administration route.

Absorption

When theophylline is given as an oral solution or a rapid-release tablet, it's absorbed rapidly and completely.

Gastric measures

Absorption of some of theophylline's slow-release forms depends on the gastric pH. Food can alter absorption.

Distribution

Theophylline is approximately 60% protein-bound in adults and 36% protein-bound in the neonate. It readily crosses the placental barrier and is secreted in breast milk.

Metabolism and excretion

Theophylline is metabolized primarily in the liver. In adults and children, about 10% of a dose is excreted unchanged in the urine. Because infants have immature livers with reduced metabolic functioning, as much as one-half a dose may be excreted unchanged in their urine.

Pharmacodynamics (how drugs act)

Methylxanthines act in a number of ways.

Relax and breathe deeply

Methylxanthines decrease airway reactivity and relieve bronchospasm by relaxing bronchial smooth muscle. Their specific mechanism of action in reversible obstructive airway disease such as asthma isn't completely understood. (See *Other drugs to relieve bronchospasm.*)

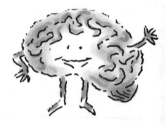

Xanthines stimulate my medulla and the central nervous system to decrease airway reactivity, relax bronchial smooth muscle, and stimulate breathing.

A stimulating conversation

In nonreversible obstructive airway disease (chronic bronchitis, emphysema, and apnea), methylxanthines appear to increase the sensitivity of the brain's respiratory center to carbon dioxide and to stimulate the respiratory drive.

Pumping you up

In chronic bronchitis and emphysema, these drugs decrease fatigue of the diaphragm, the respiratory muscle that separates the abdomen from the thoracic cavity. They also improve ventricular function and, therefore, the heart's pumping action.

Pharmacotherapeutics (how drugs are used)

Theophylline and its salts are used to treat:
- asthma (as second or third-line drugs)
- chronic bronchitis
- emphysema. (See *Other asthma drugs*.)

Other drugs to relieve bronchospasm

Short-acting beta$_2$-adrenergic agonists and anticholinergics (such as ipratropium bromide) act on the sympathetic nerves to relax bronchial smooth muscle and relieve bronchospasm. These drugs may be used alone or in combination with theophylline or steroid therapy.

Timing is everything
Beta$_2$-adrenergic agonists have a rapid onset of action and last from 3 to 6 hours. Anticholinergics have a slower onset of action, but their effects last longer than the beta$_2$-adrenergic agonists.

Other asthma drugs

Other asthma drugs include pirbuterol and cromolyn sodium.

Pirbuterol
An aerosolized bronchodilator, pirbuterol acetate (Maxair) acts as a beta$_2$-adrenergic receptor agonist. Stimulation of beta$_2$ receptors causes the smooth muscle of the bronchi to relax. Pirbuterol prevents bronchospasm, including that caused by asthma. It may be used alone or with theophylline or steroid therapy.

Adverse reactions
Nervousness, tremors, headache, palpitations, rapid heart rate, chest pain or tightness, nausea, diarrhea, and dry mouth may occur after pirbuterol administration.

Cromolyn sodium
Cromolyn sodium prevents the release of histamine and slow-reacting substances of anaphylaxis by stabilizing the mast cell membrane. As a result, the stimulus for bronchospasm is reduced and bronchospasm is relieved.

Cromolyn sodium is used primarily to prevent bronchial asthma. It isn't useful, however, in treating acute asthma attacks or status asthmaticus (a severe, prolonged asthma attack). Because it's absorbed poorly when given orally, cromolyn sodium is given by inhalation to improve breathing.

Adverse reactions
Bronchospasm, sneezing, wheezing, cough, nasal congestion, and throat irritation may occur after cromolyn sodium administration. Dizziness, painful or difficult urination, joint swelling and pain, nausea, headache, and skin rash may also occur.

A newborn use?

While investigation by the Food and Drug Administration is still ongoing, theophylline has been used in clinical trials to treat neonatal apnea (periods of not breathing in the newborn).

Drug interactions

Theophylline and its salts may interact with other drugs:
• Smoking cigarettes or marijuana increases theophylline elimination, decreasing its serum concentrations and effectiveness.
• Taking adrenergic stimulants or drinking beverages that contain caffeine may result in additive adverse reactions to theophylline or signs and symptoms of methylxanthine toxicity.
• Phenobarbital, phenytoin, rifampin, and carbamazepine reduce serum theophylline levels. Charcoal and ketoconazole may decrease theophylline levels.
• Receiving halothane, enflurane, isoflurane, and methoxyflurane with theophylline and theophylline derivatives increases the risk of cardiac toxicity.
• Theophylline and its derivatives may reduce the effects of lithium by increasing its rate of excretion.
• Thyroid hormones may reduce theophylline levels; antithyroid drugs may increase theophylline levels.

Toxic topics

Theophylline levels may be elevated, increasing the risk of theophylline toxicity, when the following drugs are taken with methylxanthines: cimetidine, erythromycin, corticosteroids, interferon, mexiletine, clarithromycin, troleandomycin, allopurinol (high dose), disulfiram, thiabendazole, oral contraceptives, beta blockers, ciprofloxacin, norfloxacin, enoxacin, and zileuton. (See *Adverse reactions to methylxanthines*.)

> Smoking increases the elimination of theophylline, which reduces its effectiveness.

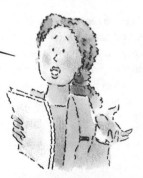

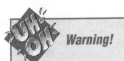

Warning!

Adverse reactions to methylxanthines

Adverse reactions to methylxanthines may be transient or symptomatic of toxicity.

Gut reactions
Adverse GI system reactions include:
• nausea
• vomiting
• abdominal cramping
• epigastric pain
• anorexia
• diarrhea.

Nerve racking
Adverse central nervous system reactions include:
• headache
• irritability
• restlessness
• anxiety
• insomnia
• dizziness.

Heart of the matter
Adverse cardiovascular reactions include:
• tachycardia
• palpitations
• arrhythmias.

Expectorants

Expectorants thin mucus so it's cleared more easily out of airways. They also soothe mucous membranes in the respiratory tract.

> Expectorants thin mucus, helping me cough up clogging secretions more productively.

Guaifenesin

The most commonly used expectorant is *guaifenesin*.

Pharmacokinetics

Guaifenesin is absorbed through the GI tract, metabolized by the liver, and excreted primarily by the kidneys.

Pharmacodynamics

By increasing production of respiratory tract fluids, expectorants reduce the thickness, adhesiveness and surface tension of mucus, making it easier to clear from the airways. Expectorants also provide a soothing effect on mucous membranes of the respiratory tract.

Pharmacotherapeutics

Guaifenesin is used for the relief of coughs from:
- colds
- minor bronchial irritation
- bronchitis
- influenza
- sinusitis
- bronchial asthma
- emphysema
- other respiratory disorders.

Read the directions

Guaifenesin may also be used to relieve a dry, hacking cough and is safe if taken as directed. It may be used alone or with antitussives, analgesics, or antihistamines.

Drug interactions

Guaifenesin administered with anticoagulants may increase the risk of bleeding. (See *Adverse reactions to guaifenesin.*)

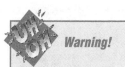
Warning!

Adverse reactions to guaifenesin

Adverse reactions to guaifenesin are rare and include:
- vomiting (if taken in large doses)
- diarrhea
- drowsiness
- nausea
- abdominal pain.

Antitussives

Antitussive drugs suppress or inhibit coughing.

> When a cough is dry, irritating, and exhausting, antitussives can bring relief.

Types of antitussives

Antitussives are typically used to treat dry, nonproductive coughs. The major antitussives include:
- benzonatate
- codeine
- dextromethorphan hydrobromide
- hydrocodone bitartrate.

Pharmacokinetics

Antitussives are absorbed well through the GI tract, metabolized in the liver, and excreted in the urine.

Pharmacodynamics

Antitussives act in slightly different ways.

Removing the sensation

Benzonatate acts by anesthetizing stretch receptors throughout the bronchi, alveoli, and pleura.

Taking direct action

Codeine, dextromethorphan, and hydrocodone suppress the cough reflex by direct action on the cough center in the medulla of the brain.

Pharmacotherapeutics

The uses of these drugs are slightly variable, but each treats a serious, nonproductive cough that interferes with a patient's ability to rest or carry out activities of daily living.

> Benzonatate can be useful during diagnostic procedures when the patient must avoid coughing.

Put it to the test

Benzonatate relieves cough caused by pneumonia, bronchitis, the common cold, and chronic pulmonary diseases such as emphysema. It also can be used during bronchial diagnostic tests such as bronchoscopy when the patient must avoid coughing.

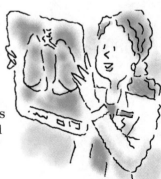

Top of the charts

Dextromethorphan is the most widely used cough suppressant in the U.S. and may provide better antitussive activity than codeine. It's popularity may stem from the fact that it produces few adverse reactions.

For really tough coughs

The narcotic antitussives (typically codeine and hydrocodone) are reserved for treating intractable cough, usually associated with lung cancer.

Drug interactions

Antitussives may interact with other drugs:
• Codeine and hydrocodone may cause excitation, an extremely elevated temperature, hypertension or hypotension, and coma when taken with monoamine oxidase (MAO) inhibitors.
• Dextromethorphan use with MAO inhibitors may produce excitation, an elevated body temperature, hypotension, and coma.
• Codeine may cause increased central nervous system (CNS) depression, such as drowsiness, lethargy, stupor, respiratory depression, coma, and death, when taken with other CNS depressants, including alcohol, barbiturates, sedative-hypnotics, and phenothiazines. (See *Adverse reactions to antitussives*.)

Mucolytics

Mucolytics act directly on mucus, breaking down sticky, thick secretions so they're more easily eliminated.

Acetylcysteine

Acetylcysteine is the only thiol compound mucolytic used clinically in the United States for patients with abnormal or thick mucus.

Pharmacokinetics

Inhaled acetylcysteine is absorbed from the pulmonary epithelium. When taken orally, the drug is absorbed from the GI tract.

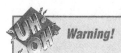
Warning!

Adverse reactions to antitussives

Benzonatate
• Dizziness
• Sedation
• Headache
• Nasal congestion
• Burning in the eyes
• GI upset or nausea
• Constipation
• Skin rash, eruptions, or itching
• Chills
• Chest numbness

Narcotic antitussives
• Pupil constriction
• Bradycardia
• Tachycardia
• Hypotension
• Stupor
• Seizures
• Circulatory collapse
• Respiratory arrest

Metabolism and excretion

Acetylcysteine is metabolized in the liver and its excretion is unknown.

Pharmacodynamics

Acetylcysteine decreases the thickness of respiratory tract secretions by altering the molecular composition of mucus. It also restores glutathione, a substance that plays an important role in oxidation-reduction processes.

Liver cleaner

Glutathione's enzymatic action in the liver reduces acetaminophen toxicity from overdose.

Pharmacotherapeutics

Mucolytics are used with other therapies to treat patients with abnormal or thick mucous secretions and may benefit patients with:

- bronchitis
- emphysema
- pulmonary complications related to cystic fibrosis
- atelectasis caused by mucous obstruction, as may occur in pneumonia, bronchiectasis, or chronic bronchitis.

Patient preparations

Mucolytics may also be used to prepare patients for bronchography and other bronchial studies.

Overdose antidote

Acetylcysteine is the antidote for acetaminophen overdose. However, it doesn't fully protect against liver damage caused by acetaminophen toxicity.

Drug interactions

Activated charcoal decreases acetylcysteine's effectiveness. When using acetylcysteine to treat acetaminophen overdose, remove activated charcoal from the stomach before administering. (See *Adverse reactions to acetylcysteine.*)

> When thick secretions overwhelm me, mucolytics thin mucus quickly so I can breathe better.

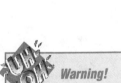

Warning!

Adverse reactions to acetylcysteine

Acetylcysteine has a "rotten egg" odor during administration that may cause nausea. With prolonged or persistent use, acetylcysteine may produce:

- bronchospasm
- drowsiness
- nausea and vomiting
- severe runny nose
- stomatitis.

Decongestants

Decongestants may be classified as systemic or topical, depending on how they're administered.

Types of decongestants

As sympathomimetic drugs, systemic decongestants stimulate the sympathetic nervous system to reduce swelling of the respiratory tract's vascular network. Systemic decongestants include:
- ephedrine
- phenylpropanolamine
- pseudoephedrine.

Topical concerns

Topical decongestants are also powerful vasoconstrictors. When applied directly to swollen mucous membranes of the nose, they provide immediate relief from nasal congestion and include:
- ephedrine, epinephrine, and phenylephrine (sympathomimetic amines)
- naphazoline, oxymetazoline, tetrahydrozoline, and xylometazoline (imidazoline derivatives of sympathomimetic amines).

Pharmacokinetics

The pharmacokinetic properties of decongestants vary.

Absorbed quickly...

When taken orally, the systemic decongestants are absorbed readily from the GI tract and widely distributed throughout the body into various tissues and fluids, including the cerebrospinal fluid, placenta, and breast milk.

...metabolized slowly

Systemic decongestants are slowly and incompletely metabolized by the liver and excreted largely unchanged in the urine within 24 hours of oral administration.

Direct action

Topical decongestants act directly on the alpha receptors of the vascular smooth muscle in the nose, causing the arterioles to constrict. As a result of this direct vasoconstriction, absorption of the drug becomes negligible.

Pharmacodynamics

The properties of systemic and topical decongestants vary slightly.

System(ic) analysis

The systemic decongestants cause vasoconstriction by directly stimulating alpha-adrenergic receptors on the blood vessels in the nasal mucosa. They also cause contraction of urinary and GI sphincters, dilation of the pupils of the eyes, and decreased secretion of insulin.

Indirect hit

These drugs may also act indirectly, resulting in the release of norepinephrine from storage sites in the body, resulting in peripheral vasoconstriction.

On topic(al)

Like systemic decongestants, topical decongestants stimulate alpha-adrenergic receptors in the smooth muscle of the blood vessels in the nose, resulting in vasoconstriction. The combination of reduced blood flow to the nasal mucous membranes and decreased capillary permeability reduces swelling. This action improves respiration by helping to drain sinuses, clear nasal passages, and open eustachian tubes.

Pharmacotherapeutics

Systemic and topical decongestants are used to relieve the symptoms of swollen nasal membranes resulting from:
- hay fever
- allergic rhinitis
- vasomotor rhinitis
- acute coryza (profuse discharge from the nose)
- sinusitis
- the common cold.

Team tactics

Systemic decongestants are frequently given with other drugs, such as antihistamines, antimuscarinics, antipyretic-analgesics, caffeine, and antitussives.

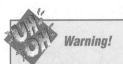

Advantage, topical

Topical decongestants provide two major advantages over systemics: minimal adverse reactions and rapid symptom relief.

Drug interactions

Because they produce vasoconstriction, which reduces drug absorption, drug interactions involving topical decongestants seldom occur. Systemic decongestants may interact with other drugs:

• Increased CNS stimulation may occur when the systemic decongestants are taken with other sympathomimetic drugs, including epinephrine, norepinephrine, dopamine, dobutamine, isoproterenol, metaproterenol, terbutaline, phenylephrine, and tyramine.

• The interaction of systemic decongestants and MAO inhibitors may cause severe hypertension or a hypertensive crisis, which can be life-threatening.

• Alkalinizing drugs may increase the effects of pseudoephedrine by reducing its urinary excretion. (See *Adverse reactions to decongestants.*)

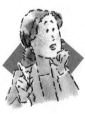

Quick quiz

1. Which adverse reaction can occur if guaifenesin is taken in larger doses than necessary?
    A.   Constipation
    B.   Vomiting
    C.   Insomnia

Answer: B. Vomiting can occur if guaifenesin is taken in abnormally large doses.

2. Which medication should patients avoid when taking dextromethorphan?
    A.   acetaminophen
    B.   guaifenesin
    C.   phenelzine

Warning!

Adverse reactions to decongestants

Most adverse reactions to decongestants result from central nervous system stimulation and include:
• nervousness
• restlessness
• insomnia
• nausea
• palpitations
• difficulty urinating
• elevations in blood pressure.

Topical decongestants
The most common adverse reaction associated with prolonged use (more than 5 days) of topical decongestants is rebound nasal congestion.

   Other reactions include:
• burning and stinging of the nasal mucosa
• sneezing
• mucosal dryness or ulceration.

Issue of sensitivity
Patients hypersensitive to other sympathomimetic amines may also be hypersensitive to decongestants.

Answer: C. MAO inhibitors such as phenelzine should be avoided in patients taking dextromethorphan; concurrent use may cause life threatening reactions.

3. Besides emphysema, acetylcysteine also may be used to treat which condition?
- A. Acetaminophen overdose
- B. Severe rhinorrhea
- C. Stomatitis

Answer: A. Acetylcysteine is an effective antidote used to treat acetaminophen overdose.

4. Which adverse reaction most commonly occurs with a decongestant such as oxymetazoline, especially if it's taken more often than the recommended frequency?
- A. Nausea
- B. Dizziness
- C. Rebound nasal congestion

Answer: C. Rebound nasal congestion commonly occurs when oxymetazoline is taken more frequently than recommended.

Scoring

☆☆☆   If you answered all four questions correctly, you're slicker than a mucolytic in action!

☆☆   If you answered two or three questions correctly, you're as relaxed as bronchial smooth muscle on xanthines.

☆   If you answered fewer than two questions correctly, you may need to clear your head with a decongestant.

8

Gastrointestinal drugs

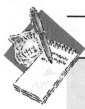

Just the facts

In this chapter, you'll review:

♦ classes of drugs used to improve GI function

♦ uses and varying actions of these drugs

♦ how these drugs are absorbed, distributed, metabolized, and excreted

♦ drug interactions and adverse reactions to these drugs.

Drugs and the GI system

The GI tract is basically a hollow, muscular tube that begins at the mouth and ends at the anus; it encompasses the pharnyx, esophagus, stomach, and the small and large intestines. Its primary functions are to digest and absorb foods and fluids and excrete metabolic waste.

Getting on tract

Classes of drugs used to improve GI function include:
• peptic ulcer drugs
• adsorbent, antiflatulent, and digestive drugs
• antidiarrheal and laxative drugs
• antiemetic and emetic drugs.

Peptic ulcer drugs

A peptic ulcer is a circumscribed lesion in the mucosal membrane, developing in the lower esophagus, stomach, duodenum, or jejunum.

Counting causes

There are three major causes of peptic ulcers:

bacterial infection with *Helicobacter pylori*

use of nonsteroidal anti-inflammatory drugs (NSAIDs)

hypersecretory states such as Zollinger-Ellison syndrome (a condition in which excessive secretion of gastric acid causes peptic ulcers).

Balancing act

Peptic ulcer drugs are aimed at either eradicating *H. pylori* or restoring the balance between acid and pepsin secretions and the GI mucosal defense. These drugs include:
- systemic antibiotics
- antacids
- Histamine-2 (H_2)–receptor antagonists
- proton pump inhibitors
- other peptic ulcer drugs, such as misoprostol and sucralfate.

Systemic antibiotics

H. pylori is a gram-negative bacteria that is thought to be a major causative factor in the formation of peptic ulcers and gastritis (inflammation of the lining of the stomach). Eradication of the bacteria promotes ulcer healing and decreases their recurrence.

Teamwork is a must

Successful treatment involves the use of two or more antibiotics in combination with other drugs. *Systemic antibiotics* used to treat *H. pylori* include:
- metronidazole
- tetracycline
- clarithromycin
- amoxicillin.

Pharmacokinetics (how drugs circulate)
Systemic antibiotics are variably absorbed from the GI tract.

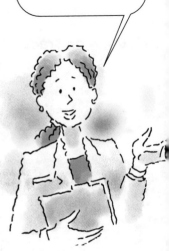

Treatment plans that use at least two antimicrobial drugs plus an antacid for 2 weeks are successful in curing up to 90% of patients with peptic ulcers.

Dairy delay

Food, especially dairy products, decreases the absorption of tetracycline but doesn't significantly delay the absorption of the other antibiotics.

Distribution and excretion

All of these antibiotics are distributed widely and are excreted primarily in the urine.

Pharmacodynamics (how drugs act)

Antibiotics act by treating the *H. pylori* infection. They're usually combined with an H_2-receptor antagonist or a proton pump inhibitor to decrease stomach acid and further promote healing.

Pharmacotherapeutics (how drugs are used)

Various combinations of antimicrobial drugs with either an H_2-receptor antagonist or a proton pump inhibitor have been clinically studied.

Successful strategy

Treatment plans that use at least two antimicrobial drugs and an antacid for 2 weeks are successful in curing up to 90% of patients with peptic ulcers.

Drug interactions

Tetracycline and metronidazole can interact with many other medications. For example, tetracycline increases digoxin levels and, when combined with methoxyflurane, increases the risk of nephrotoxicity. Metronidazole and tetracycline increase the risk of bleeding when taken with oral anticoagulants. (See *Adverse reactions to antibiotics.*)

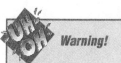

Warning!

Adverse reactions to antibiotics

Antibiotics used to improve GI tract function may lead to adverse reactions:
• Metronidazole, clarithromycin, and tetracycline commonly cause mild GI disturbances.
• Clarithromycin and metronidazole may also produce abnormal tastes.
• Amoxicillin may cause diarrhea.

Antacids

Antacids are over-the-counter (OTC) medications. They're used alone or with other drugs to treat peptic ulcers and include:
• magnesium hydroxide and aluminum hydroxide
• simethicone
• magaldrate (aluminum-magnesium complex)
• calcium carbonate.

Pharmacokinetics

Antacids work locally in the stomach by neutralizing gastric acid. They don't need to be absorbed to treat peptic ulcers.

Distribution and excretion

Antacids are distributed throughout the GI tract and are eliminated primarily in the feces.

Pharmacodynamics

The acid-neutralizing action of antacids reduces the total amount of acid in the GI tract, allowing peptic ulcers time to heal.

The more it works, the sooner it rests

Because pepsin acts more effectively when the stomach is highly acidic, as acidity drops, pepsin action is also reduced. Contrary to popular belief, antacids don't work by coating peptic ulcers or the lining of the GI tract.

Pharmacotherapeutics

Antacids, used alone or with other drugs, are primarily prescribed to relieve pain and promote healing in peptic ulcer disease.

Settling the GI system

Antacids also relieve symptoms of acid indigestion, heartburn, dyspepsia (burning or indigestion), or gastroesophageal reflux disease (GERD), where the contents of the stomach and duodenum flow back into the esophagus.

In critical situations

Antacids may also be used to prevent stress ulcers and GI bleeding in critically ill patients during times of severe physical stress. They may be used to control hyperphosphatemia (elevated blood phosphate levels) in kidney failure. Because calcium binds with phosphate in the GI tract, calcium carbonate antacids prevent phosphate absorption.

Drug interactions

All antacids can interfere with the absorption of oral drugs given at the same time. Absorption of digoxin, iron

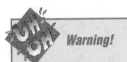

Warning!

Adverse reactions to antacids

All adverse reactions to antacids are dose related and include:
• diarrhea
• constipation
• electrolyte imbalances.

salts, isoniazid, quinolones, and tetracyclines may be reduced if taken within 2 hours of antacids. (See *Adverse reactions to antacids.*)

H₂-receptor antagonists

H₂-receptor antagonists are commonly prescribed antiulcer drugs in the United States and include:
- cimetidine
- nizatidine
- ranitidine
- famotidine.

Pharmacokinetics

Cimetidine, nizatidine, and ranitidine are absorbed rapidly and completely from the GI tract. Famotidine isn't completely absorbed. Food and antacids may reduce the absorption of H₂-receptor antagonists.

Distribution, metabolism, and excretion

H₂-receptor antagonists are distributed widely throughout the body, metabolized by the liver, and excreted primarily in the urine.

Pharmacodynamics

H₂-receptor antagonists block histamine from stimulating the acid-secreting parietal cells of the stomach.

The acid test

Acid secretion in the stomach depends on the binding of gastrin, acetylcholine, and histamine to receptors on the parietal cells. If the binding of any one of these substances is blocked, acid secretion is reduced. The H₂-receptor antagonists, by binding with H₂ receptors, block the action of histamine in the stomach and reduce acid secretion.

Pharmacotherapeutics

H₂-receptor antagonists are used therapeutically to:
- promote healing of duodenal and gastric ulcers
- provide long-term treatment of pathologic GI hypersecretory conditions such as Zollinger-Ellison syndrome

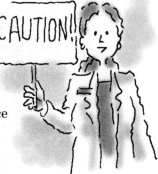

It's important to note that antacids can interfere with the absorption of other orally administered drugs.

CAUTION!

• reduce gastric acid production and prevent stress ulcers in severely ill patients and in those with reflux esophagitis or upper GI bleeding.

Drug interactions

H_2-receptor antagonists may interact with antacids and other drugs:
• Antacids reduce the absorption of cimetidine, nizatidine, ranitidine, and famotidine.
• Cimetidine may increase the blood levels of oral anticoagulants, propranolol (and possibly other beta blockers), benzodiazepines, tricyclic antidepressants, theophylline, procainamide, quinidine, lidocaine, phenytoin, calcium channel blockers, cyclosporine, carbamazepine, and narcotic analgesics by reducing their metabolism in the liver and subsequent excretion.
• Cimetidine taken with carmustine increases the risk of bone marrow toxicity.
• Cimetidine inhibits metabolism of ethyl alcohol in the stomach, resulting in higher blood alcohol levels. (See *Adverse reactions to H_2-receptor antagonists*.)

Proton pump inhibitors

Proton pump inhibitors disrupt chemical binding in stomach cells to reduce acid production, lessening irritation and allowing peptic ulcers to better heal. They include:
• rabeprazole
• pantoprazole
• omeprazole
• lansoprazole.

Pharmacokinetics

Proton pump inhibitors are given orally in enteric-coated formulas to bypass the stomach because they're highly acid labile (easily disarranged). When in the small intestine, they dissolve and absorption is rapid.

Metabolism and excretion

These medications are highly protein-bound and are extensively metabolized by the liver to inactive compounds, then eliminated in urine.

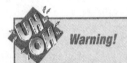

Warning!

Adverse reactions to H_2-receptor antagonists

Use of H_2-receptor antagonists may lead to adverse reactions:
• Cimetidine and ranitidine may produce headache, dizziness, malaise, muscle pain, nausea, diarrhea or constipation, rashes, itching, loss of sexual desire, and impotence.
• Famotidine and nizatidine produce few adverse reactions, with headache being the most common, followed by constipation or diarrhea and rash.

Pharmacodynamics

Proton pump inhibitors block the last step in the secretion of gastric acid by combining with hydrogen, potassium, and adenosine triphosphate in the parietal cells of the stomach.

Pharmacotherapeutics

Proton pump inhibitors are indicated for:
- short-term treatment of active gastric ulcers
- active duodenal ulcers
- erosive esophagitis
- symptomatic GERD that isn't responsive to other therapies
- active peptic ulcers associated with *H. pylori* infection, in combination with antibiotics
- long-term treatment of hypersecretory states such as Zollinger-Ellison syndrome.

Drug interactions

Proton pump inhibitors may interfere with the metabolism of diazepam, phenytoin, and warfarin, causing increased half-lives and elevated plasma concentrations of these drugs.

Absorbing talk

Proton pump inhibitors also may interfere with the absorption of drugs that depend on gastric pH for absorption, such as ketoconazole, digoxin, ampicillin, and iron salts. (See *Adverse reactions to proton pump inhibitors.*)

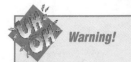

Warning!

Adverse reactions to proton pump inhibitors

- Abdominal pain
- Diarrhea
- Nausea and vomiting

Other peptic ulcer drugs

Research continues on the usefulness of other drugs in treating peptic ulcer disease. Two other peptic ulcer drugs currently in use are:
- misoprostol
- sucralfate.

Pharmacokinetics

Each of these drugs has slightly different pharmacokinetic properties.

Absorption, metabolism, and excretion

After an oral dose, misoprostol is absorbed extensively and rapidly. It's metabolized to misoprostol acid, which is clinically active, meaning it's able to produce a pharmacologic effect. Misoprostol acid is highly protein-bound and is excreted primarily in the urine.

Sucralfate is minimally absorbed from the GI tract and is excreted in the feces.

Pharmacodynamics

The actions of these drugs vary.

Naysaying NSAIDs

Misoprostol protects against peptic ulcers caused by NSAIDs by reducing the secretion of gastric acid and by boosting the production of gastric mucus, a natural defense against peptic ulcers.

Ulcer protection?

Sucralfate works locally in the stomach, rapidly reacting with hydrochloric acid to form a thick, pastelike substance that adheres to the gastric mucosa and, especially, to ulcers. By binding to the ulcer site, sucralfate actually protects the ulcer from the damaging effects of acid and pepsin to promote healing.

Pharmacotherapeutics

Each of these drugs has its own therapeutic use.

Making it less complicated

Misoprostol prevents gastric ulcers caused by NSAIDs in patients at high risk for complications resulting from gastric ulcers.

In the short run

Sucralfate is used for short-term treatment (up to 8 weeks) of duodenal or gastric ulcers, and prevention of recurrent ulcers or stress ulcers.

Drug interactions

Both misoprostol and sucralfate may interact with other drugs.

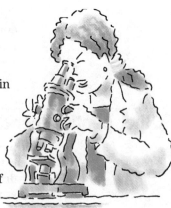

Sucralfate reacts with hydrochloric acid to form a pastelike substance that adheres to ulcer sites, reducing pain and promoting healing.

• Antacids may bind with misoprostol or decrease its absorption. However, this effect doesn't appear to be clinically significant.
• Some drugs bind with sucralfate in the GI tract, decreasing their absorption.
• Antacids may reduce the binding of sucralfate to the gastric and duodenal mucosa, reducing its effectiveness. (See *Adverse reactions to other peptic ulcer drugs.*)

Adsorbent, antiflatulent, and digestive drugs

Adsorbent, antiflatulent, and digestive drugs are used to fight undesirable toxins, acids, and gases in the GI tract, aiding healthy GI function.

Adsorbent drugs

Natural and synthetic *adsorbents* are prescribed as antidotes for the ingestion of toxins, substances that can lead to poisoning or overdose.

Charcoal sketch

The most commonly used clinical adsorbent is activated charcoal, a black powder residue obtained from the distillation of various organic materials.

Pharmacokinetics

Activated charcoal must be administered soon after toxic ingestion because activated charcoal can only bind with drugs or poisons that haven't yet been absorbed from the GI tract.

Vicious cycle

After initial absorption, some poisons move back into the intestines, where they're reabsorbed. Activated charcoal may be administered repeatedly to break this cycle.

Absorption, metabolism, and excretion
Activated charcoal, which isn't absorbed or metabolized by the body, is excreted unchanged in the feces.

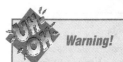

Warning!

Adverse reactions to other peptic ulcer drugs

Misoprostol
• Diarrhea (common)
• Abdominal pain
• Gas
• Indigestion
• Nausea
• Vomiting

Sucralfate
• Constipation
• Nausea
• Metallic taste

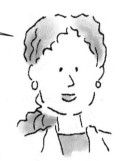

When a patient has swallowed an overdose or poison, activated charcoal helps to adsorb toxins not yet digested by binding with them…

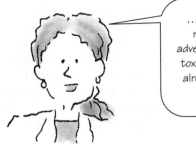

…but it can't reverse the adverse effects of toxins that have already entered the body.

Pharmacodynamics

Because adsorbents attract and bind toxins in the intestine, they inhibit toxins from being absorbed from the GI tract. However, this binding doesn't change any toxic effects caused by earlier absorption of the poison.

Pharmacotherapeutics

Activated charcoal is a general-purpose antidote used for many types of acute oral poisoning. It isn't indicated in acute poisoning from cyanide, ethanol, methanol, iron, sodium chloride alkalies, inorganic acids, or organic solvents.

Drug interactions

Drugs to induce vomiting such as syrup of ipecac have traditionally been given before administering activated charcoal. That is because vomiting enhances activated charcoal's effectiveness by decreasing the amount of toxin in the GI tract to be absorbed and giving ipecac with activated charcoal will cause the ipecac to be made inactive through absorption. However, the use of ipecac is currently discouraged because charcoal administration shouldn't be delayed. (See *Adverse reactions to activated charcoal*.)

Antiflatulent drugs

Antiflatulents disperse gas pockets in the GI tract. They're available alone or in combination with antacids. A major antiflatulent drug currently in use is simethicone.

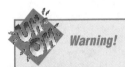

Warning!

Adverse reactions to activated charcoal

Activated charcoal turns stools black and may cause constipation.

Teaming up
A laxative such as sorbitol usually is given with activated charcoal to prevent constipation.

Pharmacokinetics

Antiflatulents aren't absorbed from the GI tract. They're distributed only in the intestinal lumen and are eliminated intact in the feces.

Pharmacodynamics

Antiflatulents provide defoaming action in the GI tract. By producing a film in the intestines, simethicone disperses mucus-enclosed gas pockets and helps prevent their formation.

Pharmacotherapeutics

Antiflatulents are prescribed to treat conditions in which excess gas is a problem, such as:
• functional gastric bloating
• postoperative gaseous bloating
• diverticular disease
• spastic or irritable colon
• air swallowing.

Drug interactions

Simethicone doesn't interact significantly with other drugs and doesn't cause any known adverse reactions.

Digestive drugs

Digestive drugs (digestants) aid digestion in patients who are missing enzymes or other substances needed to digest food. Digestants that function in the GI tract, liver, and pancreas include:
• dehydrocholic acid
• pancreatin and pancrelipase (pancreatic enzymes).

Pharmacokinetics

Digestants aren't absorbed; they act locally in the GI tracts and are excreted in feces.

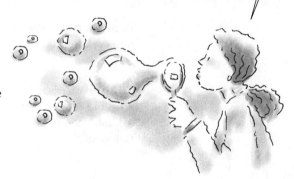

Antiflatulence drugs, such as simethicone, create a film in the intestines that collapses and disperses gas bubbles.

Pharmacodynamics

The action of digestants resembles the action of the body substances they replace. Dehydrocholic acid, a bile acid, increases the output of bile in the liver. The pancreatic enzymes pancreatin and pancrelipase replace normal pancreatic enzymes.

Breaking it down

These drugs contain trypsin to digest proteins, amylase to digest carbohydrates, and lipase to digest fats.

Pharmacotherapeutics

Because their action resembles the action of the body substances they replace, each digestant has its own indication.

Mirror images

Dehydrocholic acid, a bile acid, provides temporary relief from constipation and promotes the flow of bile.

Pancreatic enzymes are administered to patients with insufficient levels of pancreatic enzymes, such as those with pancreatitis and cystic fibrosis. They may also be used to treat steatorrhea (disorder of fat metabolism characterized by fatty, foul-smelling stools).

Drug interactions

Antacids reduce the effects of pancreatin and pancrelipase and shouldn't be given at the same time. (See *Adverse reactions to digestive drugs*.)

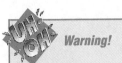

Warning!

Adverse reactions to digestive drugs

Dehydrocholic acid
- Abdominal cramping
- Biliary colic (with gallstone obstruction of biliary duct)
- Diarrhea

Pancreatic enzymes
- Diarrhea
- Nausea

Antidiarrheal and laxative drugs

Diarrhea and constipation represent the two major symptoms related to disturbances of the large intestine.

Stop!

Antidiarrheals act systemically or locally and include:
- opioid-related drugs
- kaolin and pectin (a combination drug and the only one that acts locally).

Loosen up!

Laxatives stimulate defecation and include:
- hyperosmolar drugs
- dietary fiber and related bulk-forming substances
- emollients
- stimulants
- lubricants.

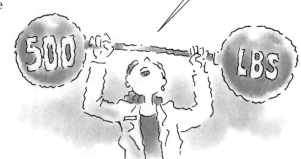

Although many nonprescription laxatives are available, diet and lifestyle changes are probably the best first line of defense against constipation.

Opioid-related drugs

Opioid-related drugs decrease peristalsis (involuntary, progressive wavelike intestinal movement that pushes fecal matter along) in the intestines and include:
- difenoxin
- diphenoxylate
- loperamide.

Pharmacokinetics

Difenoxin with atropine and diphenoxylate with atropine are readily absorbed from the GI tract. However, loperamide isn't absorbed well after oral administration.

Distribution, metabolism, and excretion

All three medications are distributed in the serum, metabolized in the liver, and excreted primarily in the feces. Diphenoxylate is metabolized to difenoxin, its biologically active major metabolite.

Pharmacodynamics

Difenoxin, diphenoxylate, and loperamide slow GI motility by depressing the circular and longitudinal muscle action (peristalsis) in the large and small intestines. These drugs also decrease expulsive contractions throughout the colon.

Pharmacotherapeutics

Difenoxin, diphenoxylate, and loperamide are used to treat acute, nonspecific diarrhea. Loperamide also is used to treat chronic diarrhea.

Drug interactions

Difenoxin, diphenoxylate, and loperamide may enhance the depressant effects of barbiturates, alcohol, narcotics, tranquilizers, and sedatives. (See *Adverse reactions to opioid-related drugs*.)

Kaolin and pectin

Kaolin and *pectin* mixtures are locally acting OTC antidiarrheals. They work by adsorbing irritants and soothing the intestinal mucosa.

Pharmacokinetics

Kaolin and pectin aren't absorbed and, therefore, aren't distributed throughout the body. They are excreted in the feces.

Pharmacodynamics

Kaolin and pectin act as adsorbents, binding with bacteria, toxins, and other irritants on the intestinal mucosa. Pectin decreases the pH in the intestinal lumen and provides a soothing effect on the irritated mucosa.

Pharmacotherapeutics

Kaolin and pectin are used to relieve mild to moderate acute diarrhea. They also may be used to temporarily relieve chronic diarrhea until the cause has been determined and definitive treatment begun.

Drug interactions

These antidiarrheals can interfere with the absorption of digoxin or other drugs from the intestinal mucosa if administered at the same time. (See *Adverse reactions to kaolin and pectin*.)

Hyperosmolar laxatives

Hyperosmolar laxatives work by drawing water into the intestine, thereby promoting bowel distention and peristalsis. They include:
• glycerin

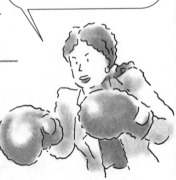

Kaolin and pectin give diarrhea the one-two punch by adsorbing irritants and soothing the intestinal mucosa.

• lactulose
• saline compounds (magnesium salts, sodium biphosphate, sodium phosphate, polyethylene glycol [PEG] and electrolytes).

Pharmacokinetics

The pharmacokinetic properties of the hyperosmolar laxatives vary.

Direct placement

Glycerin is placed directly into the colon by enema or suppository and isn't absorbed systemically.

Minimal absorption

Lactulose enters the GI tract orally and is minimally absorbed. As a result, the drug is distributed only in the intestine. It's metabolized by bacteria in the colon and excreted in the feces.

Introducing ions

After saline compounds are introduced into the GI tract orally or as an enema, some of their ions are absorbed. Absorbed ions are excreted in the urine, the unabsorbed drug in the feces.

Pegging PEG

PEG is a nonabsorbable solution that acts as an osmotic drug but doesn't alter electrolyte balance.

Pharmacodynamics

Hyperosmolar laxatives produce a bowel movement by drawing water into the intestine. Fluid accumulation distends the bowel and promotes peristalsis and a bowel movement.

Pharmacotherapeutics

The uses of hyperosmolar laxatives vary:
• Glycerin is helpful in bowel retraining.
• Lactulose is used to treat constipation and help reduce ammonia production and absorption from the intestines in liver disease.
• Saline compounds are used when prompt and complete bowel evacuation is required.

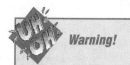 **Warning!**

Adverse drug reactions to kaolin and pectin

Kaolin and pectin mixtures cause few adverse reactions. However, constipation may occur, especially in elderly or debilitated patients or with overdose or prolonged use.

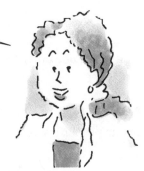

Hyperosmolar laxatives help the colon draw the water necessary for distention, peristalsis, and eventual movement.

Drug interactions

Hyperosmolar laxatives don't interact significantly with other drugs. However, oral drugs given 1 hour before administering PEG will be flushed from the GI tract unabsorbed. (See *Adverse reactions to hyperosmolar laxatives.*)

Dietary fiber and related bulk-forming laxatives

A high-fiber diet is the most natural way to prevent or treat constipation. *Dietary fiber* is the part of plants not digested in the small intestine.

Bulking up

The *bulk-forming laxatives,* which resemble dietary fiber, contain natural and semisynthetic polysaccharides and cellulose. These laxatives include:
- methylcellulose
- polycarbophil
- psyllium hydrophilic mucilloid.

Pharmacokinetics

Dietary fiber and bulk-forming laxatives aren't absorbed systemically. The polysaccharides in these drugs are converted by intestinal bacterial flora into osmotically active metabolites that draw water into the intestine.

Excretion

Dietary fiber and bulk-forming laxatives are excreted in the feces.

Pharmacodynamics

Dietary fiber and bulk-forming laxatives increase stool mass and water content, promoting peristalsis.

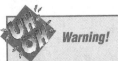

Warning!

Adverse reactions to hyperosmolar laxatives

Adverse reactions to hyperosmolar laxatives involve fluid and electrolyte imbalances.

Glycerin
- Weakness
- Fatigue

Lactulose
- Abdominal distention, gas, and abdominal cramps
- Nausea and vomiting
- Diarrhea
- Hypokalemia
- Hypovolemia
- Increased blood glucose level

Saline compounds
- Weakness
- Lethargy
- Dehydration
- Hypernatremia
- Hypermagnesemia
- Hyperphosphatemia
- Hypocalcemia
- Cardiac arrhythmias
- Shock

Polyethylene glycol
- Nausea
- Abdominal fullness
- Explosive diarrhea
- Bloating

Pharmacotherapeutics

Bulk-forming laxatives are used:
• to treat simple cases of constipation, especially constipation resulting from a low-fiber or low-fluid diet
• to aid patients recovering from acute myocardial infarction (MI) or cerebral aneurysms who need to avoid Valsalva's maneuver (forced expiration against a closed airway) and maintain soft feces
• to manage patients with irritable bowel syndrome and diverticulosis.

> A diet high in fiber is the best way to prevent constipation. Fiber increases stool mass and helps draw water into the intestine to support peristalsis.

Drug interactions

Decreased absorption of digoxin, warfarin, and salicylates occurs if these drugs are taken within 2 hours of fiber or bulk-forming laxatives. (See *Adverse reactions to dietary fiber and related bulk-forming laxatives.*)

Emollient laxatives

Emollients — also known as stool softeners — include the calcium, potassium, and sodium salts of docusate.

Pharmacokinetics

Administered orally, emollients are absorbed and excreted through bile in the feces.

Pharmacodynamics

Emollients soften the stool and make bowel movements easier by emulsifying the fat and water components of feces in the small and large intestines. This detergent action allows water and fats to penetrate the stool, making it softer and easier to eliminate.

Stimulating talk

Emollients also stimulate electrolyte and fluid secretion from intestinal mucosal cells.

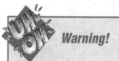

Warning!

Adverse reactions to dietary fiber and related bulk-forming laxatives

Adverse reactions to dietary fiber and related bulk-forming laxative include:
• gas
• a sensation of abdominal fullness
• intestinal obstruction
• fecal impaction (hard stool that can't be removed from the rectum)
• esophageal obstruction (if sufficient liquid hasn't been administered with the drug)
• severe diarrhea.

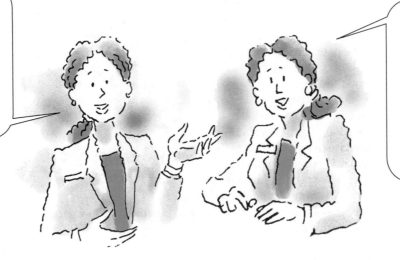

By allowing water to penetrate the fecal matter, emollients help soften the stool, easing the strain of defecation.

This makes emollients an excellent therapeutic tool for patients coming off surgery who need to avoid muscular straining.

Pharmacotherapeutics

Emollients are the drugs of choice for softening stools in patients who should avoid straining during a bowel movement, including those with:
- recent MI or surgery
- disease of the anus or rectum
- increased intracranial pressure (ICP)
- hernias.

Drug interactions

Taking oral doses of mineral oil with oral emollients increases the systemic absorption of mineral oil and may result in tissue deposits of the oil.

Caution

Because emollients may enhance the absorption of many oral drugs, drugs with low margins of safety (narrow therapeutic index) should be administered cautiously with emollients. (See *Adverse reactions to emollient laxatives*.)

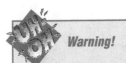
Warning!

Adverse reactions to emollient laxatives

Although adverse reactions to emollients seldom occur, they may include:
- a bitter taste
- diarrhea
- throat irritation
- mild, transient abdominal cramping.

Stimulant laxatives

Stimulant laxatives, also known as irritant cathartics, include:
- bisacodyl
- cascara sagrada
- castor oil
- phenolphthalein
- senna.

Pharmacokinetics

Stimulant laxatives are minimally absorbed and are metabolized in the liver. The metabolites are excreted in the urine and feces.

Pharmacodynamics

Stimulant laxatives stimulate peristalsis and produce a bowel movement by irritating the intestinal mucosa or stimulating nerve endings of the intestinal smooth muscle.

No job is too small

Castor oil and phenolphthalein also increase peristalsis in the small intestine.

Pharmacotherapeutics

Stimulant laxatives are the preferred drugs for emptying the bowel before general surgery, sigmoidoscopic or proctoscopic procedures, and radiologic procedures, such as barium studies of the GI tract.

Freeing you up in other situations

Stimulant laxatives also are used to treat constipation caused by prolonged bed rest, neurologic dysfunction of the colon, and constipating drugs such as narcotics.

Drug interactions

No significant drug interactions occur with the stimulant laxatives. However, because stimulant laxatives produce increased intestinal motility, they reduce the absorption of other oral drugs administered at the same time, especially sustained-release forms. (See *Adverse reactions to stimulant laxatives*.)

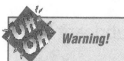

Warning!

Adverse reactions to stimulant laxatives

Adverse reactions to stimulant laxatives include:
- weakness
- nausea
- abdominal cramps
- mild inflammation of the rectum and anus.

Lubricant laxatives

Mineral oil is the main *lubricant laxative* in current clinical use.

Pharmacokinetics

In its nonemulsified form, mineral oil is minimally absorbed; the emulsified form is about half absorbed. Absorbed mineral oil is distributed to the mesenteric lymph nodes, intestinal mucosa, liver, and spleen.

Metabolism and excretion

Mineral oil is metabolized by the liver and excreted in the feces.

Pharmacodynamics

Mineral oil lubricates the stool and the intestinal mucosa and prevents water reabsorption from the lumen of the bowel. The increased fluid content of the feces increases peristalsis. Rectal administration by enema also produces distention.

Pharmacotherapeutics

Mineral oil is used to treat constipation and maintain soft stools when straining is contraindicated, such as after recent MI (to avoid Valsalva's maneuver), eye surgery (to prevent increased pressure in the eye), or cerebral aneurysm repair (to avoid increased ICP).

Impacting impaction

Administered orally or by enema, this lubricant laxative is also used to treat patients with fecal impaction.

Drug interactions

Mineral oil has few interactions with other drugs:
• Mineral oil may impair the absorption of many oral medications, including fat-soluble vitamins, oral contraceptives, and anticoagulants.
• Mineral oil may interfere with the antibacterial activity of nonabsorbable sulfonamides. (See *Adverse reactions to mineral oil.*)

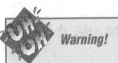

Warning!

Adverse reactions to mineral oil

Adverse reactions to mineral oil include:
• nausea
• vomiting
• diarrhea
• abdominal cramping.

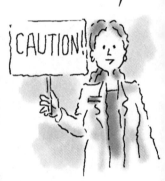

One important thing to remember about all laxatives: they have the potential for abuse, particularly by patients with eating disorders. This is a very serious health hazard.

Antiemetic and emetic drugs

Antiemetics and *emetics* represent two groups of drugs with opposing actions. Emetic drugs, which are derived from plants, produce vomiting. Antiemetic drugs decrease nausea, reducing the urge to vomit.

Antiemetics

The major antiemetics include:
• antihistamines, including dimenhydrinate, diphenhydramine hydrochloride, buclizine hydrochloride, cyclizine hydrochloride, hydroxyzine hydrochloride, hydroxyzine pamoate, meclizine hydrochloride, and trimethobenzamide hydrochloride
• phenothiazines, including chlorpromazine hydrochloride, perphenazine, prochlorperazine maleate, promethazine hydrochloride, and thiethylperazine maleate
• serotonin receptor antagonists, including ondansetron and granisetron.

Top of the charts

Ondansetron is currently the antiemetic of choice in the United States.

Pharmacokinetics

The pharmacokinetic properties of antiemetics may slightly vary.

Absorption, metabolism, and excretion

Oral antihistamine antiemetics are absorbed well from the GI tract and are metabolized primarily by the liver. Their inactive metabolites are excreted in the urine.

Phenothiazine antiemetics and serotonin receptor antagonists are absorbed well, extensively metabolized by the liver, and excreted in the urine and feces.

Pharmacodynamics

The action of antiemetics may vary.

> Some antiemetics work by blocking the vomiting center in my medulla or nearby areas that stimulate vomiting.

Other antiemetics

Here are other antiemetics currently in use.

Benzquinamide

Benzquinamide hydrochloride is used to prevent or treat nausea and vomiting caused by anesthesia and surgery. This drug may be preferred in some circumstances because it doesn't produce central nervous system or respiratory depression. Plus, benzquinamide doesn't produce the extrapyramidal effects (abnormal involuntary movements) or hypotension that may occur with the phenothiazines.

Scopolamine

Scopolamine prevents motion sickness, but its use is limited because of its sedative and anticholinergic effects. One scopolamine transdermal preparation, Transderm-Scōp, is highly effective without producing the usual adverse effects.

Metoclopramide

Metoclopramide hydrochloride has been used for many years in Europe to prevent motion sickness and is being used in the U.S. to prevent chemotherapy–induced nausea and vomiting.

Diphenidol

Diphenidol effectively prevents vertigo (whirling sensation), in addition to preventing or treating generalized nausea and vomiting. However, its use is limited because of the auditory and visual hallucinations, confusion, and disorientation that may occur.

Dronabinol

Dronabinol, a purified derivative of the cannabis, is a schedule II drug (meaning it has a high potential for abuse) used to treat the nausea and vomiting resulting from cancer chemotherapy in patients who don't respond adequately to conventional antiemetics. It's also been used to stimulate appetite in patients with acquired immunodeficiency syndrome. However, dronabinol can accumulate in the body, and the patient can develop tolerance or physical and psychological dependence.

What's going on here?

The mechanism of action that produces the antiemetic effect of antihistamines is unclear.

Don't pull the trigger!

Phenothiazines produce their antiemetic effect by blocking the dopaminergic receptors in the chemoreceptor trigger zone in the brain. (This area of the brain, near the medulla, stimulates the vomiting center in the medulla, causing vomiting). These drugs may also directly depress the vomiting center.

Stopping serotonin stimulation

The serotonin receptor antagonists block serotonin stimulation centrally in the chemoreceptor trigger zone and peripherally in the vagal nerve terminals, both of which stimulate vomiting.

Pharmacotherapeutics

The uses of the antiemetics may vary.

Lend me your ear

With the exception of trimethobenzamide, the antihistamines are specifically used for nausea and vomiting caused by inner ear stimulation. As a consequence, these drugs prevent or treat motion sickness. They usually prove most effective when given before activities that produce motion sickness and are much less effective when nausea or vomiting has already begun.

Severe cases

Phenothiazine antiemetics and serotonin receptor antagonists control severe nausea and vomiting from various causes. They're used when vomiting becomes severe and potentially hazardous, such as postsurgical or viral nausea and vomiting. Both types of drugs are also prescribed to control the nausea and vomiting resulting from cancer chemotherapy and radiotherapy. (See *Other antiemetics*.)

Drug interactions

Antiemetics may have many significant interactions:
• Antihistamines and phenothiazines can produce additive central nervous system (CNS) depression and sedation when taken with CNS depressants, such as barbiturates, tranquilizers, antidepressants, alcohol, and opioids.
• Antihistamines can cause additive anticholinergic effects such as constipation, dry mouth, vision problems, and urine retention when taken with anticholinergic drugs, including tricyclic antidepressants, phenothiazines, and antiparkinsonian drugs.
• Phenothiazine antiemetics taken with anticholinergic drugs increase the anticholinergic effect and decrease the antiemetic effects.
• Phenothiazine antiemetics taken with lithium may increase the risk of neurologic toxicity.
• Droperidol plus phenothiazine antiemetics increase the risk of extrapyramidal (abnormal involuntary movements) effects. (See *Adverse reactions to antiemetics*.)

Emetics

Emetics are used to induce vomiting in a person who has ingested toxic substances. *Ipecac syrup* is the emetic of

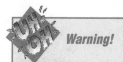

Warning!

Adverse reactions to antiemetics

Use of these antiemetic drugs may lead to adverse reactions.
• Antihistamine and phenothiazine antiemetics produce drowsiness; paradoxical central nervous system (CNS) stimulation may also occur.
• CNS effects associated with phenothiazine and serotonin receptor antagonist antiemetics include confusion, anxiety, euphoria, agitation, depression, headache, insomnia, restlessness, and weakness.
• The anticholinergic effect of the antiemetics may cause constipation, dry mouth and throat, painful or difficult urination, urine retention, impotence, and vision and auditory disturbances.
• Hypotension and orthostatic hypotension with a rise in heart rate, fainting, and dizziness are common adverse reactions to the phenothiazine antiemetics.

choice because it's the most effective and least likely to cause problems.

Controversy?

The use of ipecac syrup has become controversial, however, because it delays the use of charcoal.

Pharmacokinetics

Little information exists concerning the absorption, distribution, and excretion of ipecac syrup. After administration of ipecac syrup, vomiting occurs within 10 to 30 minutes.

Measuring success

The success of treatment is directly linked to fluid intake with ipecac administration.

Pharmacodynamics

Ipecac syrup induces vomiting by stimulating the vomiting center located in the brain's medulla.

Pharmacotherapeutics

Ipecac syrup is considered the therapy of choice for emptying the stomach because of its effectiveness and low incidence of adverse effects.

Drug interactions

Because ipecac syrup is used only in acute situations, drug interactions rarely occur. If poisoning results from ingestion of a phenothiazine, the phenothiazine's antiemetic effect may decrease the emetic effect of ipecac syrup. (See *Adverse reactions to ipecac syrup*.)

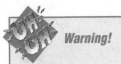

Warning!

Adverse reactions to ipecac syrup

Ipecac syrup rarely produces adverse reactions when used in the recommended dosages. However, prolonged vomiting for more than 1 hour or repeated vomiting involving more than six episodes in 1 hour, lethargy, and diarrhea may occur.

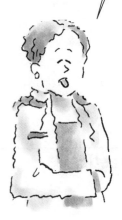

After administration of ipecac syrup, vomiting occurs within 10 to 30 minutes.

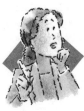

Quick quiz

1. A patient is puzzled about why he's taking antibiotics for an ulcer. The doctor explains that antibiotics will:
    A.   destroy the bacteria causing the ulcer.
    B.   destroy the virus causing the ulcer.
    C.   prevent infection from entering through open areas in the gastric mucosa.

Answer: A. Antibiotics destroy bacteria responsible for ulcer formation.

2. What is a common adverse reaction to misoprostol?
    A.   Indigestion
    B.   Diarrhea
    C.   Headache

Answer: B. Diarrhea is a common adverse reaction to misoprostol.

3. How does simethicone relieve GI tract gas?
    A.   It disperses and prevents gas pocket formation.
    B.   It facilitates expulsion of gas pockets.
    C.   It neutralizes gastric contents and reduces gas.

Answer: A. Simethicone relieves GI tract gas by producing a film in the intestines that disperses mucous-enclosed gas pockets and helps prevent their formation.

4. The antiemetic drug that would probably be best for a patient who experiences motion sickness on airplanes is:
    A.   chlorpromazine hydrochloride.
    B.   dronabinol.
    C.   dimenhydrinate.

Answer: C. An antihistamine, such as dimenhydrinate, is the most effective antiemetic for a patient who experiences motion sickness during air travel.

5. To prevent a postsurgical patient from straining during a bowel movement, the doctor is most likely to prescribe the laxative:

A. docusate sodium.
B. magnesium citrate.
C. bisacodyl.

Answer: A. Docusate sodium is commonly prescribed to prevent straining during a bowel movement after surgery.

Scoring

☆☆☆ If you answered all five questions correctly, well done! You digested this GI information admirably!

☆☆ If you answered three or four questions correctly, keep up the good work (preferably without emetics).

☆ If you answered fewer than three questions correctly, you may need extra stimulation to move through this chapter.

9

Anti-infective drugs

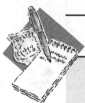

Just the facts

In this chapter, you'll review:

♦ classes of drugs that act as anti-infectives

♦ uses and varying actions of these drugs

♦ how these drugs are absorbed, distributed, metabolized, and excreted

♦ drug interactions and adverse reactions to these drugs.

Selecting an antimicrobial drug

Selecting an appropriate antimicrobial drug to treat a specific infection involves several important factors:

☝ First, the microorganism must be isolated and identified—generally achieved through growing a culture.

✌ Then its susceptibility to various drugs must be determined. Because culture and sensitivity results take 48 hours, treatment usually starts at assessment and then is reevaluated when test results are obtained.

🖐 The location of the infection must be considered. For therapy to be effective, an adequate concentration of the antimicrobial must be delivered to the infection site.

🖐 Finally, the cost of the drug must be considered, as well as its potential adverse effects and the possibility of patient allergies.

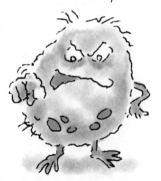

Because I'm a sensitive guy, I'm only responsive to certain drugs.

Clinical controversy

The rise of the resistance movement

Indiscriminate use of antimicrobial drugs has serious consequences. Unnecessary exposure of organisms to these drugs encourages emergence of resistant strains. These resistant strains are likely to do far more damage than their predecessors.

Make reservations
Use of antimicrobial drugs should be reserved for patients with infections caused by susceptible organisms and should be used in high enough doses and for an appropriate period of time. New antimicrobial drugs should be reserved for severely ill patients with serious infections that don't respond to conventional drugs.

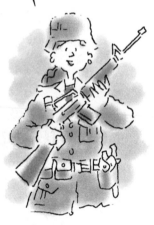

It's war out there, so choose your weapons carefully. Wise use of antimicrobials helps prevent resistance.

Preventing pathogen resistance

The usefulness of antimicrobial drugs is limited by pathogens that may develop resistance to a drug's action.

Mutants!

Resistance is the ability of a microorganism to live and grow in the presence of an antimicrobial drug that is usually bacteriostatic (inhibits the growth or multiplication of bacteria) or bactericidal (kills bacteria). Resistance usually results from genetic mutation of the microorganism. (See *The rise of the resistance movement*.)

Antibacterial drugs

Antibacterial drugs are used mainly to treat systemic (involving the whole body rather than a localized area) bacterial infections. The antibacterial classes include:
- aminoglycosides
- penicillins
- cephalosporins
- tetracyclines
- clindamycin and lincomycin
- macrolides
- vancomycin

- carbapenems
- monobactams
- fluoroquinolones
- sulfonamides
- nitrofurantoin.

Aminoglycosides

Aminoglycosides provide effective bactericidal activity against:
- aerobic gram-negative bacilli
- some aerobic gram-positive bacteria
- mycobacteria
- some protozoa.

Common aminoglycosides

Aminoglycosides currently in use include:
- amikacin sulfate
- gentamicin sulfate
- kanamycin sulfate
- neomycin sulfate
- netilmicin sulfate
- paromomycin sulfate
- streptomycin sulfate
- tobramycin sulfate.

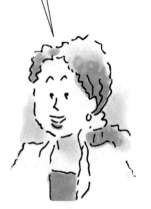

Aminoglycosides are usually given parenterally because they're poorly absorbed from the GI tract.

Pharmacokinetics (how drugs circulate)

Because aminoglycosides are absorbed poorly from the GI tract, they're usually given parenterally. After I.V. or I.M. administration, aminoglycoside absorption is rapid and complete.

Distribution

Aminoglycosides are distributed widely in extracellular fluid. They readily cross the placental barrier but don't cross the blood-brain barrier.

Metabolism and excretion

Aminoglycosides aren't metabolized. They're excreted primarily by the kidneys.

Pharmacodynamics (how drugs act)

Aminoglycosides act as bactericidal drugs (remember, this means they kill bacteria) against susceptible organisms by interrupting protein synthesis by acting on a specific ribosome in the microorganism.

Rising resistance

Bacterial resistance to an aminoglycoside may be related to:
- failure of the drug to cross the cell membrane
- altered binding to ribosomes
- destruction of the drug by bacterial enzymes.

One-two punch

Some gram-positive cocci (enterococci) resist aminoglycoside transport across the cell membrane. When penicillin is used with aminoglycoside therapy, the cell wall is altered, allowing the aminoglycoside to penetrate the bacterial cell.

Pharmacotherapeutics (how drugs are used)

Aminoglycosides are most useful in treating:
- infections caused by aerobic gram-negative bacilli
- serious nosocomial (hospital-acquired) infections, such as gram-negative bacteremia (abnormal presence of microorganisms in the bloodstream), peritonitis (inflammation of the peritoneum, the membrane that lines the abdominal cavity), and pneumonia, in critically ill patients
- urinary tract infections (UTIs) caused by enteric bacilli that are resistant to less toxic antibiotics, such as penicillins and cephalosporins
- infections of the central nervous system (CNS) and the eye (treated with local instillation).

Works well with others

Aminoglycosides are used in combination with penicillins to treat gram-positive organisms such as staphylococcal or enterococcal infections.

Inactive duty

Aminoglycosides are inactive against anaerobic bacteria.

Role call

Individual aminoglycosides may have their own particular usefulness:
• Streptomycin is active against many strains of mycobacteria, including *Mycobacterium tuberculosis*, and against gram-positive bacteria *Nocardia* and *Erysipelothrix*.
• Amikacin, gentamicin, netilmicin, and tobramycin are active against *Acinetobacter*, *Citrobacter*, *Enterobacter*, *Klebsiella*, *Proteus* (indole-positive and indole-negative), *Providencia*, *Serratia*, *Escherichia coli*, and *Pseudomonas aeruginosa*.

Drug interactions

Carbenicillin, ticarcillin, mezlocillin, and piperacillin reduce the effects of amikacin, gentamicin, kanamycin, neomycin, netilmicin, streptomycin, and tobramycin.

Putting up a blockade

Amikacin, gentamicin, kanamycin, neomycin, netilmicin, streptomycin, and tobramycin administered with neuromuscular blockers cause increased neuromuscular blockade, such as increased muscle relaxation and respiratory distress.

Kidney punch

The risk of toxicity to the kidney and neurologic system increases when aminoglycosides are given with the anesthetic methoxyflurane. When amikacin, gentamicin, kanamycin, netilmicin, or tobramycin are taken with cyclosporines, amphotericin B, or acyclovir, there is also an increased risk of kidney toxicity.

What? Say that again...

The symptoms of ototoxicity (damage to the ear) caused by aminoglycosides may be masked by antiemetic drugs. Loop diuretics taken with aminoglycosides increase the risk of ototoxicity. (See *Adverse reactions to aminoglycosides*.)

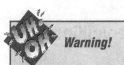

Warning!

Adverse reactions to aminoglycosides

Serious adverse reactions limit the use of aminoglycosides and include:
• neuromuscular reactions, ranging from peripheral nerve toxicity to neuromuscular blockade
• ototoxicity
• kidney toxicity.

Oral history
Adverse reactions to oral aminoglycosides include:
• nausea
• vomiting
• diarrhea.

Penicillins

Penicillins remain one of the most important and useful antibacterials, despite the availability of numerous others. The penicillins can be divided into four groups:
- natural penicillins
- penicillinase-resistant penicillins
- aminopenicillins
- extended-spectrum penicillins.

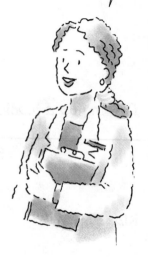

Despite the wide variety of antibacterials in use, penicillins are still among the most useful. That's because they have such a broad range of antimicrobial actions.

Pharmacokinetics

After oral administration, penicillins are absorbed mainly in the duodenum and the upper jejunum of the small intestine.

Absorb these factors

Absorption of oral penicillin varies and depends on such factors as:
- particular penicillin used
- pH of the patient's stomach and intestine
- presence of food in the GI tract.

Distribution

Penicillins are distributed widely to most areas of the body, including the lungs, liver, kidneys, muscle, bone, and placenta. High concentrations also appear in the urine, making penicillins useful in treating UTIs.

Metabolism and excretion

Penicillins are metabolized to a limited extent in the liver to inactive metabolites and are excreted 60% unchanged by the kidneys. Nafcillin also is excreted in bile.

Pharmacodynamics

Penicillins usually are bactericidal in action. They bind reversibly to several enzymes outside the bacterial cytoplasmic membrane.

Playing with PBPs

These enzymes, known as penicillin-binding proteins (PBPs), are involved in cell-wall synthesis and cell division. Interference with these processes inhibits cell-wall synthesis, causing rapid destruction of the cell.

Pharmacotherapeutics

No other class of antibacterial drugs provides as wide a spectrum of antimicrobial activity as the penicillins.

Oral option

Penicillin is given by I.M. injection when oral administration is inconvenient or a patient's compliance is questionable. Because long-acting preparations of penicillin G (penicillin G benzathine and penicillin G procaine) are relatively insoluble, they must be administered by the I.M. route.

Drug interactions

Penicillins may interact with various drugs:
• Probenecid increases the plasma concentration of penicillins.
• Penicillins reduce tubular secretion of methotrexate in the kidney, increasing the risk of methotrexate toxicity.
• Tetracyclines and chloramphenicol reduce the bactericidal action of penicillins.
• Neomycin decreases the absorption of penicillin V.
• The effectiveness of oral contraceptives is reduced when they're taken with penicillin V and ampicillin.

Acting against aminoglycosides

High dosages of penicillin G and extended-spectrum penicillins (carbenicillin, mezlocillin, piperacillin, and ticarcillin) inactivate aminoglycosides. Moreover, penicillins shouldn't be mixed in the same I.V. solutions with aminoglycosides. (See *Adverse reactions to penicillins.*)

Cephalosporins

Many antibacterial drugs introduced for clinical use in recent years have been *cephalosporins.*

Through the generations

Cephalosporins are grouped into generations according to their effectiveness against different organisms, their characteristics, and their development:
• First-generation cephalosporins include cefadroxil, cefazolin sodium, cephalexin monohydrate, and cephradine.

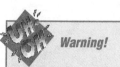

Warning!

Adverse reactions to penicillins

Hypersensitivity reactions are the major adverse reactions to penicillins and include:
• anaphylactic reactions
• serum sickness (a hypersensitivity reaction occurring 1 to 2 weeks after injection of a foreign serum)
• drug fever
• various skin rashes.

Oral penicillins
Adverse GI reactions are associated with oral penicillins and include:
• tongue inflammation
• nausea or vomiting
• diarrhea.

Aminopenicillins and extended-spectrum penicillins
The aminopenicillins and extended-spectrum penicillins can produce pseudomembranous colitis (diarrhea caused by a change in the flora of the colon or an overgrowth of a toxin-producing strain of *Clostridium difficile*).

Oxacillin
Oxacillin therapy may cause liver toxicity.

• Second-generation cephalosporins include cefaclor, cefamandole nafate, cefmetazole sodium, cefprozil, ceftibuten, cefuroxime axetil, and cefuroxime sodium.
• Third-generation cephalosporins include cefdinir, cefixime, cefoperazone sodium, cefotaxime sodium, cefpodoxime proxetil, ceftazidime, ceftizoxime sodium, and ceftriaxone sodium.
• Fourth-generation cephalosporins include cephalosporin and cefepime hydrochloride.

Kissing cousin

Loracarbef is a synthetic beta-lactam antibiotic that belongs to a new class of drugs known as the carbacephen antibiotics. Because it's similar to second-generation cephalosporins, it's included with the cephalosporins.

A sensitive issue

Because penicillins and cephalosporins are chemically similar (they both have what is called a beta-lactam molecular structure), some cross-sensitivity occurs. This means that someone who has had a reaction to penicillin is also at risk for a reaction to cephalosporins.

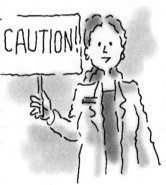

Be careful! A person who has had a reaction to penicillin may also have a reaction to cephalosporins.

Pharmacokinetics

Many cephalosporins are administered parenterally because they aren't absorbed from the GI tract; some cephalosporins are absorbed from the GI tract and can be administered orally, but food usually delays the absorption of these oral cephalosporins.

Distribution

After absorption, cephalosporins are distributed widely, although most aren't distributed in the CNS.

Generational divide

Cefuroxime (second-generation), along with the third-generation drugs cefotaxime, ceftizoxime, ceftriaxone, and ceftazidime, does cross the blood-brain barrier. Cefepime (fourth-generation) also crosses the blood-brain barrier, but it isn't known to what extent.

Metabolism

Many cephalosporins, including loracarbef, aren't metabolized at all. Cephalothin sodium, cephapirin sodium, and cefotaxime sodium are metabolized to the nonacetyl forms, which provide less antibacterial activity than the parent compounds. To a small extent, ceftriaxone is metabolized in the intestines to inactive metabolites, which are excreted via the biliary system.

Excretion

All cephalosporins are excreted primarily unchanged by the kidneys with the exception of cefoperazone and ceftriaxone, which are excreted in the feces via bile.

Pharmacodynamics

Cephalosporins inhibit cell-wall synthesis by binding to the bacterial enzymes known as PBPs, located on the cell membrane. After the drug damages the cell wall by binding with the PBPs, the body's natural defense mechanisms destroy the bacteria. (See *How cephalosporins attack bacteria*, page 198.)

Pharmacotherapeutics

The four generations of cephalosporins have particular therapeutic uses:
• First-generation cephalosporins, which act primarily against gram-positive organisms, can be used as alternative therapy in patients allergic to penicillin. They're also used to treat staphylococcal and streptococcal infections, including pneumonia, cellulitis (skin infection), and osteomyelitis (bone infection).
• Second-generation cephalosporins act against gram-negative bacteria. Cefoxitin and cefotetan are the only cephalosporins effective against anaerobes (organisms that live without oxygen).
• Third-generation cephalosporins, which act primarily against gram-negative organisms, are the drugs of choice for infections caused by *Enterobacter*, *P. aeruginosa*, and anaerobic organisms.
• Fourth-generation cephalosporins are active against a wide range of gram-positive and gram-negative bacteria.

Drug interactions

Patients receiving cefamandole, cefoperazone, or moxalactam who drink alcoholic beverages with or up to 72 hours after taking a dose may experience acute alcohol

How cephalosporins attack bacteria

The antibacterial action of cephalosporins depends on their ability to penetrate the bacterial wall and bind with proteins on the cytoplasmic membrane, as shown below.

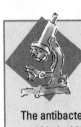

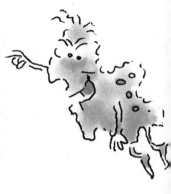

Cephalosporins penetrate and bind. That's how they wipe me out.

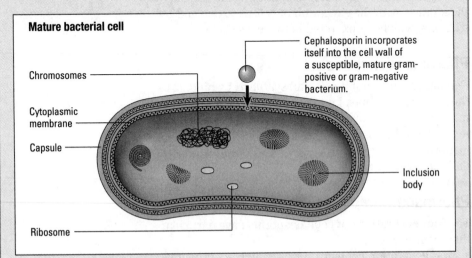

Mature bacterial cell

Chromosomes

Cytoplasmic membrane

Capsule

Ribosome

Cephalosporin incorporates itself into the cell wall of a susceptible, mature gram-positive or gram-negative bacterium.

Inclusion body

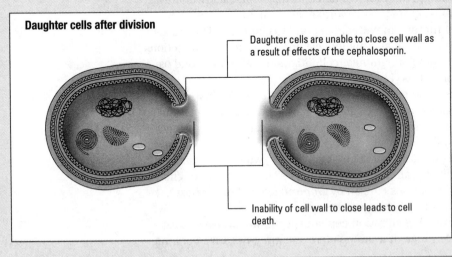

Daughter cells after division

Daughter cells are unable to close cell wall as a result of effects of the cephalosporin.

Inability of cell wall to close leads to cell death.

intolerance, with such signs and symptoms as headache, flushing, dizziness, nausea, vomiting, or abdominal cramps within 30 minutes of alcohol ingestion.

In use with uricosurics

Uricosurics (drugs to relieve gout), such as probenecid and sulfinpyrazone, can reduce kidney excretion of some cephalosporins, including loracarbef. Probenecid is used therapeutically to increase and prolong cephalosporin plasma concentrations. (See *Adverse reactions to cephalosporins.*)

Tetracyclines

Tetracyclines are broad-spectrum antibiotics. They may be classified as:
• short-acting compounds such as chlortetracycline hydrochloride
• intermediate-acting compounds such as demeclocycline hydrochloride
• long-acting compounds such as doxycycline hyclate and minocycline hydrochloride.

Pharmacokinetics

Tetracyclines are absorbed from the duodenum when taken orally.

Distribution and excretion

Tetracyclines are distributed widely into body tissues and fluids, concentrated in bile, and excreted primarily by the kidneys. Doxycycline is also excreted in the feces. Minocycline undergoes enterohepatic recirculation. The excretion of chlortetracycline is unknown.

Pharmacodynamics

All tetracyclines are primarily bacteriostatic, meaning they inhibit the growth or multiplication of bacteria. The tetracyclines penetrate the bacterial cell by an energy-dependent process. Within the cell, they bind primarily to a subunit of the ribosome, inhibiting the protein synthesis required for maintaining the bacterial cell.

Pharmacotherapeutics

Tetracyclines provide a broad spectrum of activity against:

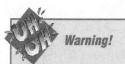
Warning!

Adverse reactions to cephalosporins

Adverse reactions to cephalosporins include:
• confusion
• seizures
• bleeding
• nausea
• vomiting
• diarrhea.

An issue of sensitivity

Hypersensitivity reactions are the most common systemic adverse reactions to cephalosporins and include:
• hives
• itching
• rash that appears like the measles
• serum sickness (reaction after injection of a foreign serum characterized by edema, fever, hives, and inflammation of the blood vessels and joints)
• anaphylaxis (in rare cases).

- gram-positive and gram-negative aerobic and anaerobic bacteria
- spirochetes
- mycoplasmas
- rickettsiae
- chlamydiae
- some protozoa.

Longer equals broader

The long-acting compounds doxycycline and minocycline provide more action against various organisms than other tetracyclines.

Taking aim

Tetracyclines are used to treat Rocky Mountain spotted fever, Q fever, and Lyme disease. They're the drugs of choice for treating nongonococcal urethritis caused by *Chlamydia* and *Ureaplasma urealyticum*. Combination therapy with a tetracycline and streptomycin is the most effective treatment for brucellosis.

Zit zapper

Tetracyclines in low dosages effectively treat acne because they can decrease the fatty acid content of sebum.

Drug interactions

Tetracyclines can reduce the effectiveness of oral contraceptives and the bactericidal action of penicillin. Other interactions often affect the ability of tetracyclines to move through the body.
- Aluminum, calcium, and magnesium antacids reduce the absorption of oral tetracyclines.
- Iron salts, bismuth subsalicylate, and zinc sulfate reduce absorption of doxycycline, oxytetracycline, and tetracycline.
- Barbiturates, carbamazepine, and phenytoin increase the metabolism and reduce the antibiotic effect of doxycycline.

Be wary of dairy

These drugs, with the exception of doxycycline and minocycline, may also interact with milk and milk products, which bind with the drugs and prevent their absorption. (See *Adverse reactions to tetracyclines*.)

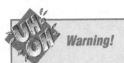

Warning!

Adverse reactions to tetracyclines

Tetracyclines produce many of the same adverse reactions as other antibacterials, such as:
- superinfection (overgrowth of resistant organisms)
- nausea
- vomiting
- abdominal distress and distention
- diarrhea.

Watch the sun

Other adverse reactions include:
- photosensitivity reactions (red rash on areas exposed to sunlight)
- liver toxicity
- kidney toxicity.

Clindamycin

Due to its high potential for serious adverse effects, *clindamycin* is another antibacterial prescribed only when there is no therapeutic alternative.

Pharmacokinetics

When taken orally, clindamycin is absorbed well and distributed widely in the body. It's metabolized by the liver and excreted by the kidney and biliary pathways.

Pharmacodynamics

Clindamycin inhibits bacterial protein synthesis. It may also inhibit the binding of bacterial ribosomes. At therapeutic concentrations, clindamycin is primarily bacteriostatic against most organisms.

Pharmacotherapeutics

Because of its potential for serious toxicity and pseudomembranous colitis (characterized by severe diarrhea, abdominal pain, fever, and mucus and blood in the stools), clindamycin is limited to a few clinical situations in which safer alternative antibacterials aren't available:
• It's potent against most aerobic gram-positive organisms, including staphylococci, streptococci (except *Enterococcus faecalis*), and pneumococci.
• It's effective against most of the clinically important anaerobes and is used primarily to treat anaerobic intra-abdominal, pleural, or pulmonary infections caused by *Bacteroides fragilis*. It's also used as an alternative to penicillin in treating *Clostridium perfringens* infections.
• It may also be used as an alternative to penicillin in treating staphylococcal infections in a patient with penicillin allergy.

Drug interactions

Clindamycin may block neuromuscular transmission and may enhance the action of neuromuscular blockers. (See *Adverse reactions to clindamycin*, page 202.)

Macrolides

Macrolides are used to treat a number of common infections. They include erythromycin derivatives, such as:
- erythromycin
- erythromycin estolate
- erythromycin ethylsuccinate
- erythromycin gluceptate
- erythromycin lactobionate
- erythromycin stearate.

These aren't derivatives

Other macrolides include:
- azithromycin
- clarithromycin.

Pharmacokinetics

Because erythromycin is acid-sensitive, it must be buffered or have enteric coating to prevent destruction by gastric acid. In the duodenum, erythromycin is absorbed. It's distributed to most tissues and body fluids (except for cerebrospinal fluid).

Metabolism and excretion

Erythromycin is metabolized by the liver and excreted in bile in high concentrations; small amounts are excreted in the urine. It also crosses the placental barrier and is secreted in breast milk.

Pharmacodynamics

Macrolides inhibit ribonucleic acid (RNA)–dependent protein synthesis by acting on a small portion of the ribosome, much like clindamycin.

Pharmacotherapeutics

Erythromycin has a range of therapeutic uses:
- It provides a broad spectrum of antimicrobial activity against gram-positive and gram-negative bacteria, including *Mycobacterium*, *Treponema*, *Mycoplasma*, and *Chlamydia*.
- It's also effective against pneumococci and group A streptococci. *Staphylococcus aureus* is sensitive to ery-

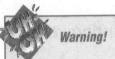

Warning!

Adverse reactions to clindamycin

Pseudomembranous colitis may occur with clindamycin. This syndrome can be fatal and requires prompt discontinuation of the drug. Although this is the most serious reaction to clindamycin and limits its use, other reactions may also occur, such as:
- diarrhea
- stomatitis (mouth inflammation)
- nausea
- vomiting
- hypersensitivity reactions.

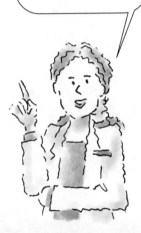

Erythromycin is acid-sensitive, so it needs to be buffered or coated to prevent contact with stomach acids.

thromycin; however, resistant strains may appear during therapy.
• Erythromycin is the drug of choice for treating *Mycoplasma pneumoniae* infections as well as pneumonia caused by *Legionella pneumophila*.

A pal to penicillin

In patients who are allergic to penicillin, erythromycin is effective for infections produced by group A beta-hemolytic streptococci or *Streptococcus pneumoniae*. It also may be used to treat gonorrhea and syphilis in patients who can't tolerate penicillin G or the tetracyclines. Erythromycin may also be used to treat minor staphylococcal infections of the skin.

Ranging wide and far...

Azithromycin provides a broad spectrum of antimicrobial activity against gram-positive and gram-negative bacteria, including *Mycobacterium*, *S. aureus*, *Haemophilus influenzae*, *Moraxella catarrhalis*, and *Chlamydia*. It's also effective against pneumococci and groups C, F, and G streptococci.

Clarithromycin is a broad-spectrum antibacterial drug that is active against gram-positive aerobes, such as *S. aureus*, *S. pneumoniae*, and *Streptococcus pyogenes*; gram-negative aerobes, such as *H. influenzae* and *M. catarrhalis*; and other aerobes such as *M. pneumoniae*.

Drug interactions

Macrolides may interact with other drugs:
• Erythromycin, azithromycin, and clarithromycin can increase theophylline levels in patients receiving high dosages of theophylline, increasing the risk of theophylline toxicity.
• Clarithromycin may increase the concentration of carbamazepine when used together. (See *Adverse reactions to macrolides*.)

Vancomycin

Vancomycin hydrochloride is used increasingly to treat methicillin-resistant *S. aureus*, which has become a major concern in the United States and other parts of the

> The macrolides are broad-spectrum antibiotics used to treat a number of common infections.

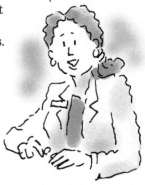

UH OH! *Warning!*

Adverse reactions to macrolides

Although erythromycin produces few adverse effects, it may produce:
• epigastric distress
• nausea
• vomiting
• diarrhea (especially with large doses)
• rashes
• fever
• eosinophilia (an increase in the number of eosinophils, a type of white blood cell)
• anaphylaxis.

world. Because of the emergence of vancomycin-resistant enterococci, vancomycin must be used judiciously.

Pharmacokinetics

Because vancomycin is absorbed poorly from the GI tract, it must be given I.V. to treat systemic infections. Vancomycin diffuses well into pleural (around the lungs), pericardial (around the heart), synovial (joint), and ascitic (in the peritoneal cavity) fluids.

Metabolism and excretion

The metabolism of vancomycin is unknown. Approximately 85% of the dose is excreted unchanged in urine within 24 hours. A small amount may be eliminated through the liver and biliary tract.

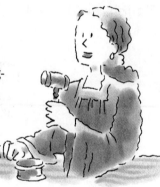

Vancomycin must be used judiciously because of the emergence of vancomycin-resistant enterococci.

Pharmacodynamics

Vancomycin inhibits bacterial cell-wall synthesis, damaging the bacterial plasma membrane. When the bacterial cell wall is damaged, the body's natural defenses can attack the organism.

Pharmacotherapeutics

Vancomycin is active against gram-positive organisms, such as *Staphylococcus aureus*, *S. epidermidis*, *S. pyogenes*, *Enterococcus*, and *S. pneumoniae*.

In the I.V. league

I.V. vancomycin is the therapy of choice for patients with serious resistant staphylococcal infections who are hypersensitive to penicillins.

Oral history

Orally administered, vancomycin is used for patients with antibiotic-associated *Clostridium difficile* colitis who are unable to take metronidazole or have responded poorly to metronidazole.

The 1 in the 1-2 punch

Vancomycin, when used with an aminoglycoside, is also the treatment of choice for *E. faecalis* endocarditis in patients who are allergic to penicillin.

Drug interactions

Vancomycin may increase the risk of toxicity when administered with other drugs toxic to the kidneys and organs of hearing, such as aminoglycosides, amphotericin B, cisplatin, bacitracin, colistin, and polymyxin B. (See *Adverse reactions to vancomycin.*)

Carbapenems

Carbapenems are a class of beta-lactam antibacterials that includes:
- imipenem-cilastatin sodium (a combined drug)
- meropenem.

The Broadway of antibacterials

The antibacterial spectrum of activity for imipenem-cilastatin is broader than that of any other antibacterial studied to date.

Pharmacokinetics

The pharmacokinetic properties of carbapenems slightly vary.

Distribution, metabolism, and excretion

Imipenem must be given with cilastatin because imipenem alone is rapidly metabolized in the tubules of the kidneys, rendering it ineffective. After parenteral administration, imipenem-cilastatin is distributed widely. It's metabolized by several mechanisms and excreted primarily in the urine.

Mostly unchanged

After parenteral administration meropenem is distributed widely, including to the CNS. Metabolism is insignificant. 70% of the drug is excreted unchanged in the urine.

Pharmacodynamics

Imipenem and meropenem usually are bactericidal. They exert antibacterial activity by inhibiting bacterial cell-wall synthesis.

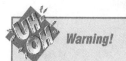

Warning!

Adverse reactions to vancomycin

Adverse reactions to vancomycin, although rare, include:
- hypersensitivity and anaphylactic reactions
- drug fever
- eosinophilia (an increased number of eosinophils, a type of white blood cell [WBC])
- neutropenia (reduced number of neutrophils, another type of WBC).

Rash behavior
Severe hypotension may occur with rapid I.V. administration of vancomycin and may be accompanied by a red rash with flat and raised lesions on the face, neck, chest, and arms.

Pharmacotherapeutics

Imipenem has the broadest spectrum of activity of currently available beta-lactam antibiotics:
• It's effective against aerobic gram-positive species, such as *Streptococcus*, *S. aureus*, and *S. epidermidis*.
• Most *Enterobacter* species are inhibited by imipenem.
• It also inhibits *P. aeruginosa* (including strains resistant to piperacillin and ceftazidime) and most anaerobic species, including *B. fragilis*.

Lone ranger

It also may be used alone for mixed aerobic and anaerobic infections, as therapy for serious nosocomial (hospital-acquired) infections or infections in immunocompromised hosts.

Don't forget the other carbapenem

Meropenem is indicated in the treatment of intra-abdominal infections as well as for management of bacterial meningitis caused by susceptible organisms.

Drug interactions

Carbapenems may interact with other drugs:
• Taking probenecid with imipenem-cilastatin or meropenem increases the serum concentration of cilastatin, but only slightly increases the serum concentration of imipenem.
• Probenecid may cause meropenem to accumulate to toxic levels.
• The combination of imipenem-cilastatin and an aminoglycoside acts synergistically against *E. faecalis*. (See *Adverse reactions to carbapenems*.)

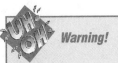

Monobactams

Aztreonam is the first member in the class of *monobactam antibiotics*. It's a synthetic monobactam with a narrow spectrum of activity that includes many gram-negative aerobic bacteria.

Pharmacokinetics

After parenteral administration, aztreonam is rapidly and completely absorbed and distributed widely. It's metabolized partially and excreted primarily in the urine as unchanged drug.

Pharmacodynamics

Aztreonam's bactericidal activity results from inhibition of bacterial cell-wall synthesis. It preferentially binds to the PBP-3 of susceptible gram-negative bacteria. As a result, division of the cell wall is inhibited and lysis occurs.

Pharmacotherapeutics

Aztreonam is indicated in a range of therapeutic situations:
• It's effective against a wide variety of gram-negative aerobic organisms, including *P. aeruginosa*.
• It's effective against most strains of the following organisms: *E. coli, Enterobacter, Klebsiella pneumoniae, K. oxytoca, Proteus mirabilis, Serratia marcescens, H. influenzae,* and *Citrobacter.*
• It's also used to treat complicated and uncomplicated UTIs, septicemia, and lower respiratory tract, skin and skin-structure, intra-abdominal, and gynecologic infections caused by susceptible gram-negative aerobic bacteria.
• It's usually active against gram-negative aerobic organisms that are resistant to antibiotics hydrolyzed by beta-lactamases. (Beta-lactamase is an enzyme that makes an antibiotic ineffective.)

It can need help

Aztreonam shouldn't be used alone as empiric therapy in seriously ill patients if the infection may be caused by gram-positive bacteria or if a mixed aerobic-anaerobic bacterial infection is suspected.

Drug interactions

Aztreonam may interact with several other drugs:
• Probenecid increases serum levels of aztreonam by prolonging the tubular secretion rate of aztreonam in the kidneys.
• Synergistic or additive effects occur when aztreonam is used with aminoglycosides or other antibiotics, such as cefoperazone, cefotaxime, clindamycin, and piperacillin.

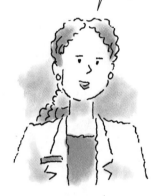

Aztreonam inhibits bacterial cell-wall synthesis, preventing cell-wall division.

• Potent inducers of beta-lactamase production (cefoxitin, imipenem) may inactivate aztreonam.
• Taking aztreonam with clavulanic acid may produce synergistic or antagonistic effects, depending on the organism involved. (See *Adverse reactions to aztreonam*.)

Fluoroquinolones

Fluoroquinolones are structurally similar synthetic antibiotics. They are primarily administered to treat UTIs as well as upper respiratory infections, pneumonia, and gonorrhea and include:
• alatrofloxacin mesylate
• ciprofloxacin
• enoxacin
• gatifloxacin
• levofloxacin
• lomefloxacin
• moxifloxacin
• norfloxacin
• sparfloxacin
• trovafloxacin.

Pharmacokinetics

After oral administration, fluoroquinolones are absorbed well.

Metabolism and excretion

Fluoroquinolones aren't highly protein-bound, are minimally metabolized in the liver, and are excreted primarily in the urine. Sparfloxacin is excreted equally in the urine and feces; trovafloxacin is primarily eliminated in feces.

Pharmacodynamics

Fluoroquinolones work by interrupting deoxyribonucleic acid (DNA) synthesis during bacterial replication. As a result, the bacteria are prevented from replicating.

Pharmacotherapeutics

Fluoroquinolones can be used to treat a wide variety of UTIs. Each drug in this class also has specific indications:

Warning!

Adverse reactions to aztreonam

• Diarrhea
• Hypersensitivity and skin reactions
• Hypotension
• Nausea and vomiting
• Transient electrocardiogram changes (including ventricular arrhythmias)
• Transient increases in serum liver enzymes.

Fluoroquinolones are commonly used to treat UTIs.

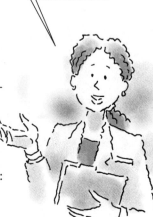

- Ciprofloxacin is used to treat lower respiratory tract infections, infectious diarrhea, and skin, bone, or joint infections.
- Trovafloxacin mesylate and its I.V. form alatrofloxacin mesylate are used to treat community and hospital-acquired pneumonia, sinusitis, gonorrhea, and complicated diabetic foot ulcers.
- Sparfloxacin is used to treat bronchitis and community-acquired pneumonia.
- Lomefloxacin also is used to treat lower respiratory tract infections and to prevent UTIs in patients who are undergoing procedures through the urethra (the tube from the bladder to the outside of the body).
- Ofloxacin also is used to treat selected sexually transmitted diseases, lower respiratory infections, skin and skin-structure infections, and prostatitis (inflammation of the prostate gland).
- Levofloxacin is also indicated for treatment of lower respiratory infections.

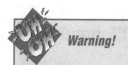

Warning!

Adverse reactions to fluoroquinolones

Well tolerated by most patients, fluoroquino-lones produce few adverse reactions, but may produce:
- nausea
- vomiting
- diarrhea
- abdominal pain.

Drug interactions

Several drug interactions may occur with the fluoro-quinolones:
- Administration with antacids that contain magnesium or aluminum hydroxide results in decreased absorption of the fluoroquinolone.
- With the exception of lomefloxacin and levofloxacin, the fluoroquinolones also interact with xanthine derivatives, such as aminophylline or theophylline, increasing the plasma theophylline concentration and the risk of theophylline toxicity.
- Giving ciprofloxacin, norfloxacin, or lomefloxacin with probenecid results in decreased kidney elimination of these fluoroquinolones, increasing their serum concentrations and half-lives.
- Enoxacin increases the anticoagulant effect or oral anticoagulants.
- Enoxacin may increase serum digoxin and cyclosporine levels in some patients.
- Drugs that prolong the QT interval are contraindicated during sparfloxacin therapy. (See *Adverse reactions to fluoroquinolones*.)

Sulfonamides

Sulfonamides were the first effective systemic antibacterial drugs and include:
- co-trimoxazole
- sulfadiazine
- sulfamethoxazole
- sulfisoxazole.

Pharmacokinetics

Most sulfonamides are absorbed well and distributed widely in the body. They're metabolized in the liver to inactive metabolites and excreted by the kidneys.

Pharmacodynamics

Sulfonamides are bacteriostatic drugs that prevent the growth of microorganisms by inhibiting folic acid production. The decreased folic acid synthesis decreases the number of bacterial nucleotides and inhibits bacterial growth.

Pharmacotherapeutics

Sulfonamides are frequently used to treat acute UTIs. With recurrent or chronic UTIs, the infecting organism may not be susceptible to sulfonamides. Therefore, the choice of therapy should be based on bacteria susceptibility tests.

Infectious behavior

Sulfonamides also are used to treat infections caused by *Nocardia asteroides, Toxoplasma gondii,* and *Pneumocystis carinii.* Sulfonamides exhibit a wide spectrum of activity against gram-positive and gram-negative bacteria.

Drug interactions

Sulfonamides have few significant interactions:
- They increase the hypoglycemic affects of the sulfonylureas (oral antidiabetic drugs), increasing the tendency for low blood glucose levels.
- When taken with methenamine they may lead to the development of crystals in the urine.

• Co-trimoxazole may increase the anticoagulant effect of coumarin anticoagulants.
• Co-trimoxazole plus cyclosporine increases the risk kidney toxicity. (See *Adverse reactions to sulfonamides*.)

Nitrofurantoin

Nitrofurantoin is used primarily to treat acute and chronic UTIs.

Pharmacokinetics

After oral administration, nitrofurantoin is absorbed rapidly and well from the GI tract. Taking the drug with food enhances the bioavailability of nitrofurantoin.

Distribution

The drug is 20% to 60% protein-bound. Nitrofurantoin crosses the placental barrier and is secreted in breast milk. It's also distributed in bile.

Metabolism and excretion

Nitrofurantoin is partially metabolized by the liver, and 30% to 50% is excreted unchanged in the urine.

Pharmacodynamics

Usually bacteriostatic, nitrofurantoin may become bactericidal, depending on its urinary concentration and the susceptibility of the infecting organisms.

Reduces power?

Although the exact mechanism of action is unknown, the drug appears to inhibit formation of acetyl coenzyme A from pyruvic acid, thereby inhibiting the energy production of the infecting organism. Nitrofurantoin also may disrupt bacterial cell-wall formation.

Pharmacotherapeutics

Because the absorbed drug concentrates in the urine, nitrofurantoin is used to treat UTIs. It has a higher antibacterial activity in acid urine. Nitrofurantoin isn't effective against systemic bacterial infections.

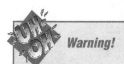

Warning!

Adverse reactions to sulfonamides

Excessively high doses of less water-soluble sulfonamides can produce crystals in the urine and deposits of sulfonamide crystals in the renal tubules. This complication isn't a problem with the newer water-soluble sulfonamides. Hypersensitivity reactions may occur and appear to increase as the dosage increases.

Is it serum sickness?
A reaction that resembles serum sickness may occur, producing fever, joint pain, hives, bronchospasm, and leukopenia (reduced white blood cell count).

Photo finish
Sulfonamides also can produce photosensitivity.

Drug interactions

Nitrofurantoin has few significant interactions:
• Probenecid and sulfinpyrazone inhibit the excretion of nitrofurantoin by the kidneys, reducing its efficacy and increasing its toxic potential.
• Antacids can decrease the extent and rate of nitrofurantoin absorption.
• Nitrofurantoin may decrease the antibacterial activity of norfloxacin and nalidixic acid. (See *Adverse reactions to nitrofurantoin*.)

Antiviral drugs

Antiviral drugs are used to prevent or treat viral infections. Major antiviral drugs used to treat systemic infections include:
• acyclovir
• ganciclovir
• famciclovir
• foscarnet
• amantadine hydrochloride
• nelfinavir
• zidovudine
• didanosine
• zalcitabine.

Antiherpesvirus drugs

Acyclovir sodium, an *antiherpesvirus drug,* is an effective antiviral drug that causes minimal toxicity to cells. A derivative of acyclovir, ganciclovir has potent antiviral activity against herpes simplex virus (HSV) and cytomegalovirus (CMV).

A prodrug drug

Famciclovir is a prodrug (a precursor of a drug) that undergoes rapid change to the active antiviral compound penciclovir. It enters viral cells (HSV types 1 and 2 and varicella zoster), where it inhibits viral replication.

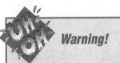

Warning!

Adverse reactions to nitrofurantoin

Adverse reactions to nitrofurantoin include:
• GI irritation
• anorexia
• nausea
• vomiting
• diarrhea
• dark yellow or brown urine
• abdominal pain
• chills
• fever
• joint pain
• anaphylaxis
• hypersensitivity reactions involving the skin, lungs, blood, and liver.

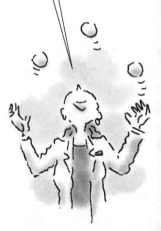

Antiviral drugs keep viruses from multiplying.

Pharmacokinetics

Each of these antiherpesvirus drugs travels its own route through the body.

Slow by mouth

When given orally, absorption of acyclovir is slow and only 15% to 30% complete. It's distributed throughout the body and metabolized primarily inside the infected cells; the majority of the drug is excreted in the urine.

I.V. only

Ganciclovir is administered I.V. because it's absorbed poorly from the GI tract. More than 90% of ganciclovir isn't metabolized and is excreted unchanged by the kidneys.

Bound? Not much

Famciclovir is less than 20% bound to plasma proteins. It's extensively metabolized in the liver and excreted in urine.

Pharmacodynamics

To be effective, acyclovir and ganciclovir must be metabolized to their active form in cells infected by the herpesvirus.

Presto-chango

Acyclovir enters virus-infected cells, where it's changed through a series of steps to acyclovir triphosphate. Acyclovir triphosphate inhibits virus-specific DNA polymerase, an enzyme necessary for viral growth, and disrupts viral replication.

On entry into CMV-infected cells, ganciclovir is converted to ganciclovir triphosphate, which is thought to produce its antiviral activity by inhibiting viral DNA synthesis.

Pharmacotherapeutics

Acyclovir is used to treat infection caused by herpes viruses, including HSV types 1 and 2 and the varicella-zoster virus. Oral acyclovir is used primarily to treat initial and recurrent HSV type 2 infections.

In the I.V. league

I.V. acyclovir is used to treat:
• severe initial HSV type 2 infections in patients with normal immune systems
• initial and recurrent skin and mucus membrane HSV type 1 and 2 infections in immunocompromised patients
• herpes zoster infections (shingles) caused by the varicella-zoster virus in immunocompromised patients
• disseminated varicella-zoster virus in immunocompromised patients
• varicella infections (chickenpox) caused by varicella-zoster virus in immunocompromised patients.

RSVP for CMV

Ganciclovir is used to treat CMV retinitis in immunocompromised patients, including those with acquired immunodeficiency syndrome (AIDS) and other CMV infections such as encephalitis.

If it keeps coming back

Famciclovir is used to treat acute herpes zoster and recurrent genital herpes.

Drug interactions

These herpesvirus drugs may interact with other drugs:
• Probenecid reduces kidney excretion and increases blood levels of ganciclovir, famciclovir, and acyclovir, increasing the risk of toxicity.
• The risk of kidney damage increases when drugs that are toxic to the kidneys are taken with acyclovir.
• Taking ganciclovir with drugs that are damaging to tissue cells, such as dapsone, pentamidine isethionate, flucytosine, vincristine, vinblastine, doxorubicin, amphotericin B, and trimethoprim-sulfa combinations, inhibits replication of rapidly dividing cells in the bone marrow, GI tract, skin, and sperm-producing cells.
• Imipenem-cilastatin increases the risk of seizures when taken with ganciclovir.
• Zidovudine increases the risk of granulocytopenia (reduced number of granulocytes, a type of white blood cell) when taken with ganciclovir. (See *Adverse reactions to antiherpesvirus drugs.*)

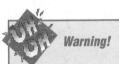

Warning!

Adverse reactions to antiherpesvirus drugs

Treatment with each of these antiherpesvirus drugs may lead to particular adverse reactions.

Acyclovir
Reversible kidney impairment may occur with rapid I.V. injection or infusion of acyclovir.

Oral history
Common reactions to oral acyclovir include headache, nausea, vomiting, and diarrhea.

Issues of sensitivity
Hypersensitivity reactions may occur with acyclovir.

Ganciclovir
The most common adverse reactions to ganciclovir are granulocytopenia and thrombocytopenia.

Famciclovir
Common adverse reactions to famciclovir include headache and nausea.

Foscarnet

The antiviral drug *foscarnet* is used to treat CMV retinitis in patients with AIDS. It's also used to treat acyclovir-resistant HSV infections in immunocompromised patients.

Pharmacokinetics

Foscarnet is poorly bound to plasma proteins. In patients with normal renal function, the majority of foscarnet is excreted unchanged in the urine.

Pharmacodynamics

Foscarnet prevents viral replication by selectively inhibiting DNA polymerases (an enzyme that helps form DNA from a precursor substance that exists in DNA).

Pharmacotherapeutics

Foscarnet's primary therapeutic use is in the treatment of CMV retinitis in patients with AIDS.

Drug interactions

Foscarnet is known to have few drug interactions:
• Foscarnet and pentamidine together increase the risk of hypocalcemia (low blood calcium levels) and toxicity to the kidneys.
• Use of foscarnet and other drugs that alter serum calcium levels may result in hypocalcemia.
• The risk of kidney impairment increases when drugs toxic to the kidneys, such as amphotericin B and aminoglycosides, are taken with foscarnet. (See *Adverse reactions to foscarnet.*)

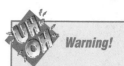

Warning!

Adverse reactions to foscarnet

Adverse reactions to foscarnet may include:
• fatigue, depression, fever, confusion, headache, numbness and tingling, dizziness, and seizures
• nausea and vomiting, diarrhea, and abdominal pain
• granulocytopenia and leukopenia
• involuntary muscle contractions, neuropathy
• difficult breathing
• rash
• altered kidney function.

Amantadine and rimantadine hydrochloride

Amantadine and its derivative *rimantadine hydrochloride* are used to prevent or treat influenza A infections.

Pharmacokinetics

After oral administration, amantadine and rimantadine are absorbed well in the GI tract and distributed widely throughout the body.

Metabolism and excretion

Amantadine is eliminated primarily in the urine; rimantadine is extensively metabolized and then excreted in urine.

Pharmacodynamics

Although the exact mechanism of action of amantadine is unknown, the drug appears to inhibit an early stage of viral replication. Rimantadine inhibits viral RNA and protein synthesis.

Pharmacotherapeutics

Amantadine and rimantadine are used to prevent and treat respiratory tract infections caused by strains of the influenza A virus. They can reduce the severity and duration of fever and other symptoms in patients already infected with influenza A.

In the meantime

They also protect patients undergoing immunization during the 2 weeks needed for immunity to develop or patients who can't take the influenza vaccine because of hypersensitivity.

Calming the shakes

Amantadine is also used to treat parkinsonism and drug-induced extrapyramidal reactions (abnormal involuntary movements).

Drug interactions

Amantadine may interact with other drugs:
• Taking anticholinergics with amantadine increases adverse anticholinergic effects.
• Amantadine given with hydrochlorothiazide-triamterene results in decreased urine excretion of amantadine, resulting in increased amantadine levels.
• Amantadine and trimethoprim levels are increased when used together.

All quiet on the rimantadine front

No drug interactions have been documented with rimantadine. (See *Adverse reactions to amantadine and rimantadine.*)

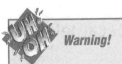

Warning!

Adverse reactions to amantadine and rimantadine

Amantadine
• Anorexia
• Anxiety
• Confusion
• Depression
• Fatigue
• Forgetfulness
• Hallucinations
• Hypersensitivity reactions
• Insomnia
• Irritability
• Nausea
• Nervousness
• Pyschosis

Rimantadine
Adverse reactions to rimantadine are similar to those for amantadine. However, they tend to be less severe.

Ribavirin

Breathe in

Ribavirin currently is available only to treat respiratory syncytial virus (RSV) infections in children.

It's administered by aerosol inhalation only, using a small-particle aerosol generator such as the Viratek Model 2.

Pharmacokinetics

Ribavirin is administered by nasal or oral inhalation and is absorbed well. It has a limited, specific distribution, with the highest concentration level found in the respiratory tract and in red blood cells (RBCs).

Metabolism and excretion

Ribavirin is metabolized in the liver and by RBCs. It's excreted primarily by the kidneys, with some excreted in the feces.

Pharmacodynamics

The mechanism of action of ribavirin isn't known completely, but the drug's metabolites inhibit viral DNA and RNA synthesis, subsequently halting viral replication.

Pharmacotherapeutics

Ribavirin therapy is used to treat severe lower respiratory tract infections caused by RSV in infants and young children.

Drug interactions

Ribavirin has few interactions with other drugs:
• Ribavirin reduces the antiviral activity of zidovudine and concomitant use of these drugs may cause blood toxicity.
• Taking ribavirin and digoxin can cause digoxin toxicity, producing such effects as GI distress, CNS abnormalities, and cardiac arrhythmias. (See *Adverse reactions to ribavirin.*)

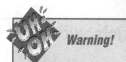

Warning!

Adverse reactions to ribavirin

• Apnea (lack of breathing)
• Cardiac arrest
• Hypotension
• Pneumothorax (air in the pleural space, causing the lung to collapse)
• Worsening of respiratory function

Nucleoside reverse transcriptase inhibitors

Didanosine, abacavir, and zalcitabine are *nucleoside reverse transcriptase inhibitors (NRTIs)* used in the treatment of advanced human immunodeficiency virus (HIV) infections.

First in the fight against AIDS

Zidovudine, another NRTI, was the first drug to receive Food and Drug Administration approval for treating AIDS or AIDS-related complex.

Pharmacokinetics

Each of the NRTIs has its own pharmacokinetic properties.

Absorbed well, distributed widely

Zidovudine is absorbed well from the GI tract, distributed widely throughout the body, metabolized by the liver, and excreted by the kidneys.

Buffer needed

Because didanosine is degraded rapidly in gastric acid, didanosine tablets and powder contain a buffering drug to increase pH. The exact route of metabolism isn't fully understood. Approximately half of an absorbed dose is excreted in the urine.

Food reduces

Oral zalcitabine is absorbed well from the GI tract when administered on an empty stomach. Absorption is reduced when the drug is given with food. Zalcitabine penetrates the blood-brain barrier.

Into space

Abacavir is rapidly and extensively absorbed after oral administration. It's distributed in the extravascular space, and about 50% binds with plasma proteins. Abacavir is metabolized by the enzymes and primarily excreted in the urine with the remainder excreted in feces.

Pharmacodynamics

NRTIs must undergo conversion to their active metabolites to produce their action:

Although there is no cure for AIDS, antiretroviral drugs such as zidovudine, didanosine, and zalcitabine temporarily inactivate the human immunodeficiency virus.

- Zidovudine is converted by cellular enzymes to an active form, zidovudine triphosphate, which prevents viral DNA from replicating. (See *How zidovudine works*, page 220.)
- Didanosine and zalcitabine undergo cellular enzyme conversion to their active antiviral metabolites to block HIV replication.
- Abacavir is converted to an active metabolite that inhibits the activity of HIV-1 transcriptase by competing with a natural component and incorporating into viral DNA.

Pharmacotherapeutics

NRTIs are used in the treatment of HIV and AIDS.

In hospital

I.V. zidovudine is used to help patients who are hospitalized and unable to take oral medication. It's also used to prevent transmission of HIV from mother to fetus and to treat AIDS-related dementia.

Oral zidovudine is used as part of a multidrug regimen for treating HIV infection.

Getting a jump on HIV

Didanosine is an alternative initial treatment of HIV infection.

Part of the combo

Zalcitabine and abacavir are used in combination with other antiretroviral agents to treat HIV infection.

Drug interactions

NRTIs may be responsible for a number of drug interactions:

- An increased risk of cellular and kidney toxicity occurs when zidovudine is taken with such drugs as dapsone, pentamidine isethionate, flucytosine, vincristine, vinblastine, doxorubicin, interferon, and ganciclovir.
- Taking zidovudine with probenecid, aspirin, acetaminophen, indomethacin, cimetidine, and lorazepam increases the risk of toxicity of either drug.
- Zidovudine plus acyclovir may produce profound lethargy and drowsiness.

Zoom in

How zidovudine works

Zidovudine can inhibit replication of human immunodeficiency virus (HIV). The first two illustrations show how HIV invades cells and then replicates itself. The bottom illustration shows how zidovudine blocks viral transformation.

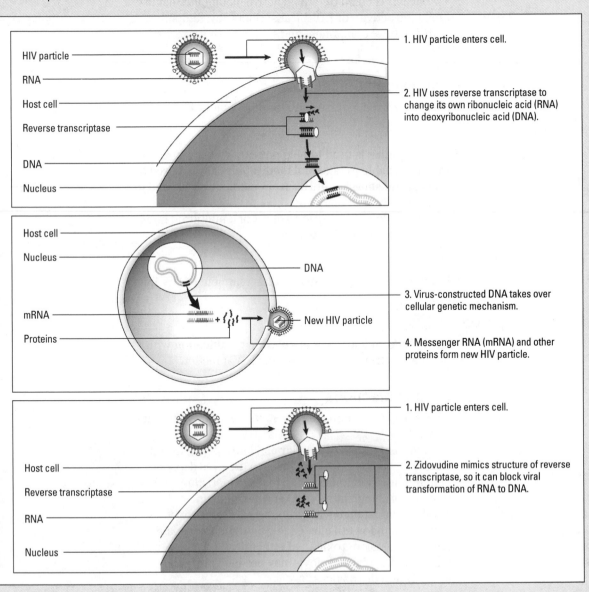

HIV particle

RNA

Host cell

Reverse transcriptase

DNA

Nucleus

1. HIV particle enters cell.

2. HIV uses reverse transcriptase to change its own ribonucleic acid (RNA) into deoxyribonucleic acid (DNA).

Host cell

Nucleus

DNA

mRNA

Proteins

New HIV particle

3. Virus-constructed DNA takes over cellular genetic mechanism.

4. Messenger RNA (mRNA) and other proteins form new HIV particle.

1. HIV particle enters cell.

Host cell

Reverse transcriptase

RNA

Nucleus

2. Zidovudine mimics structure of reverse transcriptase, so it can block viral transformation of RNA to DNA.

• Didanosine may reduce the absorption of tetracyclines, delavirdine, and fluoroquinolones.
• There is an increased risk of peripheral neuropathy (nerve degeneration or inflammation) when zalcitabine is taken with didanosine, cimetidine, chloramphenicol, cisplatin, ethionamide, gold salts, hydralazine, iodoquinol, isoniazid, metronidazole, nitrofurantoin, or vincristine.
• Zalcitabine plus pentamidine isethionate increases the risk of pancreatitis.
• Absorption of zalcitabine is reduced when taken with magnesium or aluminum antacids.
• Abacavir levels increase with alcohol consumption.
(See *Adverse reactions to NRTIs*.)

Protease inhibitors

Protease inhibitors are drugs that act against an enzyme, HIV protease, preventing the enzyme from dividing a larger viral precursor protein into the active smaller enzymes the virus needs to fully mature. The result is an immature, noninfectious cell. Drugs in this group include:
• saquinavir and saquinavir mesylate
• nelfinavir mesylate
• ritonavir
• indinavir sulfate.

Pharmacokinetics

Protease inhibitors may have different pharmacokinetic properties.

Highly bound

Saquinavir and saquinavir mesylate are poorly absorbed from the GI tract. They're widely distributed, highly bound to plasma proteins, metabolized by the liver, and excreted mainly by the kidneys.

Broken into five...

Ritonavir is well absorbed, metabolized by the liver, and broken down into at least five metabolites. It's mainly excreted in the feces, with some elimination through the kidneys.

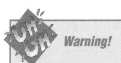

...and seven

Indinavir sulfate is rapidly absorbed and moderately bound to plasma proteins. It's metabolized by the liver into seven metabolites. The drug is excreted mainly through feces.

Availability unknown

Nelfinavir's bioavailability (the degree to which it becomes available to target tissue after administration) isn't determined. Food increases its absorption. It's highly protein bound, metabolized in the liver, and excreted primarily in the feces.

Pharmacodynamics

All of these drugs inhibit the activity of HIV protease and prevent the cleavage of viral polyproteins.

Pharmacotherapeutics

Protease inhibitors are indicated for use in combination with other for treatment of HIV infection.

Drug interactions

Protease inhibitors may interact with many drugs. Here are some common interactions:
• The action of saquinavir may be reduced by phenobarbital, phenytoin, dexamethasone, and carbamazepine.
• Ritonavir may increase the effects of alpha blockers, antiarrhythmics, antidepressants, antiemetics, antifungals, antilipemics, antimalarials, antineoplastics, beta blockers, calcium channel blockers, cimetidine, corticosteroids, erythromycin, immunosuppressants, methylphenidate, pentoxifylline, phenothiazines, and warfarin.
• Indinavir sulfate inhibits metabolism of cisapride, midazolam, and triazolam, increasing the risk of potentially fatal events such as cardiac arrhythmias.
• Buffering drugs in didanosine decrease gastric absorption of indinavir sulfate; they should be administered at least 1 hour apart.
• Rifampin markedly reduces plasma concentrations of indinavir sulfate.
• Nelfinavir may greatly increase plasma levels of amiodarone, ergot derivatives, midazolam, rifabutin, quinidine, and triazolam.

- Carbamazepine, phenobarbital, and phenytoin may reduce the effectiveness of nelfinavir.
- Indinavir and ritonavir may increase nelfinavir plasma levels. (See *Adverse reactions to protease inhibitors.*)

Antitubercular drugs

Antitubercular drugs are used to treat tuberculosis, which is caused by *Mycobacterium tuberculosis.* Not always curative, these drugs can halt the progression of a mycobacterial infection.

Myco-versatility

These drugs also are effective against less common mycobacterial infections caused by *M. kansasii, M. avium-intracellulare, M. fortuitum,* and related organisms.

Time consuming

Unlike most antibiotics, antitubercular drugs may need to be administered over many months. This creates problems, such as patient noncompliance, the development of bacterial resistance, and drug toxicity. (See *Directly observable therapy for TB*, page 224.)

Drug regimens for treating TB

Traditionally, isoniazid, rifampin, and ethambutol were the mainstays of multidrug tuberculosis (TB) therapy and successfully prevented the emergence of drug resistance.

A new regimen to combat resistance

Because of the current incidence of drug-resistant TB strains, however, a four-drug regimen is now recommended for initial treatment:

 isoniazid

 rifampin

 pyrazinamide

 streptomycin or ethambutol.

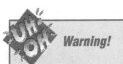

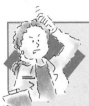

Directly observable therapy for TB

Among infectious diseases, tuberculosis (TB) remains a frequent killer worldwide. What makes treatment difficult is that it requires long-term medical therapy—often for as long as 6 to 9 months. The long length of treatment often creates problems with patient compliance, and poor compliance contributes to reactivation of the disease and the development of drug-resistant TB.

DOT on the spot

Directly observable therapy (DOT) was developed to combat these treatment issues. DOT requires that a health care worker observe a patient take every dose of medication for the duration of therapy. A controversy exists over whether every individual with TB should be observed, called universal DOT, or whether only those at risk for poor compliance should be observed; this is called selective DOT.

Who fails to comply?

Patients at risk for poor compliance include those with a previous history of poor compliance, an inability or unwillingness to follow a treatment plan, and a recent history of drug or alcohol abuse, mental illness, homelessness, incarceration, or residence in a homeless shelter. Some areas, such as Mississippi and New York City, practice universal DOT; other areas, including Massachusetts, first evaluate a patient's ability and willingness to comply.

One regimen may succeed another

Antitubercular drugs should be modified if local testing shows resistance to one or more of them. If local outbreaks of TB resistant to isoniazid and rifampin are occurring in institutions (for example, health care or correctional facilities), then five-drug or six-drug regimens are recommended as initial therapy. (See *Other antitubercular drugs.*)

Pharmacokinetics

Most antitubercular drugs are administered orally. When administered orally, these drugs are absorbed well from the GI tract and distributed widely throughout the body. They're metabolized primarily in the liver and excreted by the kidneys.

Pharmacodynamics

Antitubercular drugs are specific for mycobacteria. At usual doses, ethambutol and isoniazid are tuberculostatic, meaning they inhibit the growth of *M. tuberculosis.* In contrast, rifampin is tuberculocidal and destroys the mycobacteria. Because bacterial resistance to isoniazid and rifampin can develop rapidly, they should always be used with other antitubercular drugs.

Antireplication station

The exact mechanism of ethambutol remains unclear, but it may be related to inhibition of cell metabolism, arrest of multiplication, and cell death. Ethambutol acts only against replicating bacteria.

Breaking down walls

Although isoniazid's exact mechanism of action isn't known, it's believed that the drug inhibits the synthesis of mycolic acids, important components of the mycobacterium cell wall. This inhibition disrupts the cell wall. Only replicating, not resting, bacteria appear to be inhibited.

Synthesis stopper

Rifampin inhibits RNA synthesis in susceptible organisms. The drug is effective primarily in replicating bacteria but may have some effect on resting bacteria as well.

Acid based

The exact mechanism of action of pyrazinamide isn't known, but the antimycobacterial activity appears to be linked to the drug's conversion to the active metabolite pyrazinoic acid. Pyrazinoic acid, in turn, creates an acidic environment.

> Bring it on! And bring friends, because sometimes it can take as many as five or six drugs to wipe me out!

Other antitubercular drugs

Several other drugs are used as antitubercular drugs in combination with first-line drugs. Because these drugs have a greater incidence of toxicity, they're used primarily when resistance or allergies to less toxic drugs exist.

Fluoroquinolones

Fluoroquinolones, such as ciprofloxacin and ofloxacin, are effective against *M. tuberculosis*. Of these two drugs, ofloxacin is more potent and may be an initial choice in retreatment. These drugs are administered orally and are generally well tolerated. GI adverse reactions are most commonly reported. However, resistance to fluoroquinolones develops rapidly when these drugs are used alone or in insufficient doses.

Streptomycin

Streptomycin was the first drug recognized as effective in treating TB. Streptomycin is administered I.M. only. It appears to enhance the activity of oral antitubercular drugs and is of greatest value in the early weeks to months of therapy. However, I.M. administration limits its usefulness in long-term therapy. Rapidly absorbed from the I.M. injection site, streptomycin is excreted primarily by the kidneys as unchanged drug. Most patients tolerate streptomycin well, but those receiving large doses may exhibit eighth cranial nerve toxicity (ototoxicity).

Pharmacotherapeutics

Isoniazid usually is used with ethambutol, rifampin, or streptomycin. This is because combination therapy for TB and other mycobacterial infections can prevent or delay the development of resistance.

In uncomplicated cases

Ethambutol is used with isoniazid and rifampin to treat patients with uncomplicated pulmonary TB. The drug also is used to treat infections resulting from *M. bovis* and most strains of *M. kansasii*.

Isolating isoniazid

Although isoniazid is the most important drug for treating TB, bacterial resistance develops rapidly if it's used alone. However, resistance doesn't pose a problem when isoniazid is used alone to prevent TB in individuals who have been exposed to the disease, and no evidence exists of cross-resistance between isoniazid and other antitubercular drugs. Isoniazid is typically given orally, but may be given I.V., if necessary.

Pulmonary power

Rifampin is a first-line drug for treating pulmonary TB with other antitubercular drugs. It combats many gram-positive and some gram-negative bacteria, but is seldom used for nonmycobacterial infections because bacterial resistance develops rapidly. It's used to treat asymptomatic carriers of *Neisseria meningitidis* when the risk of meningitis is high, but it isn't used to treat *N. meningitidis* infections because of the potential for bacterial resistance.

On the TB front

Pyrazinamide is currently recommended as a first-line TB drug in combination with ethambutol, rifampin, and isoniazid. Pyrazinamide is a highly specific drug that is active only against *M. tuberculosis*. Resistance to pyrazinamide may develop rapidly when pyrazinamide is used alone.

Drug interactions

Antitubercular drugs may interact with a number of other drugs:

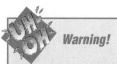

Warning!

Adverse reactions to antitubercular drugs

Here are common adverse reactions to antitubercular drugs.

Ethambutol
Itching, joint pain, GI distress, malaise, leukopenia, headache, dizziness, numbness and tingling of the extremities, and confusion may occur.

Although rare, hypersensitivity reactions to ethambutol may produce rash and fever. Anaphylaxis may also occur.

Isoniazid
Peripheral neuropathy is the most common adverse reaction.

Rifampin
The most common adverse reactions include epigastric pain, nausea, vomiting, abdominal cramps, flatulence, anorexia, and diarrhea.

Pyrazinamide
Liver toxicity is the major limiting adverse reaction. GI disturbances include nausea, vomiting, and anorexia.

• Cycloserine and ethionamide may produce additive CNS effects such as drowsiness, dizziness, headache, lethargy, depression, tremor, anxiety, confusion, and tinnitus (ringing in the ears) when administered with isoniazid.

• Isoniazid may increase levels of phenytoin, carbamazepine, diazepam, ethosuximide, primidone, theophylline, and warfarin.

• When corticosteroids and isoniazid are taken together, the effectiveness of isoniazid is reduced while the effects of corticosteroids are increased.

• Isoniazid may reduce the plasma concentration of ketoconazole, itraconazole, and oral antidiabetic agents.

• When given together, the combination of rifampin, isoniazid, ethionamide, and pyrazinamide increases the risk of hepatotoxicity.

• Pyrazinamide combined with phenytoin use may increase phenytoin levels. (See *Adverse reactions to antitubercular drugs.*)

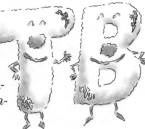

We can be treated by using two or more drugs. That's because a combination of anti-TB drugs reduces our risk of developing resistance.

Antimycotic drugs

Antimycotic, or *antifungal*, *drugs* are used to treat fungal infections and include:
• amphotericin B
• nystatin
• flucytosine
• ketoconazole
• fluconazole
• itraconazole. (See *Other antimycotic drugs*, page 228.)

Amphotericin B

Amphotericin B's potency has made it the most widely used antimycotic drug for severe systemic fungal infections.

Pharmacokinetics

After I.V. administration, amphotericin B is distributed throughout the body and excreted by the kidneys. Its metabolism isn't well defined.

Other antimycotic drugs

Several other antimycotic drugs offer alternative forms of treatment for topical fungal infections.

Clotrimazole

An imidazole derivative, clotrimazole is used:
• topically to treat dermatophyte and *Candida albicans* infections
• orally to treat oral candidiasis
• vaginally to treat vaginal candidiasis.

Griseofulvin

Griseofulvin is used to treat fungal infections of the:
• skin (tinea corporis)
• feet (tinea pedis)
• groin (tinea cruris)
• beard area of the face and neck (tinea barbae)
• nails (tinea unguium)
• scalp (tinea capitis).

Use with extreme prejudice

To prevent a relapse, griseofulvin therapy must continue until the fungus is eradicated and the infected skin or nails are replaced.

Miconazole

Available as miconazole or miconazole nitrate, this imidazole derivative is used to treat local fungal infections such as vaginal and vulvar candidiasis and topical fungal infections such as chronic candidiasis of the skin and mucous membranes.

Delivery options

Miconazole may be administered:
• I.V. or intrathecally (into the subarachnoid space) to treat fungal meningitis
• I.V. or in bladder irrigations to treat fungal bladder infections
• locally to treat vaginal infections
• topically to treat topical infections.

Other topical antimycotic drugs

Ciclopirox olamine, econazole nitrate, haloprogin, butoconazole nitrate, naftifine, tioconazole, terconazole, tolnaftate, butenafine, terbinafine, sulconazole, oxiconazole, clioquinol, triacetin, and undecylenic acid are available only as topical drugs.

Pharmacodynamics

Amphotericin B works by binding to sterol (a lipid) in the fungal cell membrane, altering cell permeability (ability to allow a substance to pass through) and allowing intracellular components to leak out.

A license to kill

Amphotericin B usually acts as a fungistatic drug (inhibiting fungal growth and multiplication) but can become fungicidal (destroying fungi) if it reaches high concentrations in the fungi.

Pharmacotherapeutics

Amphotericin B usually is administered to treat severe systemic fungal infections and meningitis caused by fungi sensitive to the drug. It's usually the drug of choice for severe infections caused by *Candida, Paracoccidioides brasiliensis, Blastomyces dermatitidis, Coccidioides immitis, Cryptococcus neoformans*, and *Sporothrix schenckii*. It's also effective against *Aspergillus fumigatus, Microsporum audouinii, Rhizopus, Candida glabrata, Trichophyton*, and *Rhodotorula*.

Last ditch effort

Because the drug is highly toxic, its use is limited to patients who have a definitive diagnosis of life-threatening infections and who are under close medical supervision.

Drug interactions

Amphotericin B may have significant interactions with many drugs:
• Because of the synergistic effects between flucytosine and amphotericin B, these two drugs commonly are combined in therapy for candidal or cryptococcal infections, especially for cryptococcal meningitis.
• The risk of kidney toxicity increases when amphotericin B is taken with aminoglycosides, cyclosporine, or acyclovir.
• Corticosteroids, extended-spectrum penicillins, and digoxin may worsen the hypokalemia (low blood potassium levels) produced by amphotericin B, possibly leading to heart problems. Moreover, the risk of digoxin toxicity is increased.
• Amphotericin B plus nondepolarizing skeletal muscle relaxants (such as pancuronium bromide) increase the muscle relaxant effects.
• Electrolyte solutions may inactivate amphotericin B when diluted in the same solution. (See *Adverse reactions to amphotericin B*.)

Nystatin

Nystatin is used only topically or orally to treat local fungal infections because it's extremely toxic when administered parenterally.

Pharmacokinetics

Oral nystatin undergoes little or no absorption, distribution, or metabolism. It's excreted unchanged in the feces. Topical nystatin isn't absorbed through the skin or mucous membranes.

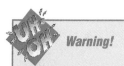
Warning!

Adverse reactions to amphotericin B

Almost all patients receiving I.V. amphotericin B, particularly at the beginning of low-dose therapy, experience:
• chills
• fever
• nausea
• vomiting
• anorexia
• muscle and joint pain
• indigestion.

Anemia
Most patients also develop normochromic (adequate hemoglobin in each red blood cell [RBC]) or normocytic anemia (too few RBCs) that significantly decreases the hematocrit. Hypomagnesemia and hypokalemia may occur, causing electrocardiographic changes requiring replacement electrolyte therapy.

Kidney concerns
Up to 80% of patients may develop some degree of kidney toxicity, causing the kidneys to lose their ability to concentrate urine.

Pharmacodynamics

Nystatin binds to sterols (lipids) in fungal cell membranes and alters the permeability of the membranes, leading to loss of cell components. Nystatin can act as a fungicidal or fungistatic drug, depending on the organism present.

Pharmacotherapeutics

Nystatin is used primarily to treat fungal skin infections. The drug is effective against *Candida.* Different forms of nystatin are available for treating different types of candidal infections.

Topical concerns

Topical nystatin is used to treat skin or mucous membrane candidal infections, such as oral thrush, diaper rash, vaginal and vulvar candidiasis, and candidiasis between skin folds.

Oral history

Oral nystatin is used to treat GI infections.

Drug interactions

Nystatin doesn't interact significantly with other drugs. (See *Adverse reactions to nystatin.*)

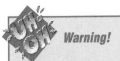

Warning!

Adverse reactions to nystatin

Reactions to nystatin seldom occur, but high dosages may produce:
- diarrhea
- nausea
- vomiting
- abdominal pain
- a bitter taste.

It can get under your skin
Topical nystatin also may cause skin irritation, and a hypersensitivity reaction may occur with oral or topical administration.

Flucytosine

Flucytosine is the only antimetabolite (a substance that closely resembles one required for normal physiologic functioning that exerts its effect by interfering with metabolism) that acts as an antimycotic (suppressing the growth of fungi). It's used primarily with another antimycotic drug such as amphotericin B to treat systemic fungal infections.

Pharmacokinetics

After oral administration, flucytosine is absorbed well from the GI tract and distributed widely. It undergoes little metabolism and is excreted primarily by the kidneys.

Memory jogger

If a drug is *fungicidal,* it destroys the fungus — *cidus* is a Latin term for "killing." If it's *fungistatic,* it prevents fungal growth and multiplication — *stasis* is a Greek term for "halting."

Pharmacodynamics

Flucytosine penetrates fungal cells where it's converted to its active metabolite fluorouracil. Fluorouracil then is incorporated into the RNA of the fungal cells, altering their protein synthesis and causing cell death.

Pharmacotherapeutics

Although amphotericin B is effective in treating candidal and cryptococcal meningitis alone, flucytosine is given with it to reduce the dosage and the risk of toxicity. This combination therapy is the treatment of choice for cryptococcal meningitis.

Standing alone

Flucytosine can be used alone to treat lower urinary tract *Candida* infections because it reaches a high urinary concentration. It's also used effectively to treat infections caused by *T. glabrata*, *Phialophora*, *Aspergillus*, and *Cladosporium*.

Drug interactions

Cytarabine may antagonize the antifungal activity of flucytosine, possibly by competitive inhibition. (See *Adverse reactions to flucytosine*.)

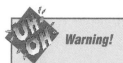

Warning!

Adverse reactions to flucytosine

Flucytosine may produce unpredictable adverse reactions, including:
- confusion
- headache
- drowsiness
- vertigo
- hallucinations
- difficulty breathing
- respiratory arrest
- rash
- nausea
- vomiting
- abdominal distention
- diarrhea
- anorexia.

Ketoconazole

Ketoconazole is an effective oral antimycotic drug with a broad spectrum of activity.

Pharmacokinetics

When given orally, ketoconazole is absorbed variably and distributed widely. It undergoes extensive liver metabolism and is excreted through the bile and feces.

Pharmacodynamics

Within the fungal cells, ketoconazole interferes with sterol synthesis, damaging the cell membrane and increasing its permeability. This leads to a loss of essential intracellular elements and inhibition of cell growth.

A license to kill

Ketoconazole usually produces fungistatic effects but also can produce fungicidal effects under certain conditions.

Pharmacotherapeutics

Ketoconazole is used to treat topical and systemic infections caused by susceptible fungi, which include dermatophytes and most other fungi.

Drug interactions

Ketoconazole may have significant interactions with other drugs:
• Use of ketoconazole with drugs that decrease gastric acidity, such as cimetidine, ranitidine, famotidine, nizatidine, antacids, and anticholinergic drugs, may decrease absorption of ketoconazole and reduce its antimycotic effects.
• Taking ketoconazole with phenytoin may alter metabolism and increase blood levels of both drugs.
• When taken with theophylline it may decrease the serum theophylline level.
• Use with other liver toxic drugs may increase the risk of liver disease.
• Combined with cyclosporine therapy it may increase cyclosporine and serum creatinine levels.
• It increases the effect of oral anticoagulants and can cause hemorrhage.
• It shouldn't be given with rifampin because serum ketoconazole concentrations can be decreased. (See *Adverse reactions to ketoconazole*.)

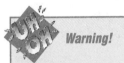

Warning!

Adverse reactions to ketoconazole

The most common adverse reactions to ketoconazole are nausea and vomiting. Less frequent reactions include:
• anaphylaxis
• joint pain
• chills
• fever
• ringing in the ears
• impotence
• photophobia.

Toxic topics
Liver toxicity is rare and reversible when the drug is stopped.

Fluconazole

Fluconazole belongs to a class of synthetic, broad-spectrum bistriazole antimycotic drugs.

Pharmacokinetics

After oral administration, fluconazole is about 90% absorbed. It's distributed into all body fluids, and over 80% of the drug is excreted unchanged in the urine.

Pharmacodynamics

Fluconazole inhibits fungal cytochrome P-450, an enzyme responsible for fungal sterol (a lipid) synthesis, causing fungal cell walls to weaken.

Pharmacotherapeutics

Fluconazole is used to treat mouth, throat, and esophageal candidiasis and serious systemic candidal infections, including UTIs, peritonitis, and pneumonia. It's also used to treat cryptococcal meningitis.

Drug interactions

Fluconazole may interact with other drugs:
• Use with warfarin may increase the risk of bleeding.
• It may increase levels of phenytoin and cyclosporine.
• It may increase the plasma concentration of oral antidiabetic drugs, such as glyburide, tolbutamide, and glipizide, increasing the risk of hypoglycemia.
• Rifampin and cimetidine enhance the metabolism of fluconazole, reducing the plasma concentration of fluconazole.
• It may increase the activity of zidovudine. (See *Adverse reactions to fluconazole*.)

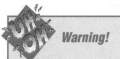

Warning!

Adverse reactions to fluconazole

• Abdominal pain
• Diarrhea
• Dizziness
• Headache
• Increase in liver enzymes
• Nausea and vomiting
• Rash

Itraconazole

Itraconazole belongs to a class of drugs known as the synthetic triazoles. It inhibits the synthesis of ergosterol, a vital component of fungal cell membranes.

Pharmacokinetics

Oral bioavailability is maximal when itraconazole is taken with food. It's bound to plasma proteins and is extensively metabolized in the liver into a large number of metabolites. It's minimally excreted in the feces.

Pharmacodynamics

Itraconazole interferes with fungal wall synthesis by inhibiting the formation of ergosterol and increasing cell-wall permeability, making the fungus susceptible to osmotic instability.

Pharmacotherapeutics

Itraconazole is used to treat blastomycosis, non-meningeal histoplasmosis, candidiasis, aspergillosis, and fungal nail disease.

Drug interactions

Itraconazole has few interactions with other drugs:
• Itraconazole may increase the risk of bleeding when combined with oral anticoagulants.
• Antacids, histamine-2–receptor antagonists, phenytoin, and rifampin lower itraconazole plasma levels. (See *Adverse reactions to itraconazole.*)

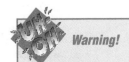

Warning!

Adverse reactions to itraconazole

• Dizziness
• Headache
• Hypertension
• Impaired liver function
• Nausea

Antimalarial and antiprotozoal drugs

Malaria is a protozoal infection of the genus *Plasmodium* that produces severe chills, fever, and profuse sweating.

Hey! It bit me!

Malaria is transmitted by the bite of the infected female *Anopheles* mosquito.

Antimalarial drugs

The major drugs used to prevent and treat malaria include:
• chloroquine hydrochloride, chloroquine phosphate, and hydroxychloroquine sulfate (4-aminoquinoline derivatives)
• mefloquine hydrochloride
• primaquine phosphate (8-aminoquinoline derivative)
• pyrimethamine
• quinidine gluconate and quinine sulfate.

Helping hands

Sulfonamides, sulfones, and tetracyclines also may be used in combination with these drugs.

Pharmacokinetics

After oral administration, antimalarial drugs are absorbed well and distributed widely throughout the body. The extent of metabolism among these drugs varies, and excretion occurs primarily in the urine.

Pharmacodynamics

The actions of these antimalarial drugs may vary.

The antithesis to synthesis

Chloroquine and hydroxychloroquine are thought to disrupt protein synthesis in the parasite. Also, these drugs may concentrate in the digestive vacuoles of the parasite, increasing pH and interfering with utilization of hemoglobin.

Power outage

Primaquine appears to affect the parasite's mitochondria (responsible for cellular energy), eventually disrupting cellular metabolism.

Folic failure

Pyrimethamine selectively inhibits the enzyme dihydrofolate reductase, which impedes folic acid reduction and ultimately disrupts parasitic reproduction. Sulfadoxine competitively inhibits dihydrofolic acid synthesis, which is necessary to convert para-aminobenzoic acid to folic acid.

DNA destruction

Quinine's antimalarial action may result from its incorporation into the DNA of the parasite, rendering it ineffective. Its action also may result from depression of oxygen uptake and carbohydrate metabolism in the parasite. In addition, quinine acts as a skeletal muscle relaxant, a local anesthetic, an antipyretic, and an analgesic, thus relieving malarial symptoms.

Following quinine's cue?

The exact mechanism of mefloquine's antimalarial effects remain unknown. Because it's a structural analogue of quinine, it may have similar pharmacodynamic effects.

Pharmacotherapeutics

The effectiveness of each antimalarial drug toward different strains of malaria varies.

Get 'em all, chloroquine!

Chloroquine remains the oral drug of choice to prevent and treat all malaria strains, except chloroquine-resistant or multidrug-resistant strains of *Plasmodium falciparum*.

Pinch hitter

Hydroxychloroquine is an alternative when chloroquine isn't available.

Resistance fighters

For treatment of malaria caused by chloroquine-resistant or multidrug-resistant strains of *P. falciparum*, quinine is the drug of choice and is given with slower-acting antimalarial drugs.

Dynamic duo

Primaquine is the drug of choice in combination with chloroquine to treat *P. malaria*, *P. vivax*, and *P. ovale*.

Prevention first

Mefloquine is used to treat malaria caused by resistant strains of *P. falciparum*. It's also administered to prevent malaria infections, including chloroquine-resistant strains of *P. falciparum*.

Parenteral practice

Quinidine is the parenteral drug of choice for the treatment of malaria in patients who can't tolerate oral therapy.

Drug interactions

Various interactions can occur between antimalarial drugs and other drugs:
• Hydroxychloroquine and quinine increase digoxin and cyclosporine levels.
• Mefloquine taken with beta blockers, quinine, quinidine, and other drugs that prolong cardiac conduction, may produce electrocardiographic abnormalities and even cardiac arrest.
• The risk of seizures increases when mefloquine is taken with chloroquine.
• Mefloquine reduces valproic acid blood levels, increasing the risk of seizures.
• Folic acid reduces the antimicrobial effect of pyrimethamine.

• Quinine may increase the effects of neuromuscular blockers (pancuronium, tubocurarine, succinylcholine), leading to breathing difficulties.
• Quinine may increase the effects of oral anticoagulants, increasing the risk of bleeding. (See *Adverse reactions to antimalarial drugs.*)

Other antiprotozoal drugs

Although many other drugs are used to treat protozoal infections, few are readily obtainable. Available *antiprotozoal drugs* include:
• atovaquone
• furazolidone
• iodoquinol
• metronidazole
• pentamidine isethionate
• trimetrexate.

Moonlighting

Amphotericin B, paromomycin, and co-trimoxazole are also used sometimes as antiprotozoals.

Pharmacokinetics

These antiprotozoal drugs may have differing pharmacokinetic properties.

Eats increase availability

After oral administration, the absorption of atovaquone varies. The bioavailability increases approximately three-fold when it's administered with meals. It's extensively bound to plasma proteins. Atovaquone isn't metabolized and is excreted primarily in the feces.

Local consequences

Iodoquinol is poorly absorbed; however, it exerts its effects locally in the lower GI tract. Its metabolism is unknown, and it's excreted primarily in the feces.

I.M. absorbed

The absorption of pentamidine is limited after aerosol administration; however, after I.M. administration it's absorbed well. Its metabolism is unknown, and it's excreted unchanged in the urine.

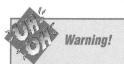
Warning!

Adverse reactions to antimalarial drugs

Here are some adverse reactions to antimalarial drugs.

Chloroquine and hydroxychloroquine
Abdominal discomfort and cramps, anorexia, nausea, vomiting, and diarrhea can occur.

Mefloquine
Vomiting, dizziness, muscle pain, nausea, fever, headache, chills, diarrhea, skin rash, abdominal pain, fatigue, loss of appetite, and ringing in the ears can occur.

Primaquine
Nausea, vomiting, and abdominal discomfort and cramps can occur.

Pyrimethamine
Anorexia, vomiting, and abdominal cramps can occur.

Quinine
Cinchonism, producing nausea, vomiting, diarrhea, sweating, blurred vision, ringing in the ears, and reduced hearing, often occur.

Intestine inactivates

After oral administration, furazolidone is absorbed poorly and is inactivated in the intestine. About 5% of an oral dose of furazolidone is excreted in the urine as unchanged drug and metabolites.

Majority if by mouth

The majority of a metronidazole dose is absorbed after oral administration. It's distributed widely, metabolized partially in the liver, and excreted in the urine and, to a lesser degree, in the feces.

Pharmacodynamics

Antiprotozoal drugs produce their effects through various actions.

Stopping traffic

Atovaquone is thought to inhibit electron transport, causing decreased activity of several enzymes of the mitochondria (recall that this is the part of the cell responsible for cellular energy metabolism). This, in turn, inhibits the synthesis of nucleic acid and adenosine triphosphate.

Getting in the way

Furazolidone may kill bacteria and protozoa by interfering with their enzyme systems and by inhibiting monoamine oxidase.

Contact killer

Iodoquinol is a contact amebicide that acts directly on protozoa in the GI tract.

DNA disruption, 1

Metronidazole destroys bacteria, amoebas, and *Trichomonas* by disrupting DNA and inhibiting nucleic acid synthesis, eventually causing cellular death.

Halting construction

Pentamidine interferes with the organism's building of DNA, RNA, phospholipids, and proteins.

DNA disruption, 2

Trimetrexate is an inhibitor of the enzyme dihydrofolate reductase. This results in disruption of DNA, RNA, and protein synthesis and, ultimately, cell death. Trimetrexate must be administered concurrently with folinic acid to protect the patient's normal cells.

Pharmacotherapeutics

Antiprotozoal drugs are used for a wide range of disorders, including *Pneumocystis carinii* infections, amebiasis, giardiasis, trichomoniasis, toxoplasmosis, African trypanosomiasis, and leishmaniasis.

Co-trimoxazole got you down?

Atovaquone is only indicated for patients with mild to moderate *P. carinii* pneumonia who can't tolerate co-trimoxazole therapy. Trimetrexate administered with folinic acid is used as an alternative for the treatment of moderate to severe *P. carinii* pneumonia in patients who can't tolerate or don't respond to co-trimoxazole, or for whom co-trimoxazole therapy is contraindicated.

Drug interactions

Antiprotozoal drugs have interactions with other drugs:
• Furazolidone and metronidazole produce a disulfiram-like reaction when taken with alcohol, causing flushing, weakness, light-headedness, and sweating.
• Furazolidone increases meperidine levels
• Furazolidone may increase blood levels of tricyclic antidepressants, leading to hypertension, fever, seizures, a rapid heart rate, and psychosis.
• Metronidazole increases the effects of oral anticoagulants, increasing the tendency for bleeding.
• Taking pentamidine with aminoglycosides, cisplatin, and amphotericin B increases the risk of kidney toxicity.
• Trimetrexate plus zidovudine can produce additive toxicity; these drugs shouldn't be administered together. (See *Adverse reactions to antiprotozoal drugs.*)

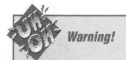 *Warning!*

Adverse reactions to antiprotozoal drugs

Antiprotozoal drugs may result in a variety of adverse reactions.

Atovaquone
• Rash
• Nausea and vomiting
• Diarrhea
• Headache
• Fever
• Cough

Furazolidone
• Nausea and vomiting

Iodoquinol
• Anorexia
• Vomiting
• Diarrhea
• Abdominal cramps
• Constipation
• Itching around the anus

Pentamidine
• Kidney toxicity
• Pain or hardness at the injection site
• Elevated liver function tests
• Leukopenia (reduced white blood cell count)
• Nausea
• Anorexia
• Bronchospasm and cough

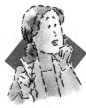

Quick quiz

1. Which rationale best justifies administration of different antitubercular drugs concurrently in treating active tuberculosis?
    A. They're second-line drugs and only effective together.
    B. Rifampin increases the activity of isoniazid.
    C. Combination therapy can prevent or delay bacterial resistance.

Answer: C. Combination therapy can prevent or delay bacterial resistance to antitubercular drugs.

2. Which adverse reaction do most patients experience when receiving I.V. amphotericin B?
    A. Anuria
    B. Coagulation defects
    C. Normochromic or normocytic anemia

Answer: C. Normochromic or normocytic anemia are common adverse reactions to I.V. amphotericin B.

3. What is the oral drug of choice for most strains of malaria?
    A. chloroquine
    B. primaquine
    C. mefloquine

Answer: A. Chloroquine is the oral drug of choice for most strains of malaria.

Scoring

 If you answered three questions correctly, extraordinary! You're more than a match for unwanted microbes!

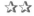 If you answered two questions correctly, congratulations. You're winning the battle against bacteria.

 If you answered fewer than two questions correctly, dig in! The war with drugs continues for five more chapters!

10

Anti-inflammatory drugs, anti-allergy drugs, and immunosuppressants

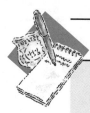

Just the facts

In this chapter, you'll review:

♦ classes of drugs that modify immune or inflammatory responses

♦ uses and varying actions of these drugs

♦ how these drugs are absorbed, distributed, metabolized, and excreted

♦ drug interactions and adverse reactions to these drugs.

Drugs and the immune system

Immune and inflammatory responses protect the body from invading foreign substances. These responses can be modified by certain classes of drugs:

• Antihistamines block the effects of histamine on target tissues.

• Corticosteroids suppress immune responses and reduce inflammation.

• Noncorticosteroid immunosuppressants prevent rejection of transplanted organs and can be used to treat autoimmune disease.

• Uricosurics prevent or control the frequency of gouty arthritis attacks.

Antihistamines

Antihistamines primarily act to block histamine effects that occur in an immediate (type I) hypersensitivity reaction, commonly called an allergic reaction. They're available alone or in combination products by prescription or over the counter.

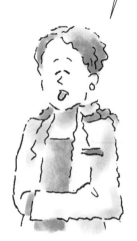

Antihistamines relieve the symptoms of an allergic reaction, such as nasal congestion and rhinitis. They don't give the body immunity to the allergy itself.

Histamine-1–receptor antagonists

The term antihistamine refers to drugs that act as histamine-1 (H_1)–receptor antagonists; that is, they compete with histamine for binding to H_1-receptor sites throughout the body. However, they don't displace histamine already bound to the receptor.

It's all about chemistry

Based on chemical structure, antihistamines are categorized into six major classes:
• Ethanolamines include clemastine fumarate, dimenhydrinate, diphenhydramine hydrochloride, and phenyltoloxamine citrate.
• Ethylenediamines include pyrilamine maleate, tripelennamine citrate, and tripelennamine hydrochloride.
• Alkylamines include brompheniramine maleate, chlorpheniramine maleate, dexchlorpheniramine maleate, and triprolidine hydrochloride.
• Phenothiazines include methdilazine hydrochloride, promethazine hydrochloride, and trimeprazine tartrate.
• Piperidines include azatadine maleate, cyclizine lactate, cyproheptadine hydrochloride, fexofenadine hydrochloride, loratadine, meclizine hydrochloride, and phenindamine tartrate.
• Miscellaneous drugs, such as hydroxyzine hydrochloride and hydroxyzine pamoate, also act as antihistamines.

Pharmacokinetics (how drugs circulate)

H_1-receptor antagonists are absorbed well after oral or parenteral administration. Some can also be given rectally.

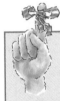

Memory jogger

Anti- is a familiar prefix meaning "opposing." That is exactly what antihistamines do: They oppose histamine effects (or allergic reactions).

Distribution

Antihistamines are distributed widely throughout the body and central nervous system (CNS), with the exception of loratadine.

Exceptional antihistamines

Fexofenadine and loratadine, nonsedating antihistamines, minimally penetrate the blood-brain barrier so that little of the drug is distributed in the CNS, producing fewer effects there than other antihistamines.

Metabolism and excretion

Antihistamines are metabolized by liver enzymes and excreted in the urine, with small amounts secreted in breast milk. Fexofenadine, mainly excreted in feces, is an exception.

Pharmacodynamics (how drugs act)

H_1-receptor antagonists compete with histamine for H_1 receptors on effector cells (the cells that cause allergic symptoms), blocking histamine from producing its effects. (See *How chlorpheniramine stops an allergic response*, page 244.)

Antagonizing tactics

H_1-receptor antagonists produce their effects by:
• blocking the action of histamine on the small blood vessels
• decreasing dilation of arterioles and engorgement of tissues
• reducing the leaking of plasma proteins and fluids out of the capillaries (capillary permeability), thereby lessening edema
• inhibiting most smooth-muscle responses to histamine (in particular, blocking the constriction of bronchial, GI, and vascular smooth muscle)
• relieving symptoms by acting on the terminal nerve endings in the skin that flare and itch when stimulated by histamine
• suppressing adrenal medulla stimulation, autonomic ganglia stimulation, and exocrine gland secretion, such as lacrimal and salivary secretion.

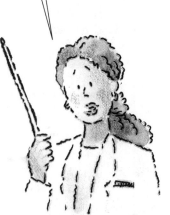

Keep in mind that although histamine binding is blocked, the overall release of histamine continues.

How chlorpheniramine stops an allergic response

Although chlorpheniramine can't reverse symptoms of an allergic response, it can stop the progression of the response. Here's what happens.

Release the mediators

When sensitized to an antigen, a mast cell reacts to repeated antigen exposure by releasing chemical mediators. One of these mediators, histamine, binds to histamine-1 (H_1)–receptors found on effector cells (the cells responsible for allergic symptoms). This initiates the allergic response that affects the respiratory, cardiovascular, GI, endocrine, and integumentary systems.

The first one there wins

Chlorpheniramine competes with histamine for H_1-receptor sites on the effector cells. By attaching to these sites first, the drug prevents more histamine from binding to the effector cells.

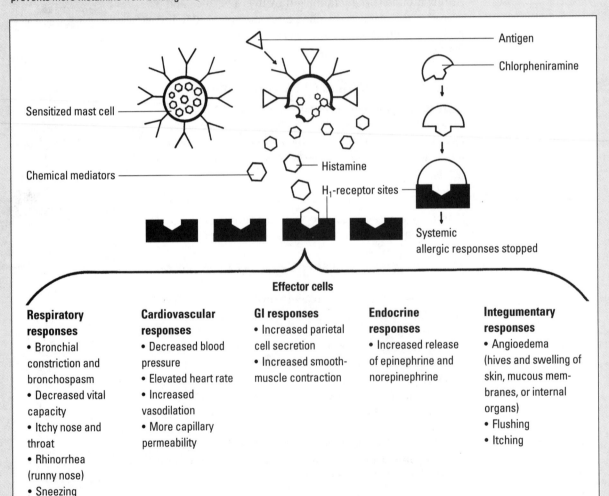

Respiratory responses
- Bronchial constriction and bronchospasm
- Decreased vital capacity
- Itchy nose and throat
- Rhinorrhea (runny nose)
- Sneezing

Cardiovascular responses
- Decreased blood pressure
- Elevated heart rate
- Increased vasodilation
- More capillary permeability

GI responses
- Increased parietal cell secretion
- Increased smooth-muscle contraction

Endocrine responses
- Increased release of epinephrine and norepinephrine

Integumentary responses
- Angioedema (hives and swelling of skin, mucous membranes, or internal organs)
- Flushing
- Itching

Going straight to the head

Several antihistamines have a high affinity for H_1 receptors in the brain and are used for their CNS effects. These drugs include diphenhydramine, dimenhydrinate, promethazine, and various piperidine derivatives.

Gut reaction

H_1-receptor antagonists don't affect parietal cell secretion in the stomach because their receptors are H_2 receptors, not H_1.

Pharmacotherapeutics (how drugs are used)

Antihistamines are used to treat the symptoms of type I hypersensitivity reactions, such as:
• allergic rhinitis (runny nose and itchy eyes caused by a local sensitivity reaction)
• vasomotor rhinitis (rhinitis not caused by allergy or infection)
• allergic conjunctivitis (inflammation of the membranes of the eye)
• urticaria (hives)
• angioedema (submucosal swelling in the hands, face, and feet).

Enlistees for other causes

Antihistamines can have other therapeutic uses:
• Many are used primarily as antiemetics (to control nausea and vomiting).
• They can also be used as adjunctive therapy to treat an anaphylactic reaction after the serious symptoms are controlled.
• Diphenhydramine can help treat Parkinson's disease and drug-induced extrapyramidal reactions (abnormal involuntary movements).
• Because of its antiserotonin qualities, cyproheptadine may be used to treat Cushing's disease, serotonin-associated diarrhea, vascular cluster headaches, and anorexia nervosa.

Drug interactions

Antihistamines may interact with many drugs, sometimes with life-threatening consequences:

• They may block or reverse the vasopressor effects of epinephrine, producing vasodilation, increased heart rate, and very low blood pressure.
• They may mask the toxic signs and symptoms of oto-toxicity (a detrimental effect on hearing) associated with aminoglycosides or large dosages of salicylates.
• They may increase the sedative and respiratory depressant effects of CNS depressants, such as tranquilizers or alcohol.
• Loratadine may cause serious cardiac effects when taken with macrolide antibiotics (such as erythromycin), fluconazole, ketoconazole, itraconazole, miconazole, cimetidine, ciprofloxacin, and clarithromycin. (See *Adverse reactions to antihistamines.*)

Corticosteroids

Corticosteroids suppress immune responses and reduce inflammation. They're available as natural or synthetic steroids.

There's no improving on nature

Natural corticosteroids are hormones produced by the adrenal cortex; most corticosteroid drugs are synthetic forms of these hormones. Natural and synthetic corticosteroids are classified according to their biological activities:
• Glucocorticoids, such as cortisone acetate and dexamethasone, affect carbohydrate and protein metabolism.
• Mineralocorticoids, such as aldosterone and fludrocortisone acetate, regulate electrolyte and water balance.

Glucocorticoids

Most *glucocorticoids* are synthetic analogues of hormones secreted by the adrenal cortex. They exert anti-inflammatory, metabolic, and immunosuppressant effects. Drugs in this class include:
• beclomethasone
• betamethasone
• cortisone
• dexamethasone
• hydrocortisone

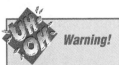

- methylprednisolone
- prednisolone
- prednisone
- triamcinolone.

Pharmacokinetics

Glucocorticoids are absorbed well when administered orally. After I.M. administration, they're absorbed completely.

Distribution

Glucocorticoids are bound to plasma proteins and distributed through the blood.

Metabolism and excretion

Glucocorticoids are metabolized in the liver and excreted by the kidneys.

Pharmacodynamics

Glucocorticoids suppress hypersensitivity and immune responses through a process not entirely understood. Researchers believe that glucocorticoids inhibit immune responses by:
- suppressing or preventing cell-mediated immune reactions
- reducing levels of leukocytes, monocytes, and eosinophils
- decreasing the binding of immunoglobulins to cell surface receptors
- inhibiting interleukin synthesis.

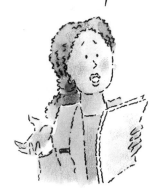

Unfortunately, when glucocorticoids inhibit the immune response they may also mask the signs and symptoms of serious infections occurring at the same time.

Taking the red (and more) out

Glucocorticoids suppress the redness, edema, heat, and tenderness associated with the inflammatory response. They start on the cellular level by stabilizing the lysosomal membrane (a structure within the cell that contains digestive enzymes) so that it doesn't release its store of hydrolytic enzymes into the cells.

What to expect from every good corticosteroid

As corticosteroids, glucocorticoids prevent leakage of plasma from capillaries, suppress the migration of polymorphonuclear leukocytes (cells that kill and digest mi-

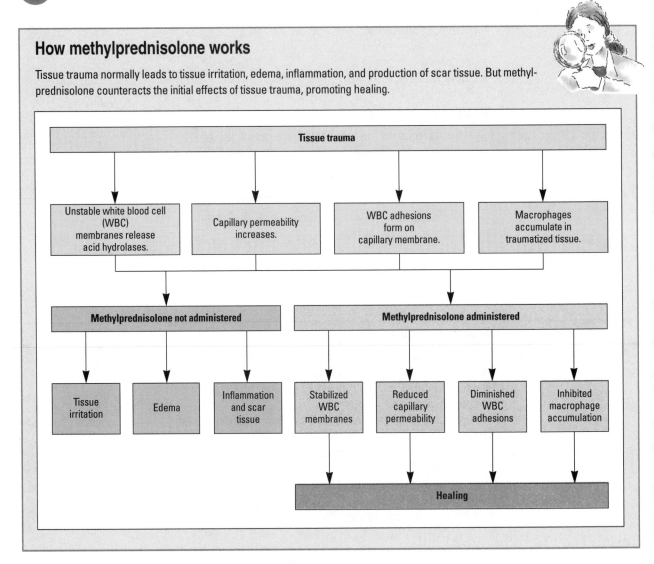

How methylprednisolone works

Tissue trauma normally leads to tissue irritation, edema, inflammation, and production of scar tissue. But methylprednisolone counteracts the initial effects of tissue trauma, promoting healing.

croorganisms), and inhibit phagocytosis (ingestion and destruction).

To ensure a job well done, glucocorticoids decrease antibody formation in injured or infected tissues and disrupt histamine synthesis, fibroblast development, collagen deposition, capillary dilation, and capillary permeability. (See *How methylprednisolone works*.)

Pharmacotherapeutics

Besides their use as replacement therapy for patients with adrenocortical insufficiency, glucocorticoids are prescribed for immunosuppression and reduction of inflammation and for their effects on the blood and lymphatic systems.

Drug interactions

Many drugs interact with corticosteroids:
• Barbiturates, phenytoin, rifampin, and aminoglutethimide may reduce their effects.
• Their potassium-wasting effects may be enhanced by amphotericin B, chlorthalidone, ethacrynic acid, furosemide, and thiazide diuretics.
• Erythromycin and troleandomycin may increase their effects by reducing their metabolism.
• They reduce the serum concentration and effects of salicylates.
• The risk of peptic ulcers associated with nonsteroidal anti-inflammatory drugs (NSAIDs) and salicylates is increased when these agents are taken with corticosteroids.
• The response to vaccines and toxoids may be reduced in a patient taking corticosteroids.
• Estrogen and oral contraceptives that contain estrogen increase the effects of corticosteroids.
• The effects of antidiabetic drugs may be reduced, resulting in increased blood glucose levels. (See *Adverse reactions to corticosteroids.*)

Mineralocorticoids

Mineralocorticoids affect electrolyte and water balance. These drugs include:
• fludrocortisone acetate, a synthetic analogue of hormones secreted by the adrenal cortex
• aldosterone, a natural mineralocorticoid (the use of which has been curtailed by high cost and limited availability).

Pharmacokinetics

Fludrocortisone acetate is absorbed well and distributed to all parts of the body.

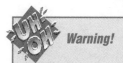

Warning!

Adverse reactions to corticosteroids

Corticosteroids affect almost all body systems. Their widespread adverse effects include:
• insomnia
• increased sodium and water retention
• increased potassium excretion
• suppressed immune and inflammatory responses
• osteoporosis
• intestinal perforation
• peptic ulcers
• impaired wound healing.

Endocrine system
Endocrine system reactions may include:
• diabetes mellitus
• hyperlipidemia
• adrenal atrophy
• hypothalamic-pituitary axis suppression
• cushingoid signs and symptoms (such as buffalo hump, moon face, and elevated blood glucose levels).

Metabolism and excretion

Fludrocortisone acetate is metabolized in the liver to inactive metabolites. The drug is excreted by the kidneys, primarily as inactive metabolites.

Pharmacodynamics

Fludrocortisone acetate affects fluid and electrolyte balance by acting on the distal renal tubule to increase sodium reabsorption and potassium and hydrogen secretion.

Pharmacotherapeutics

Fludrocortisone acetate is used as replacement therapy for patients with adrenocortical insufficiency (reduced secretion of glucocorticoids, mineralocorticoids, and androgens).

Seasoning reasoning

Fludrocortisone acetate may also be used to treat salt-losing congenital adrenogenital syndrome (characterized by a lack of cortisol and deficient aldosterone production) after the patient's electrolyte balance has been restored.

Drug interactions

As is the case with adverse reactions, the drug interactions associated with mineralocorticoids are similar to those associated with glucocorticoids.

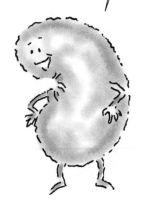

Fludrocortisone acetate gets me working harder to increase sodium reabsorption and potassium and hydrogen secretion.

Other immunosuppressants

Several drugs used for their immunosuppressant effects in patients undergoing allograft transplantation (between two people who aren't identical twins) are also used experimentally to treat autoimmune diseases (diseases resulting from an inappropriate immune response directed against the self). They include:
* azathioprine
* cyclosporine
* lymphocyte immune globulin (ATG [equine])
* muromonab-CD3
* tacrolimus.

Aiding in the battle against cancer

Cyclophosphamide, classified as an alkylating drug, also is used as an immunosuppressant, but it's used primarily to treat cancer.

Pharmacokinetics

Among immunosuppressants, different paths are taken through the body.

Absorption

When administered orally, azathioprine is absorbed readily from the GI tract, whereas absorption of cyclosporine is varied and incomplete.

Only I.V.

ATG and muromonab-CD3 are administered only by I.V. injection.

Distribution

The distribution of azathioprine isn't understood fully. Cyclosporine and muromonab-CD3 are distributed widely throughout the body. Azathioprine and cyclosporine cross the placental barrier. The distribution of ATG isn't clear, but it may be distributed to breast milk.

Metabolism and excretion

Azathioprine and cyclosporine are metabolized in the liver. Muromonab-CD3 is consumed by T cells circulating in the blood. The metabolism of ATG is unknown. Azathioprine and ATG are excreted in the urine; cyclosporine is excreted principally in the bile. How muromonab-CD3 is excreted is unknown.

Pharmacodynamics

How certain immunosuppressants achieve their desired effects has yet to be precisely determined.

What's going on here?

The exact mechanism of action of azathioprine, cyclosporine, and ATG is unknown, but may be explained by the following:
• Azathioprine antagonizes metabolism of the amino acid purine and, therefore, may inhibit ribonucleic acid and

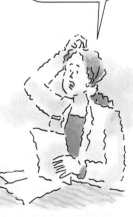

Cyclosporine may inhibit helper production of immunoglobulin and reduce the humoral response.

deoxyribonucleic acid structure and synthesis. It also may inhibit coenzyme formation and function.
• Cyclosporine is thought to inhibit helper T cells and suppressor T cells.
• ATG may eliminate antigen-reactive T cells in the blood, alter T-cell function, or both.

They do know this much...

In patients receiving kidney allografts, azathioprine suppresses cell-mediated hypersensitivity reactions and produces various alterations in antibody production. Muromonab-CD3, a monoclonal antibody, is understood to block the function of T cells.

Pharmacotherapeutics

Immunosuppressants are used mainly to prevent rejection in patients who undergo organ transplantation. (See *Cyclosporine: Miracle drug or death sentence?*)

Drug interactions

Most drug interactions with this class of drugs involve other immunosuppressant and anti-inflammatory drugs and various antibiotic and antimicrobial drugs:
• Allopurinol increases the blood levels of azathioprine.

Clinical controversy

Cyclosporine: Miracle drug or death sentence?

Organ transplantation can save a life. However, cyclosporine, an immunosuppressant drug used to reduce the risk of organ rejection, may also cause cancer.

Does cyclosporine encourage cells to become cancerous?
It has long been believed that when the immune system is weakened by immunosuppressant drugs, it loses its ability to fight and kill cancerous cells. Recent research suggests that cyclosporine may also encourage abnormal cells to become cancerous and, in addition, perhaps even grow aggressively. This research has raised obvious concern about the use of cyclosporine in organ transplantation.

A double-edged sword
However, this concern needs to be balanced against the life-threatening risk of organ rejection. Scientists are now looking for ways to block this tumor-promoting effect of cyclosporine.

• Levels of cyclosporine may be increased by ketoconazole, calcium channel blockers, cimetidine, anabolic steroids, oral contraceptives, erythromycin, and metoclopramide.
• The risk of toxicity to the kidneys is increased when cyclosporine is taken with acyclovir, aminoglycosides, and amphotericin B.
• The risk of infection and lymphoma (neoplasm of the lymph tissue, most likely malignant) is increased when cyclosporine is taken with other immunosuppressants (except corticosteroids).
• Barbiturates, rifampin, phenytoin, sulfonamides, and trimethoprim decrease plasma cyclosporine levels.
• Serum digoxin levels may be increased when cyclosporine is taken with digoxin.
• Taking ATG or muromonab-CD3 with other immunosuppressant drugs increases the risk of infection and lymphoma. (See *Adverse reactions to noncorticosteroid immunosuppressants.*)

Uricosurics and other antigout drugs

Uricosurics, along with other antigout drugs, exert their effects through their anti-inflammatory actions.

Uricosurics

The two major uricosurics are:

  probenecid

sulfinpyrazone.

Getting the gout out

Uricosurics act by increasing uric acid excretion in the urine. The primary goal in using uricosurics is to prevent or control the frequency of gouty arthritis attacks.

Pharmacokinetics

Uricosurics are absorbed from the GI tract.

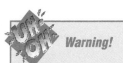

Warning!

Adverse reactions to noncorticosteroid immunosuppressants

All noncorticosteroid immunosuppressants can cause hypersensitivity reactions. Here are adverse reactions to individual drugs.

Azathioprine
• Bone marrow suppression
• Nausea and vomiting
• Liver toxicity

Cyclosporine
• Kidney toxicity
• Hyperkalemia
• Infection
• Liver toxicity
• Nausea and vomiting

Lymphocyte immune globulin
• Fever and chills
• Reduced white blood cell or platelet count
• Infection
• Nausea and vomiting

Muromonab-CD3
• Fever and chills
• Nausea and vomiting
• Tremor
• Pulmonary edema
• Infection

Distribution

Distribution of the two drugs is similar, with 75% to 95% of probenecid and 98% of sulfinpyrazone being protein-bound.

Metabolism and excretion

Metabolism of the drugs occurs in the liver, and excretion is primarily by the kidneys. Only small amounts of these drugs are excreted in the feces.

Pharmacodynamics

Probenecid and sulfinpyrazone reduce the reabsorption of uric acid at the proximal convoluted tubules of the kidneys. This results in excretion of uric acid in the urine, reducing serum urate levels.

Pharmacotherapeutics

Probenecid and sulfinpyrazone are indicated for treatment for:
* chronic gouty arthritis
* tophaceous gout (the deposition of tophi or urate crystals under the skin and into joints).

A part-time promoter

Probenecid is also used to promote uric acid excretion in patients experiencing hyperuricemia.

Substitute when acute

Probenecid and sulfinpyrazone shouldn't be given during an acute gouty attack. If taken at that time, these drugs prolong inflammation. Because these drugs may increase the chance of an acute gouty attack when therapy begins and whenever the serum urate level changes rapidly, colchicine is administered during the first 3 to 6 months of probenecid or sulfinpyrazone therapy.

Drug interactions

Many drug interactions, some potentially serious, can occur with uricosuric drugs:
* Probenecid significantly increases or prolongs the effects of cephalosporins, penicillins, and sulfonamides.
* Serum urate levels may be increased when probenecid is taken with antineoplastic drugs.

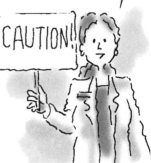

Probenecid and sulfinpyrazone aren't used to treat an acute gouty attack. In fact, these two drugs could prolong the attack.

• Probenecid increases the serum concentration of dapsone, aminosalicylic acid, and methotrexate, causing toxic reactions.
• Sulfinpyrazone increases the effectiveness of warfarin, increasing the risk of bleeding.
• Salicylates reduce the effects of sulfinpyrazone.
• The effects of oral antidiabetic agents may be increased when taken with sulfinpyrazone, increasing the risk of hypoglycemia. (See *Adverse reactions to uricosurics*.)

Other antigout drugs

Allopurinol is used to reduce production of uric acid, preventing gouty attacks, and *colchicine* is used to treat acute gouty attacks.

Pharmacokinetics

Allopurinol and colchicine take somewhat different paths through the body.

All aboard allopurinol

When given orally, allopurinol is absorbed from the GI tract. Allopurinol and its metabolite oxypurinol are distributed throughout the body except in the brain, where drug concentrations are 50% of those found in the rest of the body. It's metabolized by the liver and excreted in the urine.

Following colchicine's course

Colchicine is also absorbed from the GI tract. Colchicine is partially metabolized in the liver. The drug and its metabolites then reenter the intestinal tract through biliary secretions. After reabsorption from the intestines, colchicine is distributed to various tissues. The drug is excreted primarily in the feces and to a lesser degree in the urine.

Pharmacodynamics

Allopurinol and its metabolite oxypurinol inhibit xanthine oxidase, the enzyme responsible for the production of uric acid. By reducing uric acid formation, allopurinol eliminates the hazards of hyperuricuria.

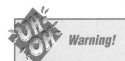
Warning!

Adverse reactions to uricosurics

Adverse reactions to uricosurics include uric acid stone formation and blood abnormalities.

Probenecid
• Headache
• Anorexia
• Nausea and vomiting
• Hypersensitivity reactions

Sulfinpyrazone
• Nausea
• Indigestion
• GI pain
• GI blood loss

Migration control

Colchicine appears to reduce the inflammatory response to monosodium urate crystals deposited in joint tissues. Colchicine may produce its effects by inhibiting migration of white blood cells (WBCs) to the inflamed joint. This reduces phagocytosis and lactic acid production by WBCs, decreasing urate crystal deposits and reducing inflammation.

Pharmacotherapeutics

Allopurinol treats primary gout, hopefully preventing acute gouty attacks. It can be prescribed with uricosurics when smaller dosages of each drug are directed. It's used to:
• treat gout or hyperuricemia that may occur with blood abnormalities and during treatment of tumors or leukemia
• treat primary or secondary uric acid nephropathy (with or without the accompanying symptoms of gout)
• treat and prevent recurrent uric acid stone formation
• treat patients who respond poorly to maximum dosages of uricosurics or who have allergic reactions or intolerance to uricosuric drugs.

Acute alert

Colchicine is used to relieve the inflammation of acute gouty arthritis attacks. If given promptly, it's especially effective in relieving pain. Also, giving colchicine during the first several months of allopurinol, probenecid, or sulfinpyrazone therapy may prevent the acute gouty attacks that sometimes accompany the use of these drugs.

Drug interactions

Colchicine doesn't interact significantly with other drugs. When allopurinol is used with other drugs, the resulting interactions can be serious:
• Allopurinol potentiates the effect of oral anticoagulants.
• Allopurinol increases the serum concentrations of mercaptopurine and azathioprine, increasing the risk of toxicity.
• Angiotensin-converting enzyme inhibitors increase the risk of hypersensitivity reactions to allopurinol.

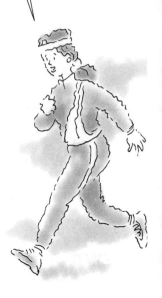

Colchicine relieves a painful gouty attack by going to work right in the joint. It can have you running smoothly again.

• Allopurinol increases serum theophylline levels.
• The risk of bone marrow depression increases when cyclophosphamide is taken with allopurinol. (See *Adverse reactions to other antigout drugs.*)

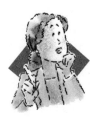

Quick quiz

1. How does diphenhydramine work?
   A.   It blocks production of histamine.
   B.   It prevents binding of histamine to receptors.
   C.   It reverses the effects of histamine.

Answer: B. Diphenhydramine prevents binding of histamine to receptors.

2. What is the most common adverse reaction to antihistamines?
   A.   Drug fever
   B.   GI distress
   C.   Sedation

Answer: C. Sedation is the most common adverse reaction to antihistamines.

3. Which of the following signs and symptoms suggest that a patient is experiencing Cushing's syndrome?
   A.   Buffalo hump, elevated blood glucose levels, and moon face
   B.   Low blood pressure, rapid heart rate, and difficulty breathing
   C.   Low blood glucose levels and reduced platelet count

Answer: A. Buffalo hump, elevated blood glucose levels, and moon face are all signs and symptoms of Cushing's syndrome. This condition can occur as an adverse reaction to corticosteroids.

4. Which of the following conditions indicates that a patient is experiencing an adverse reaction to azathioprine?
   A.   Kidney failure
   B.   Peptic ulcer
   C.   Bone marrow suppression

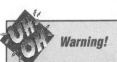

Warning!

Adverse reactions to other antigout drugs

Both allopurinol and colchicine commonly cause nausea, vomiting, diarrhea, and intermittent abdominal pain.

Allopurinol
The most common reaction to allopurinol is a rash.

Colchicine
Prolonged administration of colchicine may cause bone marrow suppression.

Answer: C. Bone marrow suppression indicates that a patient is experiencing an adverse reaction to azathioprine.

5. Which of the following is an adverse reaction to probenecid?

    A.   Edema

    B.   Vomiting

    C.   Vertigo

Answer: B. Vomiting is an adverse reaction to probenecid.

Scoring

☆☆☆   If you answered all five questions correctly, extraordinary! You certainly aren't allergic to smarts!

☆☆   If you answered three or four questions correctly, congratulations! You're taking the sting out of learning!

☆   If you answered fewer than three questions correctly, keep trying! With continued improvement, the next chapter should have you feeling better!

Psychiatric drugs

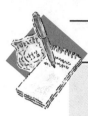

Just the facts

In this chapter, you'll review:

♦ classes of drugs that alter psychogenic behavior and promote sleep

♦ uses and varying actions of these drugs

♦ how these drugs are absorbed, distributed, metabolized, and excreted

♦ drug interactions and adverse reactions to these drugs.

Drugs and psychiatric disorders

This chapter presents drugs that are used to treat various sleep and psychogenic disorders, such as anxiety, depression, and psychotic disorders.

Sedative and hypnotic drugs

Sedatives reduce activity or excitement. Some degree of drowsiness commonly accompanies sedative use.

You're getting very sleepy...

When given in large doses, sedatives are considered hypnotics, which induce a state resembling natural sleep. The three main classes of synthetic drugs used as sedatives and hypnotics are:

 benzodiazepines

 barbiturates

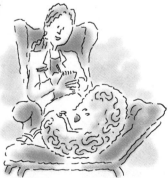

Just talking about hypnotics makes me sleepy.

nonbenzodiazepine-nonbarbiturate drugs.

And if that doesn't put you to sleep...

Other sedatives may include alcohol and over-the-counter sleep aids.

Benzodiazepines

Benzodiazepines produce many therapeutic effects, including:

- daytime sedation
- sedation before anesthesia
- sleep inducement
- relief of anxiety and tension
- skeletal muscle relaxation
- anticonvulsant activity.

Keep your eye on the hypnotic ones

Benzodiazepines are used in various clinical situations and exert either a primary or secondary sedative or hypnotic effect. Benzodiazepines used primarily for their sedative or hypnotic effects include:

- estazolam
- flurazepam hydrochloride
- lorazepam
- quazepam
- temazepam
- triazolam.

When some calm is needed

Benzodiazepines used primarily for the treatment of anxiety include:

- alprazolam
- chlordiazepoxide hydrochloride
- clorazepate dipotassium
- diazepam
- halazepam
- lorazepam
- oxazepam
- prazepam.

Pharmacokinetics (how drugs circulate)

Benzodiazepines are absorbed well from the GI tract and distributed widely in the body. Some may also be given parenterally.

Metabolism and excretion

All benzodiazepines are metabolized in the liver and excreted primarily in the urine.

Pharmacodynamics (how drugs act)

Researchers believe that benzodiazepines work by stimulating gamma-aminobutyric acid (GABA) receptors in the ascending reticular activating system (RAS) of the brain. This RAS is associated with wakefulness and attention and includes the cerebral cortex and limbic, thalamic, and hypothalamic levels of the central nervous system (CNS). (See *How benzodiazepines work*, page 262.)

Low will ease your mind

At low dosages, benzodiazepines decrease anxiety by acting on the limbic system and other areas of the brain that help regulate emotional activity. The drugs can usually calm or sedate the patient without causing drowsiness.

High will ease you into sleep

At higher dosages, benzodiazepines induce sleep, probably because they depress the RAS of the brain.

Zzzzzzzzzzzz...

Benzodiazepines increase total sleep time and produce a deep, refreshing sleep. In most cases, benzodiazepines decrease the time spent in rapid-eye-movement (REM) sleep, the state of sleep in which brain activity resembles the activity it shows when awake; the body's muscles relax, and the eyes move rapidly.

Flurazepam hydrochloride (in low dosages) and temazepam, however, don't diminish REM sleep significantly. Benzodiazepines that do decrease total REM sleep time also allow for more frequent REM cycles later in the sleep period.

Pharmacotherapeutics (how drugs are used)

Clinical indications for benzodiazepines include:
• relaxing the patient during the day of or before surgery

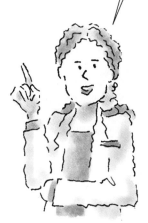

At low dosages, benzodiazepines decrease anxiety without causing drowsiness.

How benzodiazepines work

These illustrations show how benzodiazepines work at the cellular level.

Speed and passage

The speed of impulses from a presynaptic neuron across a synapse is influenced by the amount of chloride ions in the post-synaptic neuron. The passage of chloride ions into the postsynaptic neuron depends on the inhibitory neurotransmitter called gamma-aminobutyric acid, or GABA.

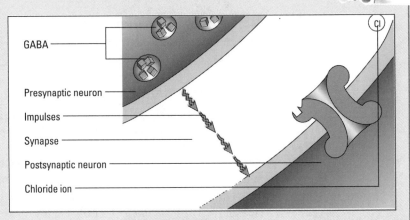

GABA

Presynaptic neuron

Impulses

Synapse

Postsynaptic neuron

Chloride ion

It binds

When GABA is released from the pre-synaptic neuron, it travels across the synapse and binds to GABA receptors on the postsynaptic neuron. This binding opens the chloride channels, allowing chloride ions to flow into the postsynaptic neuron and causing the nerve impulses to slow down.

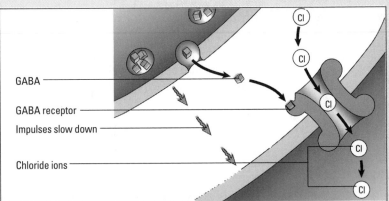

GABA

GABA receptor

Impulses slow down

Chloride ions

The result is another kind of depression

Benzodiazepines bind to receptors on or near the GABA receptor, enhancing the effect of GABA and allowing more chloride ions to flow into the postsynaptic neuron. This depresses the nerve impulses, causing them to slow down or stop.

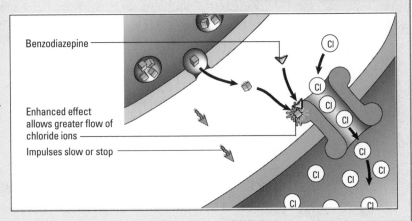

Benzodiazepine

Enhanced effect allows greater flow of chloride ions

Impulses slow or stop

- treating insomnia
- producing I.V. anesthesia
- treating alcohol withdrawal symptoms
- treating anxiety and seizure disorders
- producing skeletal muscle relaxation.

Drug interactions

Except for other CNS depressants, few drugs interact with benzodiazepines.

Deep sleep

When benzodiazepines are taken with other CNS depressants (including alcohol and anticonvulsants), the result is enhanced sedative and CNS depressant effects, including reduced level of consciousness, reduced muscle coordination, respiratory depression, and death.

Oral history

Oral contraceptives may reduce the metabolism of flurazepam hydrochloride, increasing the risk of toxicity. (See *Adverse reactions to benzodiazepines*.)

Barbiturates

The major pharmacologic action of *barbiturates* is to reduce overall CNS alertness. Barbiturates used primarily as sedatives and hypnotics include:

- amobarbital
- aprobarbital
- butabarbital sodium
- mephobarbital
- pentobarbital sodium
- phenobarbital
- secobarbital sodium.

On the dose

Low doses of barbiturates depress the sensory and motor cortex in the brain, causing drowsiness. High doses may cause respiratory depression and death because of their ability to depress all levels of the CNS.

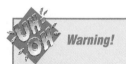

Warning!

Adverse reactions to benzodiazepines

Benzodiazepines may cause:
- amnesia
- fatigue
- muscle weakness
- mouth dryness
- nausea and vomiting
- dizziness
- ataxia (impaired ability to coordinate movement).

Getting groggy

Unintentional daytime sedation, hangover effect (residual drowsiness and impaired reaction time on awakening), and rebound insomnia may also occur.

One more may be one too many

Benzodiazepines have a potential for abuse, tolerance, and physical dependence.

Pharmacokinetics

Barbiturates are absorbed well from the GI tract, distributed rapidly, metabolized by the liver, and excreted in the urine.

Pharmacodynamics

As sedative-hypnotics, barbiturates depress the sensory cortex of the brain, decrease motor activity, alter cerebral function, and produce drowsiness, sedation, and hypnosis.

We interrupt this transmission...

These drugs appear to act throughout the CNS; however, the RAS of the brain, which is responsible for wakefulness, is a particularly sensitive site.

Pharmacotherapeutics

Barbiturates have many clinical indications, including:
• daytime sedation (for short periods only, typically less than 2 weeks)
• hypnotic effects for patients with insomnia
• preoperative sedation and anesthesia
• relief of anxiety
• anticonvulsant effects.

The decline of the barbiturates

With prolonged use of barbiturates, the patient can develop drug tolerance as well as psychological and physical dependence. In comparison, benzodiazepines are relatively effective and safe and, for these reasons, have replaced barbiturates as the sedatives and hypnotics of choice.

Drug interactions

Barbiturates may interact with many other drugs:
• They may reduce the effects of beta blockers (metoprolol, propranolol), chloramphenicol, corticosteroids, doxycycline, oral anticoagulants, oral contraceptives, quinidine, tricyclic antidepressants, metronidazole, theophylline, and cyclosporine.
• Hydantoins, such as phenytoin, reduce the metabolism of phenobarbital, resulting in increased toxic effects.

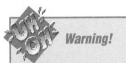

Warning!

Adverse reactions to barbiturates

Barbiturates may have widespread adverse effects.

S.O.S. for CNS
Central nervous system (CNS) reactions include:
• drowsiness
• lethargy
• headache
• depression.

Heart of the matter
Cardiovascular and respiratory effects include:
• mild bradycardia
• hypotension
• hypoventilation
• spasm of the larynx (voice box) and bronchi
• reduced rate of breathing
• severe respiratory depression.

All the rest
Other reactions include:
• vertigo
• nausea and vomiting
• diarrhea
• epigastric pain
• allergic reactions.

- Their use with methoxyflurane may stimulate production of methoxyflurane metabolites that are toxic to the kidneys.
- Their use with other CNS depressants may cause excessive CNS depression.
- Valproic acid may increase barbiturate levels.
- Monoamine oxidase (MAO) inhibitors inhibit metabolism of barbiturates, increasing their sedative effects.
- When they're taken with acetaminophen, an increased risk of liver toxicity results. (See *Adverse reactions to barbiturates*.)

Nonbenzodiazepines-nonbarbiturates

Nonbenzodiazepine-nonbarbiturate drugs act as hypnotics for short-term treatment of simple insomnia. These drugs, which offer no special advantages over other sedatives, include:
- chloral hydrate
- ethchlorvynol
- zolpidem.

Diminishing returns

With the exception of zolpidem, which may be effective for up to 35 days, nonbenzodiazepines-nonbarbiturates lose their effectiveness by the end of the 2nd week.

Pharmacokinetics

Nonbenzodiazepines-nonbarbiturates are absorbed rapidly from the GI tract, metabolized in the liver, and excreted in the urine.

Pharmacodynamics

The mechanism of action for nonbenzodiazepines-nonbarbiturates isn't fully known, but they produce depressant effects similar to barbiturates.

Pharmacotherapeutics

Nonbenzodiazepines-nonbarbiturates are typically used for:
- short-term treatment of simple insomnia
- sedation before surgery
- sedation before EEG studies.

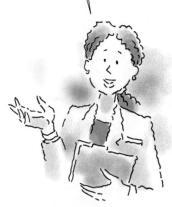

Most of these drugs lose their effectiveness after about 2 weeks.

Drug interactions

The main drug interaction involving nonbenzodiazepines-nonbarbiturates occurs when they're used with other CNS depressants, causing additive CNS depression resulting in drowsiness, respiratory depression, stupor, coma, and death.

A chlorus of interactions

Chloral hydrate may increase the risk of bleeding in patients taking oral anticoagulants. Use with I.V. furosemide may produce sweating, flushing, variable blood pressure, and uneasiness.

Ethchlorvynol reduces the effectiveness of oral anticoagulants, increasing the risk of clotting. (See *Adverse reactions to nonbenzodiazepines-nonbarbiturates.*)

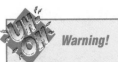

Warning!

Adverse reactions to nonbenzodiazepines-nonbarbiturates

The most common dose-related adverse reactions involving nonbenzodiazepines-nonbarbiturates include:
• nausea and vomiting
• gastric irritation
• hangover effects (possibly leading to respiratory depression or even respiratory failure).

Antidepressant and antimanic drugs

Antidepressant and *antimanic drugs* are used to treat affective disorders—disturbances in mood, characterized by depression or elation.

Pole positions

Unipolar disorders, characterized by periods of clinical depression, are treated with:
• MAO inhibitors
• tricyclic antidepressants
• other antidepressants.

Lithium is used to treat bipolar disorders, characterized by alternating periods of manic behavior and clinical depression.

MAO inhibitors

MAO inhibitors are divided into two classifications based on chemical structure:

☝ hydrazines, which include phenelzine sulfate

✌ nonhydrazines, comprised of a single drug, tranylcypromine sulfate.

Pharmacokinetics

MAO inhibitors are absorbed rapidly and completely from the GI tract and are metabolized in the liver to inactive metabolites. These metabolites are excreted mainly by the GI tract and to a lesser degree by the kidneys.

Pharmacodynamics

Although their exact mechanism of action is unclear, MAO inhibitors appear to work by inhibiting monoamine oxidase, the enzyme that normally metabolizes the neurotransmitters norepinephrine and serotonin, making more norepinephrine and serotonin available to the receptors and thereby relieving the symptoms of depression.

Pharmacotherapeutics

MAO inhibitors are the treatment of choice for atypical depression, which produces signs opposite of those of typical depression. For example, the patient gains weight, lacks suicidal tendencies, and has increased sexual drive.

It tackles typical depression, too

MAO inhibitors may be used to treat typical depression resistant to other therapies or when other therapies are contraindicated. Other uses include the treatment for:
• phobic anxieties
• neurodermatitis (an itchy skin disorder seen in anxious, nervous people)
• hypochondriasis (abnormal concern about health)
• refractory narcolepsy (sudden sleep attacks).

Drug interactions

MAO inhibitors interact with a wide variety of drugs:
• Taking MAO inhibitors with amphetamines, methylphenidate, levodopa, sympathomimetics, nonamphetamine appetite suppressants, and fenfluramine may increase catecholamine release, causing hypertension.
• Using them with fluoxetine, tricyclic antidepressants, clomipramine, trazodone, sertraline, paroxetine, and fluvoxamine may result in an elevated body temperature, excitation, and seizures.
• When taken with doxapram they may cause hypertension and arrhythmias and may increase the adverse reactions to doxapram.

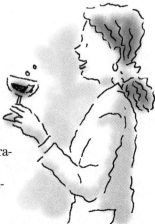

Tyramine-rich foods, such as red wine, can produce severe reactions if taken with MAO inhibitors.

• They may enhance the hypoglycemic effects of antidiabetic drugs.
• Administering them with meperidine may result in excitation, hypertension or hypotension, extremely elevated body temperature, and coma.

Forbidden fruit (and other foods)

Certain foods can interact with MAO inhibitors and produce severe reactions. The most serious reactions involve tyramine-rich foods, such as red wines, aged cheese, and fava beans, and sympathomimetic drugs. Foods with moderate tyramine contents—for example, yogurt and ripe bananas—may be eaten occasionally, but with care. (See *Adverse reactions to MAO inhibitors*.)

Tricyclic antidepressants

Tricyclic antidepressants are used to treat depression. They include:
• amitriptyline hydrochloride
• amitriptyline pamoate
• amoxapine
• clomipramine hydrochloride
• desipramine hydrochloride
• doxepin hydrochloride
• imipramine hydrochloride
• imipramine pamoate
• nortriptyline hydrochloride
• protriptyline hydrochloride
• trimipramine maleate.

Pharmacokinetics

All of the tricyclic antidepressants are active pharmacologically, and some of their metabolites are also active. They're absorbed completely when taken orally but undergo first-pass effect.

Distribution, metabolism, and excretion

With first-pass effect, a drug passes from the GI tract to the liver, where it's partially metabolized before entering the circulation. Tricyclic antidepressants are metabolized extensively in the liver and eventually excreted as inactive compounds (only small amounts of active drug are excreted) in the urine.

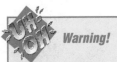

Warning!

Adverse reactions to MAO inhibitors

Adverse reactions to monoamine oxidase (MAO) inhibitors include:
• hypertensive crisis
• orthostatic hypertension
• restlessness
• drowsiness
• dizziness
• headache
• insomnia
• constipation
• anorexia
• nausea and vomiting
• weakness
• joint pain
• dry mouth
• blurred vision
• peripheral edema
• urine retention
• transient impotence
• rash
• skin and mucous membrane hemorrhage.

They just melt in fat

The extreme fat solubility of these drugs accounts for their wide distribution throughout the body, slow excretion, and long half-lives.

Pharmacodynamics

Researchers believe that tricyclic antidepressants increase the amount of norepinephrine, serotonin, or both by preventing their reuptake into the storage granules in the presynaptic nerves.

The upside to preventing reuptake

After a neurotransmitter has performed its job, several fates are possible, including rapidly reentering the neuron from which it was released (or reuptake). Preventing reuptake results in increased levels of these neurotransmitters in the synapses, relieving depression.

Pharmacotherapeutics

Tricyclic antidepressants are used to treat episodes of major depression. They're especially effective in treating depression of insidious onset accompanied by weight loss, anorexia, or insomnia. Physical signs and symptoms may respond after 1 to 2 weeks of therapy; psychological symptoms, after 2 to 4 weeks.

Problem patients

Tricyclic antidepressants are much less effective in patients with hypochondriasis, atypical depression, or depression accompanied by delusions. However, they may be helpful in treating acute episodes of depression.

The research goes on

Tricyclic antidepressants also are being investigated for use in preventing migraine headaches and in treating phobias, urinary incontinence, attention deficit disorder, duodenal or peptic ulcer disease, and diabetic neuropathy.

Drug interactions

Tricyclic antidepressants interact with several commonly used drugs:

- They increase the catecholamine effects of amphetamines and sympathomimetics, leading to hypertension.
- Barbiturates increase the metabolism of tricyclic antidepressants and decrease their blood levels.
- Cimetidine impairs metabolism of tricyclic antidepressants by the liver, increasing the risk of toxicity.
- Their concurrent use with MAO inhibitors may cause an extremely elevated body temperature, excitation, and seizures.
- An increased anticholinergic effect, such as dry mouth, urine retention, and constipation, is seen when anticholinergic drugs are taken with them.
- They reduce the antihypertensive effects of clonidine and guanethidine. (See *Adverse reactions to tricyclic antidepressants.*)

Selective serotonin reuptake inhibitors

Developed to treat depression with fewer adverse effects, *selective serotonin reuptake inhibitors,* commonly referred to as SSRIs, are chemically different from tricyclic antidepressants and MAO inhibitors. Some of the SSRIs currently available are:
- citalopram hydrobromide
- fluoxetine hydrochloride
- fluvoxamine maleate
- paroxetine hydrochloride
- sertraline hydrochloride.

Pharmacokinetics

SSRIs are absorbed almost completely after oral administration and are highly protein bound.

Metabolism and excretion

SSRIs are primarily metabolized in the liver and are excreted in the urine.

Pharmacodynamics

SSRIs inhibit the neuronal reuptake of the neurotransmitter serotonin.

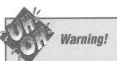
Warning!

Adverse reactions to tricyclic antidepressants

Adverse reactions to tricyclic antidepressants include:
- orthostatic hypotension (a drop in blood pressure on standing)
- sedation
- jaundice
- rashes
- photosensitivity reactions
- a fine resting tremor
- decreased sexual desire
- inhibited ejaculation
- transient eosinophilia
- reduced white blood cell count.

Special effects
Although rare, tricyclic antidepressant therapy may also lead to:
- granulocytopenia
- palpitations
- conduction delays
- rapid heartbeat.

Pharmacotherapeutics

SSRIs are used to treat the same major depressive episodes as tricyclic antidepressants and have the same degree of effectiveness. Fluvoxamine, fluoxetine, sertraline, and paroxetine are also used to treat obsessive-compulsive disorder. Paroxetine is also indicated for social anxiety disorder. (See *Putting a new stress on sertraline.*)

Don't panic, but there's more...

SSRIs may also be useful in treating panic disorders, eating disorders, personality disorders, impulse control disorders, and premenstrual syndrome.

Drug interactions

Drug interactions associated with SSRIs are associated with their ability to competitively inhibit a liver enzyme that is responsible for oxidation of numerous drugs, including tricyclic antidepressants; antipsychotics, such as clozapine and thioridazine; carbamazepine; metoprolol; flecainide; and encainide.

They don't mix with MAO inhibitors

Use of SSRIs with MAO inhibitors can cause serious, potentially fatal reactions. Individual SSRIs also have their own particular interactions:
• Use of citalopram and paroxetine with warfarin may lead to increased bleeding.
• Carbamazepine may increase clearance of citalopram.
• Fluoxetine increases the half-life of diazepam and displaces highly protein-bound drugs, leading to toxicity.
• Fluvoxamine use with diltiazem may cause bradycardia.
• Paroxetine shouldn't be used with tryptophan because this combination can cause headache, nausea, sweating, and dizziness.
• Paroxetine may increase procyclidine levels, causing increased anticholinergic effects.
• Cimetidine, phenobarbital, and phenytoin may reduce paroxetine metabolism by the liver, increasing the risk of toxicity.
• Paroxetine and sertraline may interact with other highly protein-bound drugs, causing adverse reactions to either drug. (See *Adverse reactions to SSRIs* and *Prozac peril*, page 272.)

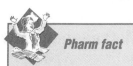

Pharm fact

Putting a new stress on sertraline

The Food and Drug Administration recently approved sertraline hydrochloride (Zoloft) as the first drug for treating posttraumatic stress disorder. Symptoms, such as intense fear, helplessness, and horror, must exist for at least 1 month and cause significant impaired functioning for use.

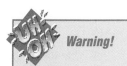

Warning!

Adverse reactions to SSRIs

Anxiety, insomnia, somnolence, and palpitations may occur with use of a serotonin selective reuptake inhibitor (SSRI).

Citalopram and paroxetine
Orthostatic hypotension may occur with citalopram and paroxetine.

Miscellaneous antidepressants

Other *antidepressants* in use today include:
• maprotiline and mirtazapine, tetracyclic antidepressants
• bupropion, a dopamine reuptake blocking agent
• venlafaxine, a serotonin-norepinephrine reuptake inhibitor
• trazodone, a triazopyridine agent
• nefazodone, a phenylpiperazine agent.

Pharmacokinetics

The paths these antidepressants take through the body may vary:
• Maprotiline and mirtazapine are absorbed from the GI tract, distributed widely in the body, metabolized by the liver, and excreted by the kidneys.
• Bupropion's absorption is unknown; it appears to be highly bound to plasma proteins. It's probably metabolized in the liver and is primarily excreted in urine.
• Venlafaxine is rapidly absorbed after oral administration, partially bound to plasma proteins, metabolized in the liver, and excreted in urine.
• Trazodone is well absorbed from the GI tract, distributed widely in the body, metabolized by the liver, and about 75% is excreted in urine. The remainder is excreted in feces.
• Nefazodone is rapidly and completely absorbed but, because of extensive metabolism, only about 20% of the drug is available. The drug is almost completely bound to plasma proteins and is excreted in the urine.

Pharmacodynamics

Much about how these drugs work has yet to be fully understood:
• Maprotiline and mirtazapine probably increase the amount of norepinephrine, serotonin, or both in the CNS by blocking their reuptake by presynaptic neurons (nerve terminals).

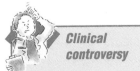

Clinical controversy

Prozac peril

Akathisia is a state of extreme agitation accompanied by suicidal thoughts, self-mutilation, and suicide attempts. The disorder can be caused by the antidepressant drug fluoxetine hydrochloride (Prozac). This adverse reaction occurs in at least 1% of patients.

Original Prozac packaging makes no mention of the link between akathisia and suicidal impulses. Health care providers are advised to be aware of the sudden onset of suicidal impulses in patients who were not previously suicidal. Meanwhile, new Prozac labels will provide a warning for Prozac users, substituting the words "suicidal ideation" for the word "depression."

• Bupropion is believed to inhibit the reuptake of the neurotransmitter dopamine.
• Venlafaxine is thought to potentiate neurotransmitter activity in the CNS by inhibiting the neural reuptake of serotonin and norepinephrine.
• Trazodone, although its effect is unknown, is thought to exert antidepressant effects by inhibiting the reuptake of norepinephrine and serotonin in the presynaptic neurons.
• Nefazodone's action isn't precisely defined. It inhibits neuronal uptake of serotonin and norepinephrine. It also occupies serotonin and alpha$_1$-adrenergic receptor sites.

Pharmacotherapeutics

These miscellaneous drugs are all used to treat depression. Trazodone may also be effective in treating aggressive behavior and panic disorder.

Drug interactions

All of these antidepressants may have serious, potentially fatal, reactions when combined with MAO inhibitors. Each of these drugs also carries its own specific risks when used with other drugs:
• Maprotiline and mirtazapine interact with CNS depressants to cause an additive effect.
• Bupropion combined with levodopa, phenothiazines, and tricyclic antidepressants increase the risk of adverse reactions, including seizures.
• Trazodone may increase serum levels of digoxin and phenytoin. Its use with antihypertensive agents may cause increased hypotensive effects. CNS depression may be enhanced if trazodone is administered with other CNS depressants.
• Nefazodone may increase the digoxin level if administered with digoxin. It increases CNS depression when combined with CNS depressants. (See *Adverse reactions to miscellaneous antidepressants.*)

Lithium

Lithium carbonate and *lithium citrate* are the drugs of choice to prevent or treat mania. The discovery of lithium was a milestone in treating mania and bipolar disorders.

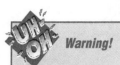

Warning!

Adverse reactions to miscellaneous antidepressants

These antidepressants may produce various adverse reactions.

Maprotiline
• Seizures
• Orthostatic hypotension
• Tachycardia
• Electrocardiographic changes

Mirtazapine
• Tremors
• Confusion
• Nausea
• Constipation

Bupropion
• Headache
• Confusion
• Tremor
• Agitation
• Tachycardia
• Anorexia
• Nausea and vomiting

Venlafaxine and nefazodone
• Headache
• Somnolence
• Dizziness
• Nausea

Trazodone
• Drowsiness
• Dizziness

Pharmacokinetics

When taken orally, lithium is absorbed rapidly and completely and is distributed to body tissues.

Metabolism and excretion

An active drug, lithium isn't metabolized and is excreted from the body unchanged.

Pharmacodynamics

In mania, the patient experiences excessive catecholamine stimulation. In bipolar disorder, the patient is affected by swings between the excessive catecholamine stimulation of mania and the diminished catecholamine stimulation of depression.

Returning to normal

Lithium may regulate catecholamine release in the CNS by:
• increasing norepinephrine and serotonin uptake
• reducing the release of norepinephrine from the synaptic vesicles (where neurotransmitters are stored) in the presynaptic neuron
• inhibiting norepinephrine's action in the postsynaptic neuron.

Getting more of the message

Researchers are also examining lithium's effects on electrolyte and ion transport. It may also modify actions of second messengers such as cyclic adenosine monophosphate.

Pharmacotherapeutics

Lithium is used primarily to treat acute episodes of mania and to prevent relapses of bipolar disorders.

Under investigation

Other uses of lithium being researched include preventing unipolar depression and migraine headaches, and treating depression, alcohol dependence, anorexia nervosa, syndrome of inappropriate antidiuretic hormone, and neutropenia.

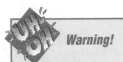

Warning!

Adverse reactions to lithium

Common adverse reactions to lithium include:
• reversible electrocardiographic changes
• thirst
• polyuria
• elevated white blood cell count.

A flood in the blood
Elevated toxic blood levels of lithium may produce:
• confusion
• lethargy
• slurred speech
• increased reflex reactions
• seizures.

No margin for error

Lithium has a narrow therapeutic margin of safety. A blood level that is even slightly higher than the therapeutic level can be dangerous.

Drug interactions

Serious interactions with other drugs can occur because of lithium's narrow therapeutic range:
• The risk of lithium toxicity increases when lithium is taken with thiazide and loop diuretics and nonsteroidal anti-inflammatory drugs.
• Administration of lithium with haloperidol, phenothiazines, and carbamazepine may produce an increased risk of neurotoxicity.
• Lithium may increase the hypothyroid effects of potassium iodide.
• Sodium bicarbonate may increase lithium excretion, reducing its effects.
• Lithium's effects are reduced when taken with theophylline.

Take this with a grain (or more) of salt

A patient on a severe salt-restricted diet is susceptible to lithium toxicity. On the other hand, an increased intake of sodium may reduce the therapeutic effects of lithium. (See *Adverse reactions to lithium*.)

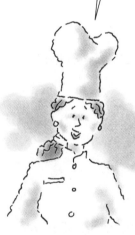

A regular salt intake helps to maintain steady lithium levels.

Antianxiety drugs

Antianxiety drugs, also called *anxiolytics*, include some of the most commonly prescribed drugs in the United States. They are used primarily to treat anxiety disorders. The three main types of antianxiety drugs are benzodiazepines (discussed in a previous section), barbiturates (also discussed in a previous section), and buspirone.

Buspirone

Buspirone hydrochloride is the first anxiolytic in a class of drugs known as azaspirodecanedione derivatives. This drug's structure and mechanism of action differ from those of other antianxiety drugs.

Advantage, buspirone

Buspirone has several advantages, including:
• less sedation
• no increase in CNS depressant effects when taken with alcohol or sedative-hypnotics
• lower abuse potential.

Pharmacokinetics

Buspirone is absorbed rapidly, undergoes extensive first-pass effect, and is metabolized in the liver to at least one active metabolite. The drug is eliminated in the urine and feces.

Pharmacodynamics

Although the mechanism of action of buspirone isn't known, it is known that buspirone doesn't affect GABA receptors like the benzodiazepines.

It's effective in the middle

Buspirone seems to produce various effects in the midbrain and acts as a midbrain modulator, possibly due to its high affinity for serotonin receptors.

Pharmacotherapeutics

Buspirone is used to treat generalized anxiety states. Patients who haven't received benzodiazepines seem to respond better to buspirone.

In case of panic

Because of its slow onset of action, buspirone is ineffective when quick relief from anxiety is needed.

Drug interactions

Unlike other antianxiety drugs, buspirone doesn't interact with alcohol or other CNS depressants. When buspirone is given with MAO inhibitors, hypertensive reactions may occur. (See *Adverse reactions to buspirone.*)

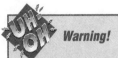

Warning!

Adverse reactions to buspirone

The most common reactions to buspirone include:
• dizziness
• light-headedness
• insomnia
• rapid heart rate
• palpitations
• headache.

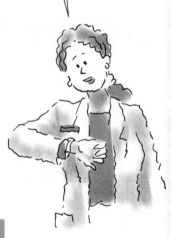

Buspirone has a slow onset, so it isn't useful for panic attacks.

Antipsychotic drugs

Antipsychotic drugs can control psychotic symptoms, such as delusions, hallucinations, and thought disorders, that can occur with schizophrenia, mania, and other psychoses.

By any other name

Drugs used to treat psychoses have several different names, including:
- antipsychotic, because they can eliminate signs and symptoms of psychoses
- major tranquilizer, because they can calm an agitated patient
- neuroleptic, because they have an adverse neurobiologic effect that causes abnormal body movements.

Two major groups

Regardless of what they're called, all antipsychotic drugs belong to one of two major groups:

typical antipsychotics, which include phenothiazines and nonphenothiazines

atypical antipsychotics, which include the newer agents, clozapine, olanzapine, and risperidone.

Typical antipsychotics

Typical antipsychotics, which include phenothiazines and nonphenothiazines, can be broken down into smaller classifications.

Different adverse reactions

Many clinicians believe that the phenothiazines should be treated as three distinct drug classes because of the differences in the adverse reactions they cause:
- Aliphatics primarily cause sedation and anticholinergic effects, and are moderately potent drugs that include chlorpromazine hydrochloride and promazine hydrochloride.
- Piperazines primarily cause extrapyramidal reactions, and include acetophenazine maleate, fluphenazine decanoate, fluphenazine enanthate, fluphenazine hydrochloride, perphenazine, and trifluoperazine hydrochloride.
- Piperidines primarily cause sedation, and include mesoridazine besylate and thioridazine hydrochloride.

Phenothiazines may produce effects up to 3 months after they're stopped.

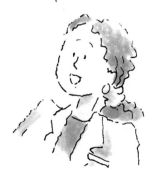

Different chemical structure

Based on their chemical structure, nonphenothiazine antipsychotics can be divided into several drug classes, including:

• butyrophenones, such as haloperidol and haloperidol decanoate
• dibenzoxazepines, such as loxapine succinate
• dihydroindolones, such as molindone hydrochloride
• diphenylbutylpiperidines, such as pimozide
• thioxanthenes, such as chlorprothixene, thiothixene, and thiothixene hydrochloride.

Pharmacokinetics

Although phenothiazines are absorbed erratically, they're very lipid soluble and highly protein-bound. Therefore, they're distributed to many tissues and are highly concentrated in the brain.

Like phenothiazines, nonphenothiazines are absorbed erratically, are lipid soluble, and are highly protein-bound. They're also distributed throughout the tissues and are highly concentrated in the brain.

Metabolism and excretion

All phenothiazines are metabolized in the liver and excreted in urine and bile. Because fatty tissues slowly release accumulated phenothiazine metabolites into the plasma, phenothiazines may produce effects up to 3 months after they're stopped.

Nonphenothiazines are also metabolized in the liver and excreted in the urine and bile.

Pharmacodynamics

Although the mechanism of action of phenothiazines isn't understood fully, researchers believe that these drugs work by blocking postsynaptic dopaminergic receptors in the brain.

The mechanism of action of nonphenothiazines resembles that of phenothiazines.

Erecting a blockade

The antipsychotic effect of phenothiazines comes about from receptor blockade in the limbic system and their antiemetic effect from the receptor blockade in the chemoreceptor trigger zone located in the brain's medulla.

Sending a charge

Phenothiazines also stimulate the extrapyramidal system (motor pathways that connect the cerebral cortex with the spinal nerve pathways).

Pharmacotherapeutics

Phenothiazines are used primarily to:
- treat schizophrenia
- calm anxious or agitated patients
- improve a patient's thought processes
- alleviate delusions and hallucinations.

Working overtime

Other therapeutic uses have been found for phenothiazines:
- They're administered to treat other psychiatric disorders, such as brief reactive psychosis, atypical psychosis, schizoaffective psychosis, autism, and major depression with psychosis.
- In combination with lithium, they're used in the treatment of patients with bipolar disorder, until the slower-acting lithium produces its therapeutic effect.
- They're prescribed to quiet mentally challenged children and agitated geriatric patients, particularly those with dementia.
- The preoperative effects of analgesics may be boosted with their addition.
- They're helpful in the management of pain, anxiety, and nausea in patients with cancer.

Solo solutions

As a group, nonphenothiazines are used to treat psychotic disorders. Thiothixene is also used to control acute agitation. Haloperidol and pimozide may be used to treat Tourette's syndrome as well.

Drug interactions

Phenothiazines interact with many different types of drugs and may have serious effects:
- Increased CNS depressant effects such as stupor may occur when they're taken with CNS depressants.

• CNS depressants may reduce phenothiazine effectiveness, resulting in increased psychotic behavior or agitation.
• Taking anticholinergic drugs with phenothiazines may result in increased anticholinergic effects such as dry mouth and constipation. By increasing phenothiazine metabolism, anticholinergic drugs may also reduce the antipsychotic effects of phenothiazines.
• Phenothiazines may reduce the antiparkinsonian effects of levodopa.
• Concurrent use with lithium increases the risk of neurotoxicity.
• Concurrent use with droperidol increases the risk of extrapyramidal effects.
• The threshold for seizures is lowered when phenothiazines are used with anticonvulsants.
• Phenothiazines may increase the serum levels of tricyclic antidepressants and beta blockers. (See *Adverse reactions to typical antipsychotics.*)

Fewer interactions

Nonphenothiazines interact with fewer drugs than phenothiazines. Their dopamine-blocking activity can inhibit levodopa and may cause disorientation in patients receiving both medications. Haloperidol may boost the effects of lithium, producing encephalopathy (brain dysfunction).

Atypical antipsychotics

Atypical antipsychotic drugs are new agents designed to treat schizophrenia. They include:
• clozapine
• olanzapine
• risperidone.

Pharmacokinetics

Atypical antipsychotics are absorbed after oral administration.

Metabolism and excretion

Atypical antipsychotics are metabolized by the liver. Metabolites of clozapine and olanzapine are inactive, whereas risperidone has an active metabolite. They're

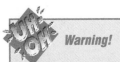

Warning!

Adverse reactions to typical antipsychotics

Neurologic reactions are the most common and serious adverse reactions associated with phenothiazines.

Extrapyramidal symptoms
Extrapyramidal symptoms (EPS) may appear after the first few days of therapy; tardive dyskinesia may occur after several years of treatment.

S.O.S! Extreme EPS!
Neuroleptic malignant syndrome is a potentially fatal condition that produces muscle rigidity, extreme EPS, severely elevated body temperature, hypertension, and rapid heart rate. If left untreated, it can result in respiratory failure and cardiovascular collapse.

Little difference
Most nonphenothiazines cause the same adverse reactions as phenothiazines.

highly plasma protein-bound and eliminated in the urine, with a small portion eliminated in feces.

Pharmacodynamics

Atypical antipsychotics typically block the dopamine receptors, but not as effectively as the typical antipsychotics, in addition to blocking serotonin receptor activity.

Putting it together

These combined actions account for the effectiveness of atypical antipsychotics against the positive and negative symptoms of schizophrenia with minimal extrapyramidal effects.

Pharmacotherapeutics

Atypical antipsychotics are indicated for schizophrenic patients who are unresponsive to typical antipsychotics.

Catching on

Because of the decreased instance of extrapyramidal effects with atypical antipsychotics, they're becoming widely prescribed.

Drug interactions

Drugs that alter the P-450 enzyme system will alter the metabolism of atypical antipsychotics.

The straight "dopa"

Atypical antipsychotics counteract the effects of levodopa and other dopamine agonists. (See *Adverse reactions to atypical antipsychotics*.)

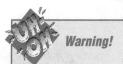
Warning!

Adverse reactions to atypical antipsychotics

Atypical antipsychotics have less extrapyramidal effects than typical antipsychotics.

Clozapine
Clozapine is associated with agranulocytosis (an abnormal decrease in white blood cells).

Olanzapine
Olanzapine places the patient at minimal risk for seizures and extrapyramidal effects.

Risperidone
Risperidone has a higher risk for extrapyramidal effects than other atypical antipsychotics and is also associated with a minimal risk for seizures and agranulocytosis.

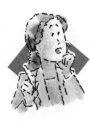

Quick quiz

1. What is the difference between a sedative and a hypnotic?

    A.   Sedatives produce physical dependence; hypnotics don't.

    B.   Sedatives reduce activity or excitement; hypnotics induce sleep.

    C.   Sedatives require larger doses than hypnotics to produce desired effects.

Answer: B. Sedatives reduce activity or excitement; hypnotics induce sleep.

2. With use of the nonbenzodiazepine-nonbarbiturate chloral hydrate, what adverse reactions are most likely?

    A.   Severe withdrawal symptoms

    B.   Hypersensitivity reactions

    C.   GI symptoms and hangover effects

Answer: C. GI symptoms and hangover effects are common adverse reactions to chloral hydrate.

3. Which of the following medications should a patient treated with lithium avoid?

    A.   Oral contraceptives

    B.   Loop diuretics

    C.   Oral antidiabetic drugs

Answer: B. Lithium shouldn't be prescribed with loop diuretics.

Scoring

    If you answered all three questions correctly, extraordinary! You definitely aren't psyched out by pharmacology!

    If you answered two questions correctly, congratulations! Your knowledge should have you feeling elated!

   If you answered fewer than two questions correctly, there's no need for anxiety! By the end of the next chapter, you'll probably have your head on straight!

12

Endocrine drugs

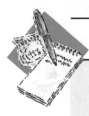

Just the facts

In this chapter, you'll review:

♦ classes of drugs that affect the endocrine system

♦ uses and varying actions of these drugs

♦ how these drugs are absorbed, distributed, metabolized, and excreted

♦ drug interactions and adverse reactions to these drugs.

Drugs and the endocrine system

The endocrine system consists of glands, which are specialized cell clusters, and hormones, the chemical transmitters secreted by the glands in response to stimulation.

Keeping well balanced

Together with the central nervous system, the endocrine system regulates and integrates the body's metabolic activities and maintains homeostasis (the body's internal equilibrium). The drug classes that treat endocrine system disorders include:
- natural hormones and their synthetic analogues
- hormonelike substances
- drugs that stimulate or suppress hormone secretion.

Antidiabetic drugs and glucagon

Insulin, a pancreatic hormone, and oral antidiabetic drugs are classified as *hypoglycemic drugs* because they lower blood glucose levels. Glucagon, another pancreatic hormone, is classified as a *hyperglycemic drug* because it raises blood glucose levels.

Sugar surplus

Diabetes mellitus, or simply diabetes, is a chronic disease of insulin deficiency or resistance. It's characterized by disturbances in carbohydrate, protein, and fat metabolism. This leads to elevated levels of the sugar glucose in the body. The disease comes in two primary forms:

☞ type 1, previously referred to as insulin-dependent diabetes mellitus

✌ type 2, previously referred to as non-insulin-dependent diabetes mellitus.

Insulin

Patients with type 1 diabetes require an external source of insulin to control blood glucose levels. *Insulin* also may be given to patients with type 2 diabetes.

Pharmacokinetics (how drugs circulate)

Insulin isn't effective when taken orally because the GI tract breaks down the protein molecule before it reaches the bloodstream.

Under the skin

All insulins, however, may be given by subcutaneous (S.C.) injection. Absorption of S.C. insulin varies according to the injection site, the blood supply, and degree of tissue hypertrophy at the injection site.

In the I.V. league

Regular insulin may also be given intravenously (I.V.) as well as in dialysate fluid infused into the peritoneal cavity for patients on peritoneal dialysis therapy.

Distribution, metabolism, and excretion

After absorption into the bloodstream, insulin is distributed throughout the body. Insulin-responsive tissues are located in the liver, adipose tissue, and muscle. Insulin is metabolized primarily in the liver, to a lesser extent in the kidneys and muscle, and is excreted in the feces and urine.

Pharmacodynamics (how drugs act)

Insulin is an anabolic, or building, hormone that promotes:
- storage of glucose as glycogen
- increase in protein and fat synthesis
- slowing of the breakdown of glycogen, protein, and fat
- balancing of fluids and electrolytes.

Insulin special effects

Although it has no antidiuretic effect, insulin can correct the polyuria (excessive urination) and polydipsia (excessive thirst) associated with the osmotic diuresis associated with hyperglycemia by decreasing the blood glucose level. Insulin also facilitates the movement of potassium from the extracellular fluid into the cell. (See *How insulin aids glucose uptake*, page 286.)

Pharmacotherapeutics (how drugs are used)

Insulin is indicated for:
- type 1 diabetes
- type 2 diabetes when other methods of controlling blood glucose levels have failed or are contraindicated
- type 2 diabetes when blood glucose levels are elevated during periods of emotional or physical stress (such as infection and surgery)
- type 2 diabetes when oral antidiabetic drugs are contraindicated because of pregnancy or hypersensitivity.

When things get complicated

Insulin is also used to treat two complications of diabetes: diabetic ketoacidosis, more common with type 1 diabetes, and hyper-

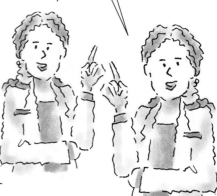

Insulin is used to treat type 1 diabetes.

It's also used to treat type 2 diabetes during periods of stress or when other methods have failed or are contraindicated.

How insulin aids glucose uptake

These illustrations show how insulin allows a cell to use glucose for energy.

1. Glucose cannot enter the cell without the aid of insulin.

2. Normally produced by the beta cells of the pancreas, insulin binds to the receptors on the surface of the target cell. Insulin and its receptor first move to the inside of the cell, which activates glucose transporter channels to move to the surface of the cell.

3. These channels allow glucose to enter the cell. The cell can then utilize the glucose for metabolism.

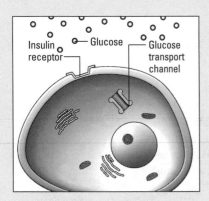
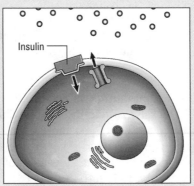
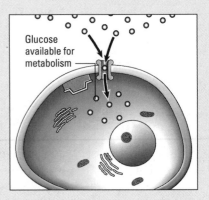

osmolar hyperglycemic nonketotic syndrome, which is more common with type 2 diabetes.

What? But I don't have diabetes...

Insulin is also used to treat severe hyperkalemia (elevated serum potassium levels) in patients without diabetes. Potassium moves with glucose from the bloodstream into the cell, lowering serum potassium levels.

Drug interactions

Some drugs interact with insulin, altering its ability to decrease the blood glucose level; other drugs directly affect glucose levels:

• Anabolic steroids, salicylates, alcohol, and monoamine oxidase (MAO) inhibitors may increase the hypoglycemic effect of insulin.

• Corticosteroids, sympathomimetic drugs, thiazide diuretics, and dextrothyroxine sodium may reduce the effects of insulin, resulting in hyperglycemia.

• Beta blockers may prolong the hypoglycemic effect of insulin and may mask signs and symptoms of hypoglycemia. (See *Adverse reactions to insulin.*)

Oral antidiabetic drugs

Most *oral antidiabetic drugs* approved for use in the United States are sulfonylureas. Types of oral antidiabetic drugs available include:
• first-generation sulfonylureas, which include acetohexamide, chlorpropamide, tolazamide, and tolbutamide
• second-generation sulfonylureas, which include glipizide and glyburide
• nonsulfonylureas, thiazolidinedione antidiabetic drugs, pioglitazone and rosiglitazone
• a biguanide drug, metformin
• an alpha-glucosidase inhibitor, acarbose.

Pharmacokinetics

Oral antidiabetic drugs are absorbed well from the GI tract and distributed via the bloodstream throughout the body.

Metabolism and excretion

Oral antidiabetic drugs are metabolized primarily in the liver and are excreted mostly in the urine, with some excreted in the bile. Glyburide is excreted equally in the urine and feces; rosiglitazone is largely excreted in both.

Pharmacodynamics

It's believed that oral antidiabetic drugs produce actions both within and outside the pancreas (extrapancreatic) to regulate blood glucose.

Pancreas partners

Oral antidiabetic drugs probably stimulate pancreatic beta cells to release insulin in a patient with a minimally functioning pancreas. Within a few weeks to a few months of starting sulfonylureas, pancreatic insulin secretion drops to pretreatment levels, but blood glucose levels remain normal or near-normal. Most likely, it's the actions of the oral anti-

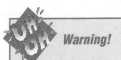

Warning!

Adverse reactions to insulin

Adverse reactions to insulin include:
• hypoglycemia (below-normal blood glucose levels)
• Somogyi effect (hypoglycemia followed by rebound hyperglycemia)
• hypersensitivity reactions
• lipodystrophy (disturbance in fat deposition)
• insulin resistance.

With all this pharmacology to learn, I sometimes feel I'm only minimally functioning. That's the least the pancreas must be doing for an oral antidiabetic drug to work.

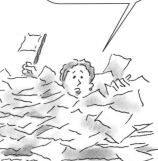

diabetic agents outside of the pancreas that maintain this glucose control.

Working beyond the pancreas

Oral antidiabetic drugs provide several extrapancreatic actions to decrease and control blood glucose. They can go to work in the liver and decrease glucose production (gluconeogenesis) there. Also, by increasing the number of insulin receptors in the peripheral tissues, they provide more opportunities for the cells to bind sufficiently with insulin, initiating the process of glucose metabolism.

Getting in on the action

Other oral antidiabetic agents produce specific actions:
• Pioglitazone and rosiglitazone improve insulin sensitivity.
• Metformin decreases liver production of glucose and intestinal absorption of glucose and improves insulin sensitivity.
• Acarbose inhibits enzymes, delaying glucose absorption.

Pharmacotherapeutics

Oral antidiabetic drugs are indicated for patients with type 2 diabetes if diet and exercise can't control blood glucose levels. These drugs aren't effective in type 1 diabetes because the pancreatic beta cells aren't functioning at a minimal level.

The old 1-2 punch

Combination oral antidiabetic drug and insulin therapy may be indicated for some patients who don't respond to either drug alone.

Drug interactions

Hypoglycemia and hyperglycemia are the main risks when oral antidiabetic drugs interact with other drugs.

Getting too low

Hypoglycemia may occur when sulfonylureas are combined with alcohol, anabolic steroids, chloramphenicol, clofibrate, gemfibrozil, MAO inhibitors, phenylbutazone, salicylates, sulfonamides, fluconazole, cimetidine, coumadin, and ranitidine. It may also occur when met-

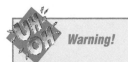

Warning!

Adverse reactions to oral antidiabetics

Hypoglycemia is a major adverse reaction common to all oral antidiabetic drugs. Here are some common oral antidiabetics and their adverse reactions.

Sulfonylureas
• Nausea
• Epigastric fullness
• Blood abnormalities
• Water retention
• Rash
• Hyponatremia
• Photosensitivity

Metformin
• Metallic taste
• Nausea and vomiting
• Abdominal discomfort

Acarbose
• Abdominal pain
• Diarrhea
• Gas

formin is combined with cimetidine, nifedipine, procainamide, ranitidine, and vancomycin.

Going too high

Hyperglycemia may occur when sulfonylureas are taken with corticosteroids, dextrothyroxine, rifampin, sympathomimetics, and thiazide diuretics. (See *Adverse reactions to oral antidiabetics*.)

Glucagon

Glucagon, a hyperglycemic drug that raises blood glucose levels, is a hormone normally produced by the alpha cells of the islets of Langerhans in the pancreas. (See *How glucagon raises glucose levels*, page 290.)

Pharmacokinetics

After S.C., I.M., or I.V. injection, glucagon is absorbed rapidly. Glucagon is distributed throughout the body, although its effect occurs primarily in the liver.

Metabolism and excretion

Glucagon is degraded extensively by the liver, kidneys, and plasma, and at its tissue receptor sites in plasma membranes. It's removed from the body by the liver and the kidneys.

Pharmacodynamics

Glucagon regulates the rate of glucose production through:
• glycogenolysis, the conversion of glycogen back into glucose by the liver
• gluconeogenesis, the formation of glucose from free fatty acids and proteins
• lipolysis, the release of fatty acids from adipose tissue for conversion to glucose.

Pharmacotherapeutics

Glucagon is used for emergency treatment of severe hypoglycemia. It's also used during radiologic examination of the GI tract to reduce GI motility.

> Glucagon can't be taken orally because it would be destroyed in the GI tract. After I.V. injection, it's absorbed rapidly to supply glucose to starving cells.

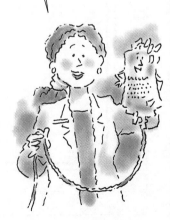

How glucagon raises glucose levels

When adequate stores of glycogen are present, glucagon can raise glucose levels in patients with severe hypoglycemia. What happens is easy to follow:

• Initially, glucagon stimulates the formation of adenylate cyclase in the liver cell.
• Adenylate cyclase then converts adenosine triphosphate (ATP) to cyclic adenosine monophosphate (cAMP).
• This product initiates a series of reactions that result in an active phosphorylated glucose molecule.

• In this phosphorylated form, the large glucose molecule can't pass through the cell membrane.
• Through glycogenolysis (the breakdown of glycogen, the stored form of glucose), the liver removes the phosphate group and allows the glucose to enter the bloodstream, raising blood glucose levels for short-term energy needs.

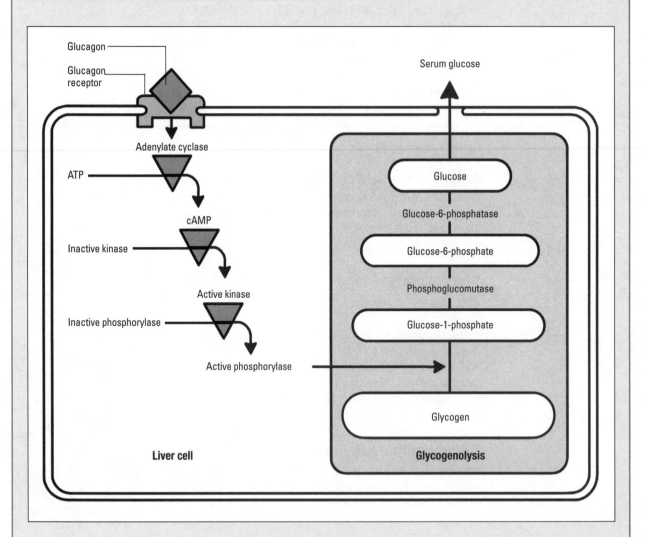

Drug interactions

Glucagon interacts adversely only with oral anticoagulants, increasing the tendency to bleed. Adverse reactions to glucagon are rare.

Thyroid and antithyroid drugs

Thyroid and antithyroid drugs function to correct thyroid hormone deficiency (hypothyroidism) and thyroid hormone excess (hyperthyroidism).

Thyroid drugs

Thyroid drugs can be natural or synthetic hormones and may contain triiodothyronine (T_3), thyroxine (T_4), or both.

All natural

Natural thyroid drugs are made from animal thyroid and include:
- thyroid USP (desiccated), which contains both T_3 and T_4
- thyroglobulin, which also contains both T_3 and T_4.

Man-made

Synthetic thyroid drugs actually are the sodium salts of the L-isomers of the hormones. These synthetic hormones include:
- levothyroxine sodium, which contains T_4
- liothyronine sodium, which contains T_3
- liotrix, which contains both T_3 and T_4.

Pharmacokinetics

Thyroid hormones are absorbed variably from the GI tract, distributed in plasma, and bound to serum proteins.

Metabolism and excretion

Thyroid drugs are metabolized through deiodination, primarily in the liver, and excreted unchanged in the feces.

Pharmacodynamics

The principal pharmacologic effect is an increased metabolic rate in body tissues. Thyroid hormones affect protein and carbohydrate metabolism and stimulate protein synthesis. They promote gluconeogenesis (the formation of glucose from free fatty acids and proteins) and increase the use of glycogen stores.

They get the heart pumping...

Thyroid hormones increase heart rate and cardiac output (the amount of blood pumped by the heart each minute). They may even increase the heart's sensitivity to catecholamines and increase the number of beta-adrenergic receptors in the heart (stimulation of beta receptors in the heart increases heart rate and contractility).

...and the blood flowing

Thyroid hormones may increase blood flow to the kidneys and increase the glomerular filtration rate (the amount of plasma filtered through the kidney each minute) in hypothyroid patients, producing diuresis.

Pharmacotherapeutics

Thyroid drugs act as replacement or substitute hormones in the following situations:
• to treat the many forms of hypothyroidism
• with antithyroid drugs to prevent goiter formation (an enlarged thyroid gland) and hypothyroidism
• to differentiate between primary and secondary hypothyroidism during diagnostic testing
• to treat papillary or follicular thyroid carcinoma.

The drug of choice

Levothyroxine is the drug of choice for thyroid hormone replacement and thyroid-stimulating hormone suppression therapy.

Drug interactions

Thyroid drugs interact with several common medications:
• They increase the effects of oral anticoagulants, increasing the tendency to bleed.
• Cholestyramine and colestipol reduce the absorption of thyroid hormones.

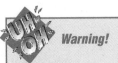

Warning!

Adverse reactions to thyroid drugs

Most adverse reactions to thyroid drugs result from toxicity.

Gut reactions
Adverse reactions in GI system include:
• diarrhea
• abdominal cramps
• weight loss
• increased appetite.

Heart of the matter
Adverse reactions in the cardiovascular system include:
• palpitations
• sweating
• rapid heart rate
• increased blood pressure
• angina
• arrhythmias.

Toxic topics
General manifestations of toxic doses include:
• headache
• tremor
• insomnia
• nervousness
• fever
• heat intolerance
• menstrual irregularities.

• Phenytoin may displace thyroxine from plasma binding sites, temporarily increasing levels of free thyroxine.
• Taking thyroid drugs with digoxin may reduce serum digoxin levels, increasing the risk of arrhythmias or heart failure.
• Carbamazepine increases metabolism of thyroid hormones, reducing their effectiveness.
• Serum theophylline levels may increase when theophylline is administered with thyroid drugs. (See *Adverse reactions to thyroid drugs.*)

Antithyroid drugs

A number of drugs act as *antithyroid drugs*, or *thyroid antagonists*. Used for patients with hyperthyroidism (thyrotoxicosis), these drugs include:
• thionamides, which include propylthiouracil and methimazole
• iodides, which include stable iodine and radioactive iodine.

Pharmacokinetics

Thionamides and iodides are absorbed through the GI tract, concentrated in the thyroid, metabolized by conjugation, and excreted in the urine.

Pharmacodynamics

Drugs used to treat hyperthyroidism work in different ways.

The antithesis to synthesis

Thionamides block iodine's ability to combine with tyrosine, thereby preventing thyroid hormone synthesis.

In Wolff(-Chaikoff)'s clothing

Stable iodine inhibits hormone synthesis through the Wolff-Chaikoff effect, in which excess iodine decreases the formation and release of thyroid hormone.

Warning: Radioactive material

Radioactive iodine reduces hormone secretion by destroying thyroid tissue through induction of acute radiation thyroiditis (inflammation of the thyroid gland) and chronic gradual thyroid atrophy. Acute radiation thyroiditis usually occurs 3 to 10 days after administering radioactive iodine. Chronic thyroid atrophy may take several years to appear.

Pharmacotherapeutics

Antithyroid drugs commonly are used to treat hyperthyroidism, especially in the form of Graves' disease (hyperthyroidism caused by autoimmunity) which accounts for 85% of all cases.

In case of removal

To treat hyperthyroidism, the thyroid gland may be removed by surgery or destroyed by radiation. Before surgery, stable iodine is used to prepare the gland for surgical removal by firming it and decreasing its vascularity.

Stable iodine is also used after radioactive iodine therapy to control symptoms of hyperthyroidism while the radiation takes effect.

If it gets too severe

Propylthiouracil, which lowers serum T_3 levels faster than methimazole, is usually used for rapid improvement of severe hyperthyroidism.

When taking them for two

Propylthiouracil is preferred over methimazole in pregnant women because its rapid action reduces transfer across the placenta and because it doesn't cause aplasia cutis (a severe skin disorder) in the fetus.

One a day keeps the trouble away

Because methimazole blocks thyroid hormone formation for a longer time, it's better suited for administration once per day to patients with mild to moderate hyperthyroidism. Therapy may continue for 12 to 24 months before remission occurs.

Drug interactions

Iodide preparations may react synergistically with lithium, causing hypothyroidism. Other interactions aren't clinically significant. (See *Adverse reactions to antithyroid drugs.*)

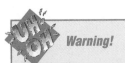 *Warning!*

Adverse reactions to antithyroid drugs

The most serious adverse reaction to thionamide therapy is granulocytopenia. Hypersensitivity reactions may also occur.

The iodides
The iodides can cause an unpleasant brassy taste and burning sensation in the mouth, increased salivation, and painful swelling of the parotid glands.

Too sensitive
Rarely, I.V. iodine administration can cause an acute hypersensitivity reaction. Radioactive iodine also can cause a rare — but acute — reaction 3 to 14 days after administration.

Pituitary drugs

Pituitary drugs are natural or synthetic hormones that mimic the hormones produced by the pituitary gland. The pituitary drugs consist of two groups:

Anterior pituitary drugs may be used diagnostically or therapeutically to control the function of other endocrine glands, such as the thyroid gland, adrenals, ovaries, and testes.

Posterior pituitary drugs may be used to regulate fluid volume and stimulate smooth-muscle contraction in selected clinical situations.

Anterior pituitary drugs

The protein hormones produced in the anterior pituitary gland regulate growth, development, and sexual characteristics by stimulating the actions of other endocrine glands. *Anterior pituitary drugs* include:
• adrenocorticotropics, which include corticotropin, corticotropin repository, corticotropin zinc hydroxide, and cosyntropin
• somatrem, a growth hormone
• gonadotropics, which include chorionic gonadotropin and menotropins
• thyrotropics, which include thyroid-stimulating hormone, thyrotropin, and protirelin.

Pharmacokinetics

Anterior pituitary drugs aren't given orally because they're destroyed in the GI tract. Some of these hormones can be administered topically, but most require injection.

Absorption, distribution, and metabolism
Usually, natural hormones are absorbed, distributed, and metabolized rapidly. Some analogues, however, are absorbed and metabolized more slowly. Anterior pituitary hormone drugs are metabolized at the receptor site and in the liver and kidneys. The hormones are excreted primarily in the urine.

Anterior pituitary drugs act on endocrine glands, such as the thyroid gland, adrenals, ovaries, and testes, to control their functions.

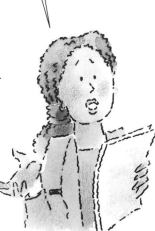

Pharmacodynamics

Anterior pituitary drugs exert a profound effect on the body's growth and development. The hypothalamus controls secretions of the pituitary gland. In turn, the pituitary gland secretes hormones that regulate secretions or functions of other glands.

Concentrate on this formula

The concentration of hormones in the blood helps determine hormone production rate. Increased hormone levels inhibit hormone production; decreased levels raise production and secretion.

Pharmacotherapeutics

The clinical indications for anterior pituitary hormone drugs are diagnostic and therapeutic:
• Corticotropin and cosyntropin are used diagnostically to differentiate between primary and secondary failure of the adrenal cortex.
• Corticotropin is also used to treat adrenal insufficiency.
• Somatrem is used to treat pituitary dwarfism.

Drug interactions

Anterior pituitary drugs interact with several different types of drugs:
• Administering immunizations to a person receiving corticotropin increases the risk of neurologic complications and may reduce the antibody response.
• Corticotropin reduces salicylate levels.
• Enhanced potassium loss may occur when diuretics are taken with corticotropins.
• Barbiturates, phenytoin, and rifampin increase the metabolism of corticotropin, reducing its effects.
• Estrogen increases the effect of corticotropin.
• Taking estrogens, amphetamines, and lithium with cosyntropin can alter results of adrenal function tests.
• Amphetamines and androgens (concurrently) administered with somatrem may promote epiphyseal (cartilaginous bone growth plate) closure.
• Concurrent use of somatrem and corticosteroids inhibits the growth-promoting action of somatrem. (See *Adverse reactions to anterior pituitary drugs.*)

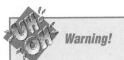

Warning!

Adverse reactions to anterior pituitary drugs

The major adverse reactions to pituitary drugs are hypersensitivity reactions.

Over the long haul
Long-term use of corticotropin can cause Cushing's syndrome.

Posterior pituitary drugs

Posterior pituitary hormones are synthesized in the hypothalamus and stored in the posterior pituitary, which, in turn, secretes the hormones into the blood. These drugs include:
• all forms of antidiuretic hormone (ADH), such as desmopressin acetate, lypressin, and vasopressin
• the oxytocic drugs oxytocin and oxytocin citrate.

Pharmacokinetics

Because enzymes in the GI tract can destroy all protein hormones, these drugs can't be given orally. Posterior pituitary drugs may be given by injection or intranasal spray.

Absorption, distribution, and metabolism

Like other natural hormones, oxytocic drugs usually are absorbed, distributed, and metabolized rapidly. Parenterally administered oxytocin is absorbed rapidly, but when it's administered intranasally, absorption is erratic.

Pharmacodynamics

Under neural control, posterior pituitary hormones affect:
• smooth-muscle contraction in the uterus, bladder, and GI tract
• fluid balance through kidney reabsorption of water
• blood pressure through stimulation of the arterial wall muscles.

Going to cAMP

ADH increases cyclic adenosine monophosphate (cAMP), which increases the permeability of the tubular epithelium in the kidneys, promoting reabsorption of water. High dosages of ADH stimulate contraction of blood vessels, increasing the blood pressure.

Desmopressin reduces diuresis and promotes clotting by increasing the plasma level of factor VIII (antihemophilic factor).

Baby talk

In pregnant women, oxytocin may stimulate uterine contractions by increasing the permeability of uterine cell

When taking certain drugs, you need to be careful to avoid diuretics such as furosemide. For example, corticotropin interacts with diuretics to enhance potassium loss.

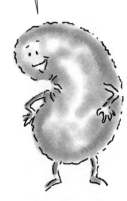

Without ADH, I can't reabsorb fluid.

membranes to sodium ions. It also can stimulate lactation through its effect on mammary glands.

Pharmacotherapeutics

ADH is prescribed for hormone replacement therapy in patients with neurogenic diabetes insipidus (an excessive loss of urine caused by a brain lesion or injury that interferes with ADH synthesis or release). However, it doesn't effectively treat nephrogenic diabetes insipidus (caused by renal tubular resistance to ADH).

The ABC's of ADH treatment

Desmopressin and lypressin are the drugs of choice for chronic ADH deficiency and are administered intranasally. These drugs are particularly useful for patients allergic or refractory to a vasopressin of animal origin.

Short-term ADH treatment is indicated for patients with transient diabetes insipidus after head injury or surgery; therapy may be lifelong for patients with idiopathic hormone deficiencies. Used for short-term therapy, vasopressin elevates blood pressure in patients with hypotension caused by lack of vascular tone. It also relieves postoperative gaseous distention.

They help with deliveries (before, during, and after)

Oxytocics are used to:
• induce labor and complete incomplete abortions
• treat preeclampsia, eclampsia, and premature rupture of membranes
• control bleeding and uterine relaxation after delivery
• hasten uterine shrinking after delivery
• stimulate lactation.

Drug interactions

Drug interactions with posterior pituitary drugs can occur with various drugs:
• Alcohol, demeclocycline, and lithium may decrease ADH activity of desmopressin, lypressin, and vasopressin.
• Chlorpropamide, clofibrate, carbamazepine, and cyclophosphamide increase ADH activity.
• Synergistic effects may occur when barbiturates or cyclopropane anesthetics are used concurrently with ADH, leading to coronary insufficiency or arrhythmias.

• Cyclophosphamide may increase the oxytocic effect of oxytocin.
• Concurrent use of vasopressors (anesthetics, ephedrine, methoxamine) and oxytocin increases the risk of hypertensive crisis and postpartum rupture of cerebral blood vessels. (See *Adverse reactions to posterior pituitary drugs.*)

Estrogens

Estrogens mimic the physiologic effects of naturally occurring female sex hormones.

To serve and protect

Estrogens are used to correct estrogen-deficient states and, along with oral contraceptives, prevent pregnancy.

Estrogen types

Estrogens that treat endocrine system disorders include:
• the natural products conjugated estrogenic substances, estradiol, and estrone
• the synthetic estrogens chlorotrianisene, dienestrol, diethylstilbestrol, diethylstilbestrol diphosphate, esterified estrogens, estradiol cypionate, estradiol valerate, ethinyl estradiol, and quinestrol.

Pharmacokinetics

Estrogens are absorbed well and distributed throughout the body. Metabolism occurs in the liver, and the metabolites are excreted primarily by the kidneys.

Pharmacodynamics

The exact mechanism of action of estrogen isn't clearly understood but it's believed to increase synthesis of deoxyribonucleic acid (DNA), ribonucleic acid (RNA), and protein in estrogen-responsive tissues in the female breast, urinary tract, and genital organs.

Pharmacotherapeutics

Estrogens are prescribed:

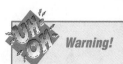
Warning!

Adverse reactions to posterior pituitary drugs

Hypersensitivity reactions are the most common adverse reactions to posterior pituitary drugs.

Natural ADH
Anaphylaxis may occur after injection. Natural antidiuretic hormone (ADH) can also cause:
• ringing in the ears
• anxiety
• hyponatremia (low serum sodium levels)
• proteins in the urine
• eclamptic attacks
• pupil dilation
• transient edema.

Synthetic ADH
Adverse reactions to synthetic ADH are rare.

Pregnant pause
Synthetic oxytocin can cause adverse reactions for pregnant women, including:
• bleeding after delivery
• GI disturbances
• sweating
• headache
• dizziness
• ringing in the ears
• severe water intoxication.

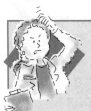

Hormone replacement therapy and heart disease

Until recently, it was believed that hormone replacement therapy (estrogen and progestin) in postmenopausal women reduced the risk of heart disease by improving blood cholesterol levels.

Those at risk
However, a recent study suggests that postmenopausal women who already have heart disease and take hormone replacement therapy may actually increase their risk of heart disease, at least during the first year of therapy. After 4 years of hormone replacement therapy, women with heart disease began to lower their risk of heart attack and chest pain.

A recommendation
Based on this research, the researchers don't recommend that postmenopausal women with heart disease start taking hormone replacement therapy. The researchers believe, however, that if a woman with heart disease has already been taking hormone replacement therapy for at least 2 years, she's probably past the danger point and is at the phase where she will begin to reduce her cardiovascular risk.

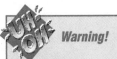

Warning!

Adverse reactions to estrogens

Adverse reactions to estrogens include:
• hypertension
• thromboembolism (blood vessel blockage caused by a blood clot)
• thrombophlebitis (vein inflammation associated with clot formation).

• primarily for hormone replacement therapy in postmenopausal women to relieve symptoms caused by loss of ovarian function (see *Hormone replacement therapy and heart disease*)
• less commonly for hormonal replacement therapy in women with primary ovarian failure or female hypogonadism (reduced hormonal secretion by the ovaries) and in patients who have undergone surgical castration
• palliatively to treat advanced, inoperable breast cancer in postmenopausal women and prostate cancer in men.

Drug interactions

Relatively few drugs interact with estrogens:
• Estrogens may decrease the effects of anticoagulants, increasing the risk of blood clots.
• Carbamazepine, barbiturates, antibiotics, phenytoin, primidone, and rifampin reduce estrogen effectiveness.
• Estrogens interfere with the absorption of dietary folic acid, which may result in a folic acid deficiency. (See *Adverse reactions to estrogens*.)

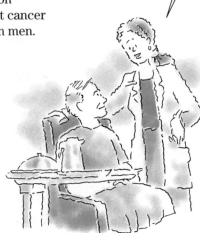

Estrogens aren't just prescribed for women. They're also used to treat prostate cancer in men.

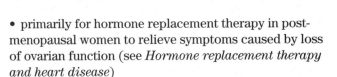

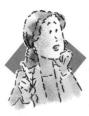

Quick quiz

1. How does insulin lower blood glucose level?
   A. It prevents glucose absorption from the GI tract.
   B. It increases glucose excretion from the GI tract.
   C. It promotes the transport of glucose into cells.

Answer: C. Insulin promotes the transport of glucose into cells.

2. Why can't glucagon be given orally?
   A. It works too slowly when given orally.
   B. It's destroyed by the GI tract.
   C. It's absorbed unpredictably.

Answer: B. Glucagon is destroyed by the GI tract.

3. Which of the following are signs that a patient taking levothyroxine is experiencing thyroid toxicity?
   A. Diarrhea and weight loss
   B. Weight gain and constipation
   C. Slow heart rate and low blood pressure

Answer: A. Diarrhea and weight loss are signs of thyroid toxicity in a patient taking levothyroxine.

4. The posterior pituitary drug used to stimulate uterine contractions is:
   A. vasopressin.
   B. oxytocin.
   C. lypressin.

Answer: B. Oxytocin stimulates uterine contractions by increasing permeability of uterine cell membranes to sodium ions. It can also stimulate lactation.

5. Estrogens are sometimes prescribed to treat which condition in men?

    A.   Prostate cancer
    B.   Testicular cancer
    C.   Colorectal cancer

Answer: A. Estrogens are sometimes prescribed for palliative treatment of prostate cancer.

Scoring

☆☆☆   If you answered all five questions correctly, extraordinary! You're hyper-knowledgeable about hyperglycemic drugs and more!

☆☆   If you answered three or four questions correctly, congratulations! You have a well-balanced understanding of pharmacology!

☆   If you answered fewer than three questions correctly, keep trying! You have two more quick quizzes to go!

⑬

Drugs for fluid and electrolyte balance

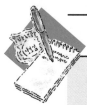

Just the facts

In this chapter, you'll review:

♦ classes of drugs that affect fluid and electrolyte balance

♦ uses and varying actions of these drugs

♦ how these drugs are absorbed, distributed, metabolized, and excreted

♦ drug interactions and adverse reactions to these drugs.

Drugs and homeostasis

Illness can easily disturb the homeostatic mechanisms that help maintain normal fluid and electrolyte balance. Such occurrences as loss of appetite, medication administration, vomiting, surgery, and diagnostic tests can also alter this delicate balance. Fortunately, numerous drugs can be used to correct these imbalances and help bring the body back toward homeostasis.

Electrolyte replacement drugs

An electrolyte is a compound or element that carries an electrical charge when dissolved in water. *Electrolyte replacement drugs* are mineral salts that increase depleted or deficient electrolyte levels, helping to maintain homeostasis, the stability of body fluid composition and volume. They include:

- potassium, the primary intracellular fluid (ICF) electrolyte
- calcium, a major extracellular fluid (ECF) electrolyte
- magnesium, an electrolyte essential for homeostasis found in ICF
- sodium, another electrolyte necessary for homeostasis found in ECF.

Potassium

Potassium is the major positively charged ion (cation) in ICF. Because the body can't store potassium, adequate amounts must be ingested daily. If this isn't possible, potassium replacement can be accomplished orally or I.V. with potassium salts, such as:

- potassium bicarbonate
- potassium chloride
- potassium gluconate
- potassium phosphate.

Pharmacokinetics (how drugs circulate)

Oral potassium is absorbed readily from the GI tract.

Absorption, metabolism, and excretion

After absorption into the ECF, almost all of the potassium passes into the ICF. Normal serum levels of potassium are maintained by the kidneys, which excrete most of the excessive potassium intake. The rest is excreted in feces and sweat.

> Because the body can't store potassium, I make sure to eat adequate amounts every day. This banana is a good source of potassium.

Pharmacodynamics (how drugs act)

Potassium moves quickly into ICF to restore depleted potassium levels and reestablish balance. It's an essential element in determining cell membrane potential and excitability.

Feel nervous about potassium?

Potassium is necessary for proper functioning of all nerve and muscle cells and for nerve impulse transmission. It's also essential for tissue growth and repair and for maintenance of acid-base balance.

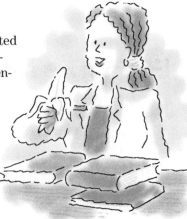

Pharmacotherapeutics (how drugs are used)

Potassium replacement therapy corrects hypokalemia, low levels of potassium in the blood. Hypokalemia is a common occurrence in conditions that increase potassium excretion or depletion, such as:
- vomiting or diarrhea
- excessive urination
- some kidney diseases
- cystic fibrosis
- burns
- excess of antidiuretic hormone (ADH) or therapy with a potassium-depleting diuretic
- alkalosis
- insufficient potassium intake from starvation
- administration of a glucocorticoid, I.V. amphotericin B, or I.V. solutions that contain insufficient potassium.

Be still my heart

Potassium is also used to decrease the toxic effects of digoxin. Because potassium inhibits the excitability of the heart, low potassium levels enhance the action of digoxin, which may result in toxicity.

Drug interactions

Potassium should be used cautiously in patients receiving potassium-sparing diuretics (such as amiloride, spironolactone, and triamterene) or angiotensin-converting enzyme inhibitors (such as captopril, enalapril, and lisinopril) to avoid hyperkalemia. (See *Adverse reactions to potassium.*)

Calcium

Calcium is a major cation in ECF. Almost all of the calcium in the body (99%) is stored in bone, where it can be mobilized if necessary. When dietary intake isn't enough to meet metabolic needs, calcium stores in bone are reduced.

Salting the body

Chronic insufficient calcium intake can result in bone demineralization. Calcium is replaced orally or I.V. with calcium salts, such as:

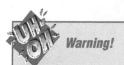

Warning!

Adverse reactions to potassium

Most adverse reactions to potassium are related to the method of administration.

Oral history
Oral potassium sometimes causes nausea, vomiting, abdominal pain, and diarrhea. Enteric-coated tablets may cause small-bowel ulceration, stenosis, hemorrhage, and obstruction.

In the I.V. league
I.V. infusion of potassium preparations can cause pain at the injection site and phlebitis (vein inflammation). Given rapidly, I.V. administration may cause cardiac arrest. Infusion of potassium in patients with decreased urine production increases the risk of hyperkalemia.

- calcium carbonate
- calcium chloride
- calcium citrate
- calcium glubionate
- calcium gluconate
- calcium lactate.

Pharmacokinetics

Oral calcium is absorbed readily from the duodenum and proximal jejunum. A pH of 5 to 7, parathyroid hormone, and vitamin D all aid calcium absorption.

Absorbed with absorption

Absorption also depends on dietary factors, such as calcium binding to fiber, phytates, and oxalates and to fatty acids, with which calcium salts form insoluble soaps.

Distribution and excretion

Calcium is distributed primarily in bone. Calcium salts are eliminated primarily in feces; the rest is excreted in urine.

Pharmacodynamics

Calcium moves quickly into ECF to restore calcium levels and reestablish balance. Calcium has several important roles in the body:
- Extracellular ionized calcium plays an essential role in normal nerve and muscle excitability.
- Calcium is integral to normal functioning of the heart, kidneys, and lungs, and it affects the blood coagulation rate as well as cell membrane and capillary permeability.
- Calcium is a factor in neurotransmitter and hormone activity, amino acid metabolism, vitamin B_{12} absorption, and gastrin secretion.
- It plays a major role in normal bone and tooth formation.

Just about all the calcium in the body can be found in the bones.

Pharmacotherapeutics

Calcium is helpful in treating magnesium intoxication. It's also helpful in strengthening myocardial tissue after defibrillation (electric shock to restore normal heart rhythm) or a poor response to epinephrine during resuscitation. Pregnancy and breast-feeding increase calcium requirements, as do periods of bone growth during childhood and adolescence.

In the I.V. league

The major clinical indication for I.V. calcium is acute hypocalcemia (low serum calcium levels), in which a rapid increase in serum calcium levels is needed. Conditions that create this need are tetany, cardiac arrest, vitamin D deficiency, parathyroid surgery, and alkalosis. I.V. calcium is also used to prevent a hypocalcemic reaction during exchange transfusions.

Oral history

Oral calcium is commonly used to supplement a calcium-deficient diet and prevent osteoporosis. Chronic hypocalcemia from such conditions as chronic hypoparathyroidism (a deficiency of parathyroid hormones), osteomalacia (softening of bones), rickets, and vitamin D deficiency is also treated with oral calcium.

Drug interactions

Calcium has few significant interactions with other drugs:
• Preparations administered with digoxin may cause cardiac arrhythmias.
• Calcium replacement drugs may reduce the response to calcium channel blockers.
• Calcium replacements may inactivate tetracyclines.
• Calcium supplements may decrease the amount of atenolol available to the tissues resulting in decreased effectiveness of the drug. (See *Adverse reactions to calcium.*)

Magnesium

Magnesium is the most abundant cation in ICF after potassium. It's essential in transmitting nerve impulses to muscle and activating enzymes necessary for carbohydrate and protein metabolism.

Officiating in the ICF

Magnesium stimulates parathyroid hormone secretion, thus regulating ICF calcium levels.

Warning!

Adverse reactions to calcium

Calcium preparations may produce hypercalcemia (elevated serum calcium levels). Early signs include:
• drowsiness
• lethargy
• muscle weakness
• headache
• constipation
• metallic taste in the mouth.

Take this to heart
Electrocardiogram changes that occur with elevated serum calcium levels include a shortened QT interval and heart block. Severe hypercalcemia can cause cardiac arrhythmias, cardiac arrest and, eventually, coma.

Traffic control

Magnesium also aids in cell metabolism and the movement of sodium and potassium across cell membranes.

A run on magnesium

Magnesium stores may be depleted by:
- malabsorption
- chronic diarrhea
- prolonged treatment with diuretics
- nasogastric suctioning
- prolonged therapy with parenteral fluids not containing magnesium
- hyperaldosteronism
- hypoparathyroidism or hyperparathyroidism
- excessive release of adrenocortical hormones.

Restocking the mineral stores

Magnesium is typically replaced in the form of magnesium sulfate.

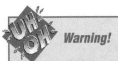

Warning!

Adverse reactions to magnesium

Adverse reactions to magnesium sulfate, which can be life-threatening, include:
- hypotension
- circulatory collapse
- flushing
- depressed reflexes
- respiratory paralysis.

Pharmacokinetics

Magnesium sulfate is distributed widely throughout the body. I.V. magnesium sulfate acts immediately, whereas after I.M. administration it acts within 30 minutes.

Metabolism and excretion

Magnesium sulfate isn't metabolized and is excreted unchanged in the urine; some is excreted in breast milk.

Pharmacodynamics

Magnesium sulfate replenishes and prevents magnesium deficiencies. It also prevents or controls seizures by blocking neuromuscular transmission.

Pharmacotherapeutics

Magnesium sulfate is the drug of choice for replacement therapy in magnesium deficiency. It's also used to treat seizures, severe toxemia, and acute nephritis in children.

Drug interactions

Magnesium has few significant interactions with other drugs:

• Magnesium used with digoxin may lead to heart block.
• Magnesium sulfate combined with alcohol, narcotics, antianxiety drugs, barbiturates, antidepressants, hypnotics, antipsychotics, or general anesthetics may increase central nervous system depressant effects.
• Magnesium sulfate combined with succinylcholine or tubocurarine potentiates and prolongs the neuromuscular blocking action of these drugs. (See *Adverse reactions to magnesium.*)

Sodium

Sodium is the major cation in ECF. Sodium performs many functions:
• It maintains the osmotic pressure and concentration of ECF, acid-base balance, and water balance.
• It contributes to nerve conduction and neuromuscular function.
• It plays a role in glandular secretion.

Don't sweat it

Sodium replacement is necessary in conditions that rapidly deplete it, such as excessive loss of GI fluids and excessive perspiration. Diuretics and tap water enemas can also deplete sodium, particularly when fluids are replaced by plain water.

The salt flats

Sodium also can be lost in trauma or wound drainage, adrenal gland insufficiency, cirrhosis of the liver with ascites, syndrome of inappropriate ADH, and prolonged I.V. infusion of dextrose in water without other solutes.

Restocking the mineral stores

Sodium is typically replaced in the form of sodium chloride.

Pharmacokinetics

Oral and parenteral sodium chloride are quickly absorbed and distributed widely throughout the body.

When I'm out jogging, I run the risk of losing important fluids through perspiration. Sodium can help me replace depleted fluids and maintain water balance.

Metabolism and excretion

Sodium chloride isn't significantly metabolized. It's eliminated primarily in urine, but also in sweat, tears, and saliva.

Pharmacodynamics

Sodium chloride solution replaces deficiencies of the sodium and chloride ions in the blood plasma.

Pharmacotherapeutics

Sodium chloride is used for water and electrolyte replacement in patients with hyponatremia from electrolyte loss or severe sodium chloride depletion.

A welcome infusion

Severe symptomatic sodium deficiency may be treated by I.V. infusion of a solution containing sodium chloride.

Drug interactions

No significant drug interactions have been reported with sodium chloride. (See *Adverse reactions to sodium.*)

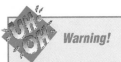

Warning!

Adverse reactions to sodium

Adverse reactions to sodium include:
• pulmonary edema (if given too rapidly or in excess)
• hypernatremia
• potassium loss.

Alkalinizing and acidifying drugs

Alkalinizing and *acidifying drugs* act to correct acid-base imbalances in the blood. These acid-base imbalances include:
• *metabolic acidosis*, a decreased serum pH caused by excess hydrogen ions in the ECF, which is treated with alkalinizing drugs
• *metabolic alkalosis*, an increased serum pH caused by excess bicarbonate in the ECF, which is treated with acidifying drugs.

Odd couple

Alkalinizing and acidifying drugs have opposite effects:
• An alkalinizing drug will increase the pH of the blood.
• An acidifying drug will decrease the pH.

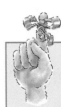

Memory jogger

Remember: a low pH means a solution is *acidic* and a high pH means it's *alkaline*. Therefore, to raise the pH, you use an *alkalinizing* drug and, likewise, to lower the pH, you use an *acidifying* drug.

Rx for o.d.

Some of these drugs also alter urine pH, making them useful in treating some urinary tract infections and drug overdoses.

Alkalinizing drugs

Four *alkalinizing drugs* are used to increase blood pH:
• sodium bicarbonate
• sodium citrate
• sodium lactate
• tromethamine.

Increasing another pH

Sodium bicarbonate is also used to increase urine pH.

Pharmacokinetics

All of the alkalinizing drugs are absorbed well when given orally.

Metabolism and excretion

Sodium citrate and sodium lactate are metabolized to the active ingredient, bicarbonate. Sodium bicarbonate isn't metabolized. Tromethamine undergoes little or no metabolism and is excreted unchanged in the urine.

Pharmacodynamics

Sodium bicarbonate separates in the blood to provide bicarbonate ions that are used in the blood buffer system to decrease the hydrogen ion concentration and raise blood pH. (Buffers prevent extreme changes in pH by taking or giving up hydrogen ions to neutralize acids or bases.) As the bicarbonate ions are excreted in the urine, urine pH rises. Sodium citrate and lactate, after conversion to bicarbonate, alkalinize the blood and urine in the same way.

Hitching up with hydrogen

Tromethamine acts by combining with hydrogen ions to alkalinize the blood; the resulting tromethamine–hydrogen ion complex is excreted in the urine.

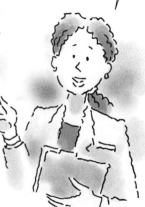

Alkalinizing drugs treat metabolic acidosis by alkalinizing the blood. They do this by decreasing the hydrogen ion concentration.

Pharmacotherapeutics

Alkalinizing drugs are commonly used to treat metabolic acidosis. Other uses include raising the urine pH to help remove certain substances, such as phenobarbital, after an overdose.

Drug interactions

The alkalinizing drugs sodium bicarbonate, sodium citrate, and sodium lactate can interact with a wide range of drugs to increase or decrease their pharmacologic effects:
• They may increase excretion and reduce the effects of ketoconazole, lithium, and salicylates.
• They may reduce the excretion and increase the effects of amphetamines, quinidine, and pseudoephedrine.
• The antibacterial effects of methenamine are reduced when taken with alkalinizing drugs. (See *Adverse reactions to alkalinizing drugs.*)

Acidifying drugs

Two *acidifying drugs* are used to correct metabolic alkalosis:

 ammonium chloride

 hydrochloric acid.

Dropping the name of another acidifier

Ascorbic acid, along with ammonium chloride, serves as a urinary acidifier.

Pharmacokinetics

The action of most acidifying drugs is immediate.

Absorption, metabolism, and excretion

Orally administered ammonium chloride is absorbed completely in 3 to 6 hours. It's metabolized in the liver to form urea, which is excreted by the kidneys, and hydrochloric acid, the acidifying drug.

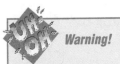

Warning!

Adverse reactions to alkalinizing drugs

Adverse reactions to alkalinizing drugs vary.

Sodium bicarbonate
• Bicarbonate overdose
• Cerebral dysfunction, tissue hypoxia, and lactic acidosis (with rapid administration for diabetic ketoacidosis)
• Water retention and edema

Sodium citrate
• Metabolic alkalosis, tetany or aggravation of existing heart disease (with overdose)
• Laxative effect (with oral administration)

Sodium lactate
• Metabolic alkalosis (with overdose)
• Extravasation
• Water retention or edema (in patient with kidney disease or heart failure)

Tromethamine
• Hypoglycemia
• Respiratory depression
• Extravasation
• Hyperkalemia
• Toxic drug levels (if given for more than 24 hours)

Break it down

After I.V. administration, hydrochloric acid is broken down into hydrogen and chloride ions. The hydrogen ions are used as the acidifying drug.

Orally administered ascorbic acid usually is absorbed well, distributed widely in body tissues, and metabolized in the liver. Its metabolites are excreted in the urine along with excess ascorbic acid, which is excreted unchanged.

Pharmacodynamics

Acidifying drugs have several actions:
• Ammonium chloride lowers the blood pH after being metabolized to urea and to hydrochloric acid, which provides hydrogen ions to acidify the blood or urine.
• Hydrochloric acid lowers blood pH directly by acidifying the blood with hydrogen ions.
• Ascorbic acid directly acidifies the urine, providing hydrogen ions and lowering urine pH.

Pharmacotherapeutics

A patient with metabolic alkalosis requires therapy with an acidifying drug that provides hydrogen ions; such a patient may need chloride ion therapy as well. Although the patient can receive both in a hydrochloric acid infusion, this infusion is difficult to prepare, and an overdose can produce severe adverse reactions.

Safe and easy

Most patients receive both types of ions in oral or parenteral doses of ammonium chloride, a safer drug that is easy to prepare.

Drug interactions

Acidifying drugs don't cause clinically significant drug interactions. However, concurrent use of ammonium chloride and spironolactone may cause increased systemic acidosis. (See *Adverse reactions to acidifying drugs*.)

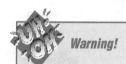

Warning!

Adverse reactions to acidifying drugs

Adverse reactions to acidifying drugs are usually mild such as GI distress. Overdose may lead to acidosis.

Ammonium chloride
• Metabolic acidosis and loss of electrolytes, especially potassium (with large doses)

Hydrochloric acid
• Metabolic acidosis (with an overdose)

Ascorbic acid
• GI distress (with high doses)
• Hemolytic anemia (in a patient with glucose-6-phosphate dehydrogenase deficiency)

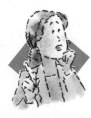

Quick quiz

1. Which drug can cause hypokalemia?
   A. digoxin
   B. amphotericin B
   C. spironolactone

Answer: B. Hypokalemia is a common occurrence in conditions that increase potassium excretion or depletion, such as administration of glucocorticoid, I.V. amphotericin B, or I.V. solutions that contain insufficient potassium.

2. Potassium should be used cautiously in patients receiving which of the following?
   A. amiloride
   B. furosemide
   C. digoxin

Answer: A. Potassium should be used cautiously in patients receiving potassium-sparing diuretics, such as amiloride, to avoid hyperkalemia.

3. How does sodium bicarbonate correct metabolic acidosis?
   A. By decreasing the hydrogen ion concentration
   B. By increasing the hydrogen ion concentration
   C. By combining with hydrogen ions to alkalinize the blood

Answer: A. Sodium bicarbonate corrects acidosis by decreasing the hydrogen ion concentration.

Scoring

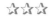   If you answered all three questions correctly, extraordinary! You're one well-balanced individual!

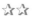   If you answered two questions correctly, congratulations. You're moving closer to complete harmony.

☆   If you answered fewer than two questions correctly, keep trying! By the end of the book, you're sure to have all your levels up!

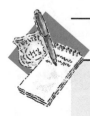

Cancer drugs

Just the facts

In this chapter, you'll review:

♦ classes of drugs used to treat cancer

♦ uses and varying actions of these drugs

♦ how these drugs are absorbed, distributed, metabolized, and excreted

♦ drug interactions and adverse reactions of these drugs.

Drugs and cancer

In the 1940s, *antineoplastic* (chemotherapeutic) *drugs* were used to treat cancer when all other therapeutic measures failed. However, most antineoplastic drugs commonly had serious adverse effects.

A brighter future

Today, many of these effects can be minimized so they aren't as devastating to the patient. In fact, many child-hood cancers are now considered curable because of the advent of chemotherapeutic drugs, many of which are now the drug of choice for different types of cancer. In addition, drugs such as interferons are being used to treat patients with cancer.

Alkylating drugs

Alkylating drugs, given alone or with other drugs, effectively act against various malignant neoplasms. These drugs fall into one of six classes:
- nitrogen mustards
- alkyl sulfonates
- nitrosoureas
- triazenes
- ethylenimines
- alkylating-like drugs.

> Alkylating drugs deactivate my DNA, cutting short my life.

Unfazed at any phase

All of these drugs produce their antineoplastic effects by deactivating deoxyribonucleic acid (DNA). They halt DNA's replication process by cross-linking its strands so that amino acids don't pair up correctly. Alkylating drugs are cell cycle–phase nonspecific. This means that their alkylating actions may take place at any phase of the cell cycle.

Nitrogen mustards

Nitrogen mustards represent the largest group of alkylating drugs. They include:
- chlorambucil
- cyclophosphamide
- estramustine
- ifosfamide
- mechlorethamine hydrochloride
- melphalan
- uracil mustard.

The first and fastest

Mechlorethamine hydrochloride was the first nitrogen mustard introduced and is still the most rapid-acting.

Pharmacokinetics (how drugs circulate)

The absorption and distribution of nitrogen mustards, as with most alkylating drugs, vary widely.

Metabolism and excretion

Nitrogen mustards are metabolized in the liver and excreted by the kidneys. Mechlorethamine undergoes metabolism so rapidly that no active drug remains after a few minutes. Most nitrogen mustards possess more intermediate half-lives than mechlorethamine.

Pharmacodynamics (how drugs act)

Nitrogen mustards form covalent bonds with DNA molecules in a chemical reaction known as alkylation. Alkylated DNA can't replicate properly, thereby resulting in cell death. Unfortunately, cells may develop resistance to the cytotoxic effects of nitrogen mustards. (See *How alkylating drugs work*, page 318.)

Pharmacotherapeutics (how drugs are used)

Because they produce leukopenia (reduced number of white blood cells [WBCs]), the nitrogen mustards are effective in treating malignant neoplasms, such as Hodgkin's disease (cancer causing painless enlargement of the lymph nodes, spleen, and lymphoid tissues) and leukemia (cancer of the blood forming tissues), that have an associated elevated WBC count.

Nitrogen bomb

Nitrogen mustards also prove effective against malignant lymphoma (cancer of the lymphoid tissue), multiple myeloma (cancer of the marrow plasma cells), melanoma (malignancy that arises from melanocytes), and cancers of the breast, ovaries, uterus, lung, brain, testes, bladder, prostate, and stomach.

Drug interactions

Nitrogen mustards interact with a wide variety of other drugs:
• Calcium-containing drugs and foods, such as antacids and dairy products, reduce absorption of estramustine.
• Taking cyclophosphamide with cardiotoxic drugs produces additive cardiac effects.
• Cyclophosphamide may reduce serum digoxin levels.
• An increased risk of ifosfamide toxicity exists when the drug is taken with allopurinol, barbiturates, chloral hydrate, or phenytoin.
• Corticosteroids reduce the effects of ifosfamide.
• The lung toxicity threshold of carmustine may be reduced when taken with melphalan.

Now I get it!

How alkylating drugs work

Alkylating drugs can attack deoxyribonucleic acid (DNA) in two ways, as shown in the illustrations below.

Bifunctional alkylation

Some drugs become inserted between two base pairs in the DNA chain, forming an irreversible bond between them. This is called *bifunctional alkylation,* which causes cytotoxic effects capable of destroying or poisoning cells.

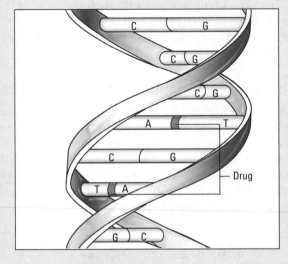

Monofunctional alkylation

Other drugs react with just one part of a pair, separating it from its partner and eventually causing it and its attached sugar to break away from the DNA molecule. This is called *monofunctional alkylation,* which eventually may cause permanent cell damage.

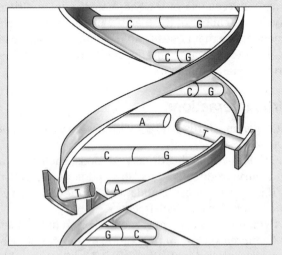

• Interferon alpha may reduce serum concentration of melphalan. (See *Adverse reactions to nitrogen mustards.*)

Alkyl sulfonates

The alkyl sulfonate *busulfan* is commonly used to treat chronic myelogenous leukemia and less commonly to treat polycythemia vera (increased red blood cell mass and increased number of WBCs and platelets) as well as other myeloproliferative (pertaining to the bone marrow) disorders.

Pharmacokinetics

Busulfan is absorbed rapidly and well from the GI tract. Little is known about its distribution.

Metabolism and excretion

Busulfan is metabolized extensively in the liver before urinary excretion. Its half-life is 2 to 3 hours.

Pharmacodynamics

As an alkyl sulfonate, busulfan forms covalent bonds with the DNA molecules in alkylation.

Pharmacotherapeutics

Busulfan primarily affects granulocytes (a type of WBC) and, to a lesser degree, platelets. Because of its action on granulocytes, it's the drug of choice for treating chronic myelogenous leukemia.

A back-up option

Busulfan is also effective in treating polycythemia vera. However, other drugs are usually used to treat polycythemia vera because busulfan can cause severe myelosuppression (halting of bone marrow function).

Drug interactions

There is an increased risk of bleeding when busulfan is taken with anticoagulants or aspirin. Concurrent use of busulfan and thioguanine may cause liver toxicity, esophageal varices (enlarged, swollen veins in the esophagus), or portal hypertension (increased pressure in the portal vein of the liver). (See *Adverse reactions to busulfan*, page 320.)

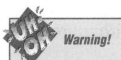
Warning!

Adverse reactions to nitrogen mustards

Many patients experience fatigue during nitrogen mustard therapy. Their use may also lead to other adverse reactions, such as:
• bone marrow suppression, leading to severe leukopenia and thrombocytopenia
• nausea and vomiting from central nervous system irritation
• stomatitis
• reversible hair loss.

Handle with care

Because nitrogen mustards are powerful local vesicants (blistering drugs), direct contact with these drugs or their vapors can cause severe reactions, especially of the skin, eyes, and respiratory tract.

Nitrosoureas

Nitrosoureas are alkylating agents that work by halting cancer cell reproduction and include:

- carmustine
- lomustine
- streptozocin.

Pharmacokinetics

When administered topically to treat mycosis fungoides (a rare skin malignancy), carmustine is 5% to 28% systemically absorbed. After oral administration, lomustine is absorbed adequately, although incompletely.

In the I.V. league

Streptozocin, which is administered I.V., doesn't undergo absorption.

Metabolism and excretion

Nitrosoureas are lipophilic (attracted to fat), distributing to fatty tissues and cerebrospinal fluid. They're metabolized extensively before urine excretion.

Pharmacodynamics

During a process called bifunctional alkylation, nitrosoureas interfere with amino acids, purines, and DNA needed for cancer cells to divide, thus halting their reproduction.

Pharmacotherapeutics

The nitrosoureas are highly lipid (fat) soluble, which allows them or their metabolites to easily cross the blood-brain barrier. Because of this ability, nitrosoureas are used to treat brain tumors and meningeal leukemias.

Drug interactions

Each of the nitrosoureas has its own interactions with other drugs. Cimetidine may increase carmustine's bone marrow toxicity. Streptozocin prolongs the elimination half-life of doxorubicin, prolonging the leukopenia and thrombocytopenia. (See *Adverse reactions to nitrosoureas.*)

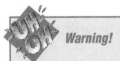

Warning!

Adverse reactions to busulfan

The major adverse reaction to busulfan is bone marrow suppression, producing severe leukopenia, anemia, and thrombocytopenia (reduced white blood cells, red blood cells, and platelets, respectively), which is usually dose-related and reversible.

Triazenes

The triazene *dacarbazine* functions as an alkylating drug after it has been activated by the liver.

Pharmacokinetics

After I.V. injection, dacarbazine is distributed throughout the body and metabolized in the liver. Within 6 hours, 30% to 46% of a dose is excreted by the kidneys (half is excreted unchanged, and half is excreted as one of the metabolites).

Dysfunction junction

In patients with kidney or liver dysfunction, the drug's half-life may increase to 7 hours.

Pharmacodynamics

Dacarbazine first must be metabolized in the liver to become an alkylating drug. It seems to inhibit ribonucleic acid (RNA) and protein synthesis. Like other alkylating drugs, dacarbazine is cell cycle–nonspecific.

Pharmacotherapeutics

Dacarbazine is used primarily to treat patients with malignant melanoma but also is used with other drugs to treat patients with Hodgkin's disease.

Drug interactions

No significant drug interactions have been reported with dacarbazine. (See *Adverse reactions to dacarbazine*, page 322.)

> After I.V. injection, dacarbazine must be metabolized by the liver before it becomes an antineoplastic drug.

Ethylenimines

Thiotepa, an *ethylenimine* derivative, is a multifunctional alkylating drug.

Pharmacokinetics

After I.V. administration, thiotepa is 100% bioavailable. Significant systemic absorption may occur when thiotepa

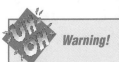

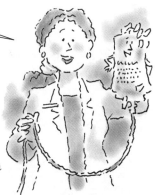

is administered into pleural (around the lungs) or peritoneal (abdominal) spaces to treat malignant effusions or is instilled into the bladder.

Metabolism and excretion

Thiotepa crosses the blood-brain barrier and is metabolized extensively in the liver. Thiotepa and its metabolites are excreted in the urine.

Pharmacodynamics

Thiotepa exerts its cytotoxic activity by interfering with DNA replication and RNA transcription. Ultimately, it disrupts nucleic acid function and causes cell death.

Pharmacotherapeutics

Thiotepa is used to treat bladder cancer. This alkylating drug is also prescribed for palliative (symptom relief) treatment of lymphomas and ovarian or breast carcinomas.

More uses?

The Food and Drug Administration (FDA) has approved thiotepa for the treatment of intracavitary effusions (accumulation of fluid in a body cavity). It may also prove useful in the treatment of lung cancer.

Drug interactions

Thiotepa may interact with other drugs:
• Concurrent use of thiotepa, anticoagulants, and aspirin may increase the risk of bleeding.
• Taking thiotepa with neuromuscular blocking drugs may prolong muscular paralysis.
• Concurrent use of thiotepa and other alkylating drugs or radiation therapy may intensify toxicity rather than enhance the therapeutic response.

It'll take your breath away

When used with succinylcholine, thiotepa may cause prolonged respirations and apnea (periods of not breathing). Thiotepa appears to inhibit the activity of cholinesterase, the enzyme that deactivates succinylcholine. (See *Adverse reactions to thiotepa.*)

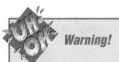

Warning!

Adverse reactions to dacarbazine

Dacarbazine use may cause some adverse reactions. These include:
• leukopenia
• thrombocytopenia
• nausea and vomiting (which begin within 1 to 3 hours after administration in most patients and may last up to 12 hours)
• phototoxicity
• flulike syndrome
• hair loss.

Alkylating-like drugs

Carboplatin and *cisplatin* are heavy metal complexes that contain platinum. Because their action resembles that of a bifunctional alkylating drug, the drugs are referred to as *alkylating–like drugs*.

Pharmacokinetics

The distribution and metabolism of carboplatin aren't defined clearly. After I.V. administration, carboplatin is eliminated primarily by the kidneys. The elimination of carboplatin is biphasic. It has an initial half-life of 1 to 2 hours and a terminal half-life of 2½ to 6 hours.

Into the lungs and peritoneum

When administered intrapleurally (into the pleural space around the lung) or intraperitoneally (into the peritoneum), cisplatin may exhibit significant systemic absorption. Highly protein-bound, cisplatin reaches high concentrations in the kidneys, liver, intestines, and testes but has poor central nervous system (CNS) penetration. The drug undergoes some liver metabolism, followed by excretion through the kidney.

Going platinum

Platinum is detectable in tissue for at least 4 months after administration.

Pharmacodynamics

Like alkylating drugs, carboplatin and cisplatin are cell cycle–nonspecific and inhibit DNA synthesis. They act like bifunctional alkylating drugs by cross-linking strands of DNA and inhibiting DNA synthesis.

Pharmacotherapeutics

These alkylating-like drugs are used in the treatment of several cancers:
• Carboplatin is used primarily to treat ovarian and lung cancer.
• Cisplatin is prescribed to treat bladder and metastatic ovarian cancer.
• Cisplatin is the drug of choice for metastatic testicular cancers.

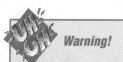

Warning!

Adverse reactions to thiotepa

The major adverse reactions to thiotepa are blood-related and include leukopenia, anemia, thrombocytopenia, and pancytopenia (deficiency of all cellular elements of the blood), which may be fatal.

Other adverse reactions include:
• nausea and vomiting (commonly)
• stomatitis and ulceration of the intestinal mucosa (especially at bone marrow transplant doses)
• hives, rash, and pruritus (occasionally).

• Cisplatin may also be used to treat head, neck, and lung cancer (although these indications are clinically accepted, they're currently unlabled uses).

Drug interactions

These alkylating-like drugs interact with a few other drugs:
• When carboplatin or cisplatin are administered with an aminoglycoside, the risk of toxicity to the kidney increases.
• Taking carboplatin or cisplatin with bumetanide, ethacrynic acid, and furosemide increase the risk of ototoxicity (damaging the organs of hearing and balance).
• Cisplatin may reduce serum phenytoin levels. (See *Adverse reactions to alkylating-like drugs.*)

Antimetabolite drugs

Because *antimetabolite drugs* structurally resemble natural metabolites, they can become involved in processes associated with the natural metabolites — that is, the synthesis of nucleic acids and proteins.

Getting specific

Antimetabolites differ sufficiently from the natural metabolites in how they interfere with this synthesis. Because the antimetabolites are cell cycle–specific and primarily affect cells that actively synthesize DNA, they're referred to as S phase–specific. Normal cells that are reproducing actively as well as the cancer cells are affected by the antimetabolites.

Each according to its metabolite

These drugs are subclassified according to the metabolite affected and include:
• folic acid analogues
• pyrimidine analogues
• purine analogues.

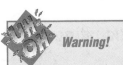

Warning!

Adverse reactions to alkylating-like drugs

Carboplatin and cisplatin produce many of the same adverse reactions as the alkylating drugs.
• Carboplatin can produce bone marrow suppression.
• Kidney toxicity may occur with cisplatin, usually after multiple courses of therapy. Carboplatin is less toxic to the kidneys.
• With long-term cisplatin therapy, neurotoxicity can occur. Neurotoxicity is less common with carboplatin.
• Tinnitus (ringing in the ears) and hearing loss, which is often permanent, may occur with cisplatin and much less commonly with carboplatin.
• Cisplatin also produces marked nausea and vomiting.

Folic acid analogues

Although researchers have developed many *folic acid analogues*, the early compound *methotrexate* remains the most commonly used.

Pharmacokinetics

Methotrexate is absorbed well and distributed throughout the body. At usual dosages, it doesn't enter the CNS readily.

Metabolism and excretion

Although methotrexate is metabolized partially, it's excreted primarily unchanged in the urine.

A disappearing act

Methotrexate exhibits a three-part disappearance from plasma; the rapid distributive phase is followed by a second phase, which reflects kidney clearance. The last phase, the terminal half-life, is 3 to 10 hours for a low dose and 8 to 15 hours for a high dose.

Pharmacodynamics

Methotrexate reversibly inhibits the action of the enzyme dihydrofolate reductase, thereby blocking normal biochemical reactions and inhibiting DNA and RNA synthesis. The result is cell death.

Pharmacotherapeutics

Methotrexate is especially useful in treating:
• acute lymphoblastic leukemia (abnormal growth of lymphocyte precursors, the lymphoblasts) in children
• choriocarcinoma (cancer that develops from the chorionic portions of the products of conception)
• osteogenic sarcoma (bone cancer)
• malignant lymphomas
• carcinomas of the head, neck, bladder, testis, and breast.

Unconventional treatment

The drug is also prescribed in low doses to treat severe psoriasis and rheumatoid arthritis that resist conventional therapy.

Drug interactions

Methotrexate interacts with several other drugs:
- Probenecid decreases methotrexate excretion, increasing the risk of methotrexate toxicity, including fatigue, bone marrow suppression, and stomatitis (mouth inflammation).
- Salicylates and nonsteroidal anti-inflammatory drugs, especially diclofenac, ketoprofen, indomethacin, and naproxen also increase methotrexate toxicity.
- Cholestyramine reduces absorption of methotrexate from the GI tract.
- Concurrent use of alcohol and methotrexate increases the risk of liver toxicity.
- Taking co-trimoxazole with methotrexate may produce blood cell abnormalities.
- Penicillin decreases renal tubular secretion of methotrexate, increasing the risk of methotrexate toxicity. (See *Adverse reactions to methotrexate*.)

Pyrimidine analogues

Pyrimidine analogues are a diverse group of drugs that inhibit production of pyrimidine nucleotides necessary for DNA synthesis. They include:
- cytarabine
- floxuridine
- fluorouracil
- gemcitabine.

Pharmacokinetics

Because pyrimidine analogues are absorbed poorly when they're given orally, they're usually administered by other routes.

Distribution, metabolism, and excretion

With the exception of cytarabine, pyrimidine analogues are distributed well throughout the body, including cerebrospinal fluid (CSF). They're metabolized extensively in the liver and are excreted in the urine.

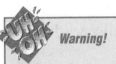

Warning!

Adverse reactions to methotrexate

Adverse reactions to methotrexate include:
- bone marrow suppression
- stomatitis
- pulmonary toxicity, exhibited as pneumonitis or pulmonary fibrosis
- skin reactions, such as photosensitivity and hair loss.

Kidney concerns
With high doses, kidney toxicity can also occur with methotrexate use. During high-dose therapy, leucovorin (folinic acid) may be used to minimize adverse reactions.

The spine of the matter
Adverse reactions to intrathecal administration (through the spinal cord into the subarachnoid space) of methotrexate may include seizures, paralysis, and death. Other less severe adverse reactions may also occur, such as headaches, fever, neck stiffness, confusion, and irritability.

Now I get it!

How pyrimidine analogues work

To understand how pyrimidine analogues work, it helps to consider the basic structure of deoxyribonucleic acid (DNA).

Climbing the ladder to understanding
DNA resembles a ladder that has been twisted. The rungs of the ladder consist of pairs of nitrogenous bases: adenine always pairs with thymine, and guanine always pairs with cytosine. Cytosine and thymine are pyrimidines; adenine and guanine are purines.

One part sugar…
The basic unit of DNA is the nucleotide. A nucleotide is the building block of nucleic acids.

It consists of a sugar, a nitrogen-containing base, and a phosphate group. It's on these components that pyrimidine analogues do their work.

In the guise of a nucleotide
After pyrimidine analogues are converted into nucleotides, they're incorporated into DNA, where they may inhibit DNA and ribonucleic acid synthesis as well as other metabolic reactions necessary for proper cell growth.

Pharmacodynamics

Pyrimidine analogues kill cancer cells by interfering with the natural function of pyrimidine nucleotides. (See *How pyrimidine analogues work.*)

Pharmacotherapeutics

Pyrimidine analogues may be used to treat many tumors. However, they're primarily indicated in the treatment of:
• acute leukemias
• GI tract adenocarcinomas (malignant epithelial cell tumors of the glands)
• carcinomas of the breast and ovaries
• malignant lymphomas.

Drug interactions

No significant drug interactions occur with pyrimidine analogues. (See *Adverse reactions to pyrimidine analogues.*)

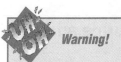

Warning!

Adverse reactions to pyrimidine analogues

Like most antineoplastic drugs, pyrimidine analogues can cause:
• fatigue and lack of energy
• inflammation of the mouth, esophagus, and throat, leading to painful ulcerations and tissue sloughing
• bone marrow suppression
• nausea and anorexia.

Gut reactions
Diarrhea may occur with fluorouracil administration.

Hair scare
Hair loss commonly occurs with fluorouracil.

Purine analogues

Purine analogues are incorporated into DNA and RNA, interfering with nucleic acid synthesis and replication. They include:
- fludarabine phosphate
- cladribine
- mercaptopurine
- thioguanine.

Pharmacokinetics

The pharmacokinetics of purine analogues aren't defined clearly. They're largely metabolized in the liver and excreted in the urine.

Pharmacodynamics

Like the other antimetabolites, fludarabine, mercaptopurine, and thioguanine first must undergo conversion to the nucleotide level to be active. The resulting nucleotides are then incorporated into DNA, where they may inhibit DNA and RNA synthesis as well as other metabolic reactions necessary for proper cell growth.

Analogous to pyrimide analogues

This conversion to nucleotides is the same process that pyrimidine analogues go through but, in this case, it's purine nucleotides that are affected. Purine analogues are cell cycle–specific as well, exerting their effect during that same S phase.

Pharmacotherapeutics

Purine analogues are used to treat acute and chronic leukemias and may be useful in the treatment of lymphomas.

Drug interactions

No significant interactions occur with cladribine or thioguanine.

A serious flub with fludarabine

Taking fludarabine and pentostatin together may cause severe pulmonary toxicity, which can be fatal.

Down to the bone

Concomitant administration of mercaptopurine and allopurinol may increase bone marrow suppression by decreasing mercaptopurine metabolism. (See *Adverse reactions to purine analogues.*)

Antibiotic antineoplastic drugs

Antibiotic antineoplastic drugs are antimicrobial products that produce tumoricidal (tumor-destroying) effects by binding with DNA. These drugs inhibit the cellular processes of normal and malignant cells. They include:
- bleomycin sulfate
- dactinomycin
- daunorubicin
- doxorubicin hydrochloride
- idarubicin hydrochloride
- mitomycin
- mitoxantrone hydrochloride
- pentostatin
- plicamycin.

Pharmacokinetics

Because antibiotic antineoplastic drugs are usually administered I.V., no absorption occurs. They're considered 100% bioavailable.

Direct deliveries

Some of the drugs are also administered directly into the body cavity being treated. Bleomycin, doxorubicin, and mitomycin are sometimes given as topical bladder instillations in which significant systemic absorption doesn't occur. When bleomycin is injected into the pleural space for malignant effusions, up to one-half of the dose is absorbed.

Distribution, metabolism, and excretion

Distribution of antibiotic antineoplastic drugs throughout the body varies as does their metabolism and elimination.

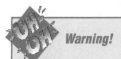

Warning!

Adverse reactions to purine analogues

Purine analogues can produce:
- bone marrow suppression
- nausea and vomiting
- anorexia
- mild diarrhea
- stomatitis
- rise in uric acid levels (a result of the breakdown of purine).

High-dose horrors
Fludarabine, when used at high doses, may cause severe neurologic effects, including blindness, coma, and death.

Pharmacodynamics

With the exception of mitomycin and pentostatin, antibiotic antineoplastic drugs intercalate, or insert themselves, between adjacent base pairs of a DNA molecule, physically separating them.

Taking the extra base

Remember, DNA looks like a twisted ladder with the rungs made up of pairs of nitrogenous bases. These drugs insert themselves between these nitrogenous bases. Then, when the DNA chain replicates, an extra base is inserted opposite the intercalated antibiotic, resulting in a mutant DNA molecule. The overall effect is cell death.

Blockage

Although the exact mechanism of pentostatin's antitumor effect is unknown, it inhibits the enzyme adenosine deaminase, blocking DNA synthesis and inhibiting RNA synthesis.

Breakage

Mitomycin is activated inside the cell to a bifunctional or even trifunctional alkylating drug. Mitomycin produces single-strand breakage of DNA. It also cross-links DNA and inhibits DNA synthesis.

Pharmacotherapeutics

Antibiotic antineoplastic drugs act against many cancers, including:
- Hodgkin's disease and malignant lymphomas
- testicular carcinoma
- squamous cell carcinoma of the head, neck, and cervix
- Wilms' tumor (a malignant neoplasm of the kidney, occurring in young children)
- osteogenic sarcoma, and rhabdomyosarcoma (malignant neoplasm composed of striated muscle cells)
- Ewing's sarcoma (a malignant tumor that originates in bone marrow, typically in long bones or the pelvis) and other soft-tissue sarcomas
- breast, ovarian, bladder, and bronchogenic carcinomas
- melanoma
- carcinomas of the GI tract
- choriocarcinoma.

Special effects

These drugs are also effective against acute leukemias and hypercalcemia.

Drug interactions

Antibiotic antineoplastic drugs interact with many other drugs:

• Pentostatin enhances the effects of vidarabine, increasing the possibility of adverse reactions to all three drugs.
• Concurrent therapy with fludarabine and pentostatin or idarubicin isn't recommended because of the risk of fatal lung toxicity.
• Bleomycin may decrease serum digoxin and serum phenytoin levels.
• Doxorubicin may reduce serum digoxin levels
• Streptozocin enhances leukopenia and thrombocytopenia (reduced number of platelets).
• Mitomycin plus vinca alkaloids may cause acute respiratory distress. (See *Adverse reactions to antibiotic antineoplastic drugs.*)

Hormonal antineoplastic drugs

Hormonal antineoplastic drugs are prescribed to alter the growth of malignant neoplasms or to manage and treat their physiological effects.

Hitting them where it hurts

Hormonal therapies prove effective against hormone-dependent tumors, such as cancers of the prostate, breast, and endometrium. Lymphomas and leukemias are usually treated with therapies that include corticosteroids because of their potential for affecting lymphocytes.

Antiestrogens

The antiestrogen *tamoxifen citrate* is the drug of choice for advanced breast cancer involving estrogen receptor–positive tumors in postmenopausal women.

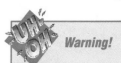

Warning!

Adverse reactions to antibiotic antineoplastic drugs

The primary adverse reaction to these drugs is bone marrow suppression. Irreversible cardiomyopathy and acute electrocardiogram changes can also occur as well as nausea and vomiting.

Extra steps
An antihistamine and antipyretic should be given before bleomycin to prevent fever and chills. Anaphylactic reactions can occur in patients receiving bleomycin for lymphoma, so test doses should be given first.

Battling bleeding
Plicamycin may produce hypotension and kidney toxicity as well as bleeding, such as nose bleed, blood during vomiting or coughing, bruising, and prolonged clotting and bleeding times.

Seeing colors
Doxorubicin may color urine red; mitoxantrone may color it blue-green.

Not tenured

Tamoxifen citrate is also used as an adjunct treatment for breast cancer and to reduce its incidence in woman at high risk.

Pharmacokinetics

After oral administration, tamoxifen is absorbed well and undergoes extensive metabolism in the liver before being excreted in the feces.

Pharmacodynamics

Estrogen receptors, found in the cancer cells of half of premenopausal and three-fourths of postmenopausal women with breast cancer, respond to estrogen to induce tumor growth.

It's bound to inhibit growth

The antiestrogen tamoxifen binds to the estrogen receptors and inhibits estrogen-mediated tumor growth. The inhibition may result because tamoxifen binds to receptors at the nuclear level or because the binding reduces the number of free receptors in the cytoplasm. Ultimately, DNA synthesis and cell growth are inhibited.

Pharmacotherapeutics

The antiestrogen tamoxifen is used in the palliative treatment of metastatic breast cancer that is estrogen receptor–positive. Tumors in postmenopausal women are more responsive to tamoxifen than those in premenopausal women. (See *Who benefits from tamoxifen?*)

Surgical aide

Tamoxifen is also used as an adjunct to surgery in postmenopausal women with axillary lymph nodes that contain cancer cells and estrogen receptor–positive tumors.

Drug interactions

Tamoxifen may interact with other drugs:
• It increases the effects of warfarin sodium, increasing the risk of bleeding.
• Bromocriptine increases the effects of tamoxifen.

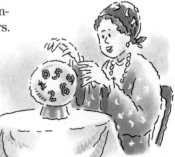

I can see that the fates of some tumors are linked with the hormones they depend on. I predict hormonal therapies will put them in grave danger.

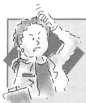

Who benefits from tamoxifen?

In 1998, the results of the "Tamoxifen Prevention Trial," sponsored by the National Cancer Institute, suggested that tamoxifen reduced the rate of breast cancer in healthy high-risk women by one-half. However, tamoxifen has serious adverse reactions that include potentially fatal blood clots and uterine cancer. The question is whether these risks are worth the benefits in healthy women.

The National Cancer Institute's report
To help answer this question, the National Cancer Institute published a report in November of 1999. They concluded that most women over age 60 would receive more harm than benefit from tamoxifen. Even though women under age 60 could benefit from taking tamoxifen, they were still at risk unless they had a hysterectomy, which eliminated the risk of uterine cancer or were in the very high-risk group for developing breast cancer.

Breaking it down further
The report also concluded that the risks of tamoxifen were greater than the benefits for black women over age 60 and almost all other women over age 60 who still had a uterus. But for older women without a uterus and with a 3.5% chance of developing breast cancer over the next 5 years, the benefits may outweigh the risks.

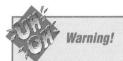

Adverse reactions to tamoxifen

Tamoxifen is a relatively nontoxic drug. The most common adverse reactions include:
• hot flashes
• nausea
• diarrhea
• fluid retention
• vomiting.

Changes in the blood
Leukopenia or thrombocytopenia (reduced white blood cell and platelets, respectively) may also occur.

Down to the bone
In patients with bone metastasis, hypercalcemia (elevated serum calcium levels) may occur as well.

• Antacids may affect its absorption in enteric-coated tablet form. (See *Adverse reactions to tamoxifen.*)

Androgens

The therapeutically useful *androgens* are synthetic derivatives of naturally occurring testosterone. They include:
• fluoxymesterone
• testolactone
• testosterone enanthate
• testosterone propionate.

Pharmacokinetics

The pharmacokinetic properties of therapeutic androgens resemble those of naturally occurring testosterone.

Absorption

Oral androgens, fluoxymesterone and testolactone, are absorbed well. The parenteral ones, testosterone enanthate and testosterone propionate, are designed specifically for slow absorption.

Distribution, metabolism, and excretion

Androgens are distributed well throughout the body, metabolized extensively in the liver, and excreted in the urine.

Checking the suspension

The duration of the parenteral forms is longer because the oil suspension is absorbed slowly. Parenteral androgens are administered one to three times per week.

Pharmacodynamics

Androgens probably act by one or more mechanisms. They may reduce the number of prolactin receptors or may bind competitively to those that are available.

Keeping its sister hormone in check

Androgens may inhibit estrogen synthesis or competitively bind at estrogen receptors. These actions prevent estrogen from affecting estrogen-sensitive tumors.

Pharmacotherapeutics

Androgens are indicated for the palliative treatment of advanced breast cancer, particularly in postmenopausal women with bone metastasis.

Drug interactions

Androgens may alter dose requirement in patients receiving insulin, oral antidiabetic drugs, or oral anticoagulants. Taking them with drugs that are toxic to the liver increases the risk of liver toxicity. (See *Adverse reactions to androgens*.)

Antiandrogens

Antiandrogens are used as an adjunct therapy with gonadotropin-releasing hormone analogues in treating advanced prostate cancer. These drugs include:
- flutamide
- nilutamide
- bicalutamide.

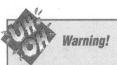

Warning!

Adverse reactions to androgens

Nausea and vomiting are the most common adverse reactions to androgens. Fluid retention caused by sodium retention may also occur.

Reactions in females
Women taking androgens may develop:
- acne
- clitoral hypertrophy
- deeper voice
- increased facial and body hair
- increased sexual desire
- menstrual irregularity.

Reactions in males
Males taking androgens may experience these effects as a result of conversion of steroids to female sex hormone metabolites:
- gynecomastia
- prostatic hypertrophy
- testicular atrophy.

Reactions in children
Children taking androgens may develop:
- premature epiphyseal closure
- secondary sex characteristic developments (especially in boys).

Pharmacokinetics

After oral administration, antiandrogens are absorbed rapidly and completely.

Metabolism and excretion

Antiandrogens are metabolized rapidly and extensively and excreted primarily in the urine.

Pharmacodynamics

Flutamide, nilutamide, and bicalutamide exert their antiandrogenic action by inhibiting androgen uptake or preventing androgen binding in cell nuclei in target tissues.

Pharmacotherapeutics

Antiandrogens are used with a gonadotropin-releasing hormone analogue, such as leuprolide, to treat metastatic prostate cancer.

A flare for their work

Concomitant administration of antiandrogens and a gonadotropin-releasing hormone analogue may help prevent the disease flare that occurs when the gonadotropin-releasing hormone analogue is used alone.

Drug interactions

Antiandrogens don't interact significantly with other drugs. However, flutamide and bicalutamide may affect the prothrombin time (a test to measure clotting factors) in a patient receiving warfarin. (See *Adverse reactions to antiandrogens.*)

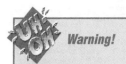

Warning!

Adverse reactions to antiandrogens

When an antiandrogen is used with a gonadotropin-releasing hormone analogue, the most common adverse reactions are:
• hot flashes
• decreased sexual desire
• impotence
• diarrhea
• nausea
• vomiting
• breast enlargement.

Progestins

Progestins are hormones used to treat various forms of cancer and include:
• hydroxyprogesterone caproate
• medroxyprogesterone acetate
• megestrol acetate.

Pharmacokinetics

When taken orally, megestrol acetate is absorbed well. After I.M. injection in an aqueous or oil suspension, hydroxyprogesterone caproate and medroxyprogesterone are absorbed slowly from their deposit sites.

Distribution, metabolism, and excretion

These drugs are distributed well throughout the body and may sequester in fatty tissue. Progestins are metabolized in the liver and excreted as metabolites in the urine.

Pharmacodynamics

The mechanism of action of progestins in treating tumors isn't completely understood. Researchers believe the drugs bind to a specific receptor to act on hormonally sensitive cells.

They're not exhibitionists

Because progestins don't exhibit a cytotoxic activity (destroying or poisoning cells), they're considered cytostatic (they keep the cells from multiplying).

Pharmacotherapeutics

Progestins are used for the palliative treatment of advanced endometrial, breast, and renal cancers. Of these drugs, megestrol is used most often.

Drug interactions

No drug interactions have been identified for megestrol. However, other progestins do have significant interactions with other drugs:
• Barbiturates, carbamazepine, and rifampin reduce the progestin effects of hydroxyprogesterone.
• Hydroxyprogesterone and medroxyprogesterone may interfere with bromocriptine's effects, causing menstruation to stop.
• Taking hydroxyprogesterone with dantrolene and other liver toxic drugs increases the risk of liver toxicity.
• Dose adjustments in oral anticoagulants may be needed when they're taken with hydroxyprogesterone.
• Aminoglutethimide and rifampin may reduce the progestin effects of medroxyprogesterone. (See *Adverse reactions to progestins*.)

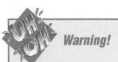
Warning!

Adverse reactions to progestins

Mild fluid retention is probably the most common reaction to progestins. Other reactions include:
• thromboemboli
• breakthrough bleeding, spotting, and changes in menstrual flow
• breast tenderness
• liver function abnormalities.

Oil issues

Patients who are hypersensitive to the oil carrier used for injection (usually sesame or castor oil) may have a local or systemic hypersensitivity reaction.

Gonadotropin-releasing hormone analogues

Gonadotropin-releasing hormone analogues are used for treatment of advanced prostate cancer. They include:
- goserelin acetate
- leuprolide acetate.

Pharmacokinetics

Goserelin is absorbed slowly for the first 8 days of therapy and rapidly and continuously thereafter. After subcutaneous injection, leuprolide is absorbed well.

Neither drug's distribution, metabolism, and excretion are defined clearly.

Pharmacodynamics

Goserelin and leuprolide act on the male's pituitary gland to increase luteinizing hormone (LH) secretion, which stimulates testosterone production. The peak testosterone level is reached about 72 hours after daily administration.

Running the reverse

With long-term administration, however, goserelin and leuprolide inhibit LH release from the pituitary and subsequently inhibit testicular release of testosterone. Because prostate tumor cells are stimulated by testosterone, the reduced testosterone level inhibits tumor growth.

Pharmacotherapeutics

Goserelin and leuprolide are used for the palliative treatment of metastatic prostate cancer. The drugs lower the testosterone level without the adverse psychological effects of castration or the adverse cardiovascular effects of diethylstilbestrol.

Drug interactions

No drug interactions have been identified with goserelin or leuprolide. (See *Adverse reactions to gonadotropin-releasing hormone analogues.*)

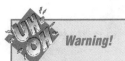 *Warning!*

Adverse reactions to gonadotropin-releasing hormone analogues

Hot flashes, impotence, and decreased sexual desire are commonly reported reactions to goserelin and leuprolide, two gonadotropin-releasing hormone analogues. Other adverse effects include:
- peripheral edema
- nausea and vomiting
- constipation
- anorexia.

Flare up

Disease symptoms and pain may worsen or flare during the first 2 weeks of goserelin or leuprolide therapy. The flare can be fatal in patients with bony vertebral metastasis.

Natural antineoplastic drugs

A subclass of antineoplastic drugs known as *natural products* includes:
- vinca alkaloids
- podophyllotoxins.

Vinca alkaloids

Vinca alkaloids are nitrogenous bases derived from the periwinkle plant. These drugs are cell cycle–specific for the M phase and include:
- vinblastine
- vincristine
- vinorelbine.

Pharmacokinetics

After I.V. administration, the vinca alkaloids are distributed well throughout the body.

Metabolism and excretion

Vinca alkaloids undergo moderate liver metabolism before being eliminated through different phases, primarily in the feces with a small percentage eliminated in the urine.

Pharmacodynamics

Vinca alkaloids may disrupt the normal function of the microtubules (structures within cells that are associated with the movement of DNA) by binding to the protein tubulin in the microtubules.

Separation anxiety

With the microtubules unable to separate chromosomes properly, the chromosomes are dispersed throughout the cytoplasm or arranged in unusual groupings. As a result, formation of the mitotic spindle is prevented, and the cells can't complete mitosis (cell division).

Under arrest

Cell division is arrested in metaphase, causing cell death. Therefore, vinca alkaloids are cell cycle–, M phase–

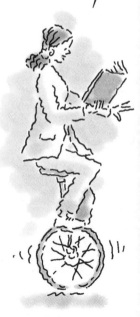

The vinca alkaloids are cell cycle–specific. They do their work during the M phase. That is the phase of mitosis, or cell division.

specific. Interruption of the microtubule function may also impair some types of cellular movement, phagocytosis (engulfing and destroying microorganisms and cellular debris), and CNS functions.

Pharmacotherapeutics

Vinca alkaloids are used in several therapeutic situations:
• Vinblastine is used to treat metastatic testicular carcinoma, lymphomas, Kaposi's sarcoma (the most common acquired immunodeficiency syndrome [AIDS]-related cancer), neuroblastoma (a highly malignant tumor originating in the sympathetic nervous system), breast carcinoma, and choriocarcinoma.
• Vincristine is used in combination therapy to treat Hodgkin's disease, malignant lymphoma, Wilms' tumor, rhabdomyosarcoma, and acute lymphocytic leukemia.
• Vinorelbine is used to treat non–small-cell lung cancer. It may also be used in the treatment of metastatic breast carcinoma, cisplatin-resistant ovarian carcinoma, and Hodgkin's disease.

Drug interactions

Vinca alkaloids have several interactions with other drugs:
• Erythromycin may increase the toxicity of vinblastine.
• Vinblastine decreases the plasma levels of phenytoin.
• Vincristine reduces the effects of digoxin.
• Asparaginase decreases liver metabolism of vincristine, increasing the risk for toxicity.
• Calcium channel blockers enhance vincristine accumulation, increasing the tendency for toxicity. (See *Adverse reactions to vinca alkaloids.*)

Podophyllotoxins

Podophyllotoxins are semisynthetic glycosides that are cell cycle–specific and act during the G2 and late S phases of the cell cycle. They include:
• etoposide
• teniposide.

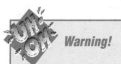
Warning!

Adverse reactions to vinca alkaloids

Nausea vomiting, constipation, and stomatitis (mouth inflammation) may occur in patients taking vinca alkaloids.

Toxic topics
Vinblastine and vinorelbine toxicities occur primarily as bone marrow suppression.

Muscle matters
Neuromuscular abnormalities frequently occur with vincristine and vinorelbine and occasionally with vinblastine therapy.

Tumor trouble
Vinblastine may produce tumor pain described as an intense stinging or burning in the tumor bed, with an abrupt onset 1 to 3 minutes after drug administration. The pain usually lasts 20 minutes to 3 hours.

Hair scare
Reversible alopecia occurs in up to one-half of patients receiving vinca alkaloids; it's more likely to occur with vincristine than vinblastine.

Outside activities

Teniposide has demonstrated some activity in treating Hodgkin's disease, lymphomas, and brain tumors.

Pharmacokinetics

When taken orally, podophyllotoxins are only moderately absorbed. Although the drugs are distributed widely throughout the body, they achieve poor CSF levels.

Metabolism and excretion

Podophyllotoxins undergo liver metabolism and are excreted primarily in the urine.

Pharmacodynamics

Although their mechanism of action aren't completely understood, podophyllotoxins produce several biochemical changes in tumor cells.

Concentrate, here's what they do

At low concentrations, these drugs block cells at the late S or G2 phase. At higher concentrations, they arrest the cells in the G2 phase.

Breaking a rung on the ladder

Podophyllotoxins can also break one of the strands of the DNA molecule. These drugs can also inhibit nucleotide transport and incorporation into nucleic acids.

Pharmacotherapeutics

Etoposide is used to treat testicular cancer and small-cell lung cancer. It may also be used to treat various lymphomas and leukemias, although these indications have not been approved by the FDA yet. Teniposide is used to treat acute lymphoblastic leukemia.

Drug interactions

Podophyllotoxins have few significant interactions with other drugs:
• Teniposide may increase the clearance and intracellular levels of methotrexate.

• Etoposide may increase the risk of bleeding in a patient taking warfarin. (See *Adverse reactions to podophyllotoxins.*)

Unclassifiable antineoplastic drugs

Many other antineoplastic drugs can't be included in existing classifications. These drugs include:
• asparaginase
• procarbazine
• hydroxyurea
• interferon
• aldesleukin
• altretamine
• paclitaxel
• docetaxel.

Asparaginases

Asparaginases are cell cycle–specific and act during the G1 phase. They include:
• asparaginase
• pegaspargase.

Pharmacokinetics

Asparaginase is administered parenterally. It's considered 100% bioavailable when administered I.V. and about 50% bioavailable when administered I.M.

Distribution and metabolism

After administration, asparaginase remains inside the blood vessels, with minimal distribution elsewhere. The metabolism of asparaginase is unknown; only trace amounts appear in urine.

Pharmacodynamics

Asparaginase and pegaspargase capitalize on the biochemical differences between normal cells and tumor cells.

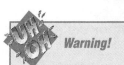

Warning!

Adverse reactions to podophyllotoxins

The majority of patients receiving podophyllotoxins experience hair loss. Other adverse reactions include:
• nausea and vomiting
• anorexia
• stomatitis
• bone marrow suppression, causing leukopenia and, less commonly, thrombocytopenia
• acute hypotension (if a podophyllotoxin is infused too rapidly by I.V.).

Tumor cells — eat your asparagine or else

Most normal cells can synthesize asparagine, but some tumor cells depend on other sources of asparagine for survival. Asparaginase and pegaspargase help to degrade asparagine to aspartic acid and ammonia. Deprived of their supply of asparagine, the tumor cells die.

Pharmacotherapeutics

Asparaginase is used primarily to induce remission in patients with acute lymphocytic leukemia.

If allergic...

Pegaspargase is used to treat acute lymphocytic leukemia in patients who are allergic to the native form of asparaginase.

Drug interactions

Asparaginase drugs may interact with other drugs. Asparaginase and pegaspargase may reduce the effectiveness of methotrexate. Concurrent use of asparaginase with prednisone or vincristine increasing the risk of toxicity. (See *Adverse reactions to asparaginase drugs.*)

Procarbazine

Procarbazine hydrochloride, a methylhydrazine derivative with monoamine oxidase (MAO) inhibiting properties, is used to treat Hodgkin's disease and primary and metastatic brain tumors. It is cell cycle–phase specific and acts on the S phase.

Pharmacokinetics

After oral administration, procarbazine is absorbed well. It readily crosses the blood-brain barrier and is well distributed into the CSF.

Metabolism and excretion

Procarbazine is metabolized rapidly in the liver and must be activated metabolically by microsomal enzymes. It's excreted in urine, primarily as metabolites. Respiratory excretion of the drug occurs as methane and carbon dioxide gas.

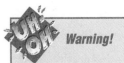

Warning!

Adverse reactions to asparaginase drugs

Many patients receiving asparaginase and pegaspargase develop nausea and vomiting. Fever, headache, abdominal pain, and liver toxicity may also occur.

Toxic topics
Asparaginase and pegaspargase can cause anaphylaxis, which is more likely to occur with intermittent I.V. dosing than with daily I.V. dosing or I.M. injections. The risk of a reaction rises with each successive treatment.

Hypersensitivity reactions may also occur.

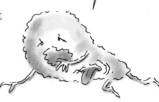

Without asparaginase, I'm finished!

Pharmacodynamics

An inert drug, procarbazine must be activated metabolically in the liver before it can produce various cell changes. It can cause chromosomal damage, suppress mitosis, and inhibit DNA, RNA, and protein synthesis. Cancer cells can develop resistance to procarbazine quickly.

Pharmacotherapeutics

Used with other antineoplastic drugs, procarbazine is most effective in the "MOPP" regimen for Hodgkin's disease, which consists of these four drugs:
- **m**echlorethamine
- **o**ncovin (vincristine)
- **p**rocarbazine
- **p**rednisone.

It can do more than just MOPP

Procarbazine is used to treat primary and metastatic brain tumors. The drug may also be useful against small-cell lung cancer, malignant lymphoma, myeloma, melanoma, and CNS tumors.

Drug interactions

Interactions with procarbazine can be significant:
- It produces an additive effect when administered with CNS depressants.
- Taken with meperidine, it may result in severe hypotension and death.

Mirroring MAO

Because of procarbazine's MAO inhibiting properties, hypertensive reactions may occur when it's administered concurrently with sympathomimetics, antidepressants, and tyramine-rich foods. (See *Adverse reactions to procarbazine*, page 344.)

Procarbazine has MAO inhibiting properties. So watch out for tyramine-rich foods!

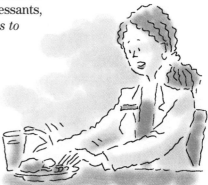

Hydroxyurea

Hydroxyurea is used most commonly for patients with chronic myelogenous leukemia.

When your neck is on the line

Hydroxyurea is also used for solid tumors and head and neck cancer.

Pharmacokinetics

Hydroxyurea is absorbed readily and distributed well into the CSF after oral administration. It reaches a peak serum level 2 hours after administration.

Metabolism and excretion

About half of a dose is metabolized by the liver to carbon dioxide, which is excreted by the lungs, or to urea, which is excreted by the kidneys. The remaining half is excreted unchanged in the urine.

Pharmacodynamics

Hydroxyurea exerts its effect by inhibiting the enzyme ribonucleotide reductase, which is necessary for DNA synthesis.

Divide and conquer

Hydroxyurea kills cells in the S phase of the cell cycle and holds other cells in the G1 phase, where they're most susceptible to irradiation.

Pharmacotherapeutics

Hydroxyurea is used to treat selected myeloproliferative disorders. It may produce temporary remissions in some patients with metastatic malignant melanomas as well.

Working with radiation

Hydroxyurea also is used in combination therapy with radiation to treat carcinomas of the head, neck, and lung.

Drug interactions

Cytotoxic drugs and radiation therapy enhance the toxicity of hydroxyurea. (See *Adverse reactions to hydroxyurea.*)

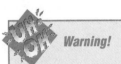

Warning!

Adverse reactions to procarbazine

Late-onset bone marrow suppression is the most common dose-limiting toxicity associated with procarbazine. Interstitial pneumonitis (lung inflammation) and pulmonary fibrosis (scarring) may also occur.

A bad start
Initial procarbazine therapy may induce a flulike syndrome, including fever, chills, sweating, lethargy, and muscle pain.

Gut reactions
GI reactions include nausea, vomiting, stomatitis, and diarrhea.

Interferons

A family of naturally occurring glycoproteins, *interferons* are so named because of their ability to interfere with viral replication. These drugs have anticancer activity as well as activity against condylomata acuminata (soft, wartlike growths on the skin and mucous membrane of the genitalia caused by a virus). The three types of interferons are:

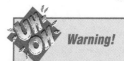

☝ *alfa interferons* derived from leukocytes

✌ *beta interferons* derived from fibroblasts (connective tissue cells)

🖐 *gamma interferons* derived from fibroblasts and lymphocytes.

Restrictions apply

Currently, only alfa interferons (alfa-2a, alfa-2b, and alfan3) are available commercially. The beta and gamma interferons are limited to investigational use.

Pharmacokinetics

After I.M. or subcutaneous administration, alfa interferons are usually absorbed well. Information about their distribution is unavailable.

Metabolism and excretion

Alfa interferons are filtered by the kidneys, where they're degraded. Liver metabolism and biliary excretion of interferons are negligible.

Pharmacodynamics

Although their exact mechanism of action is unknown, alfa interferons appear to bind to specific membrane receptors on the cell surface. When bound, they initiate a sequence of intracellular events that includes the induction of certain enzymes.

Running interference

This process may account for the ability of interferons to:
• inhibit viral replication
• suppress cell proliferation

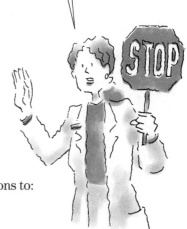

Interferons can put a stop to viral replication.

Warning!

Adverse reactions to hydroxyurea

Treatment with hydroxyurea leads to few adverse reactions. Those that do occur include:
• bone marrow suppression
• drowsiness
• headache
• nausea and vomiting
• anorexia
• elevated uric acid levels, which require some patients to take allopurinol to prevent kidney damage.

- enhance macrophage activity (engulfing and destroying microorganisms and other debris)
- increase cytotoxicity of lymphocytes for target cells.

Pharmacotherapeutics

Alfa interferons have shown their most promising activity in treating blood malignancies, especially hairy cell leukemia. Their approved indications currently include:
- hairy cell leukemia
- AIDS-related Kaposi's sarcoma
- condylomata acuminata.

Interfering in these areas as well...

Alfa interferons also demonstrate some activity against chronic myelogenous leukemia, malignant lymphoma, multiple myeloma, melanoma, and renal cell carcinoma.

Drug interactions

Interferons interact with other drugs:
- They may enhance the CNS effects of CNS depressants and substantially increase the half-life of methylxanthines (including theophylline and aminophylline).
- Concurrent use with a live virus vaccine may potentiate replication of the virus, increasing the adverse effects of the vaccine and decreasing the patient's antibody response.
- Bone marrow suppression may be increased when an interferon is used with radiation therapy or a drug that causes blood abnormalities or bone marrow suppression.
- Alfa interferons increase the risk of kidney failure from interleukin-2. (See *Adverse reactions to interferons.*)

Aldesleukin

Aldesleukin is a human recombinant interleukin-2 derivative that is used to treat metastatic renal cell carcinoma.

Pharmacokinetics

After I.V. administration of aldesleukin, about 30% is absorbed into the plasma and about 70% is absorbed rapidly by the liver, kidneys, and lungs. The drug is excreted primarily by the kidneys.

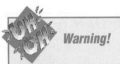

Warning!

Adverse reactions to interferons

Blood toxicity occurs in up to one-half of patients taking interferons and may produce leukopenia, neutropenia, thrombocytopenia, and anemia. Adverse GI reactions include anorexia, nausea, and diarrhea.

Alfa concerns
The most common adverse reaction to alfa interferons is a flulike syndrome that may produce fever, fatigue, muscle pain, headache, chills, and joint pain.

It catches your breath
Coughing, difficulty breathing, hypotension, edema, chest pain, and heart failure have also been associated with interferon therapy.

Pharmacodynamics

The exact antitumor mechanism of action of aldesleukin is unknown. The drug may stimulate an immunologic reaction against the tumor.

Pharmacotherapeutics

Aldesleukin is used to treat metastatic renal cell carcinoma. It may also be used in the treatment of Kaposi's sarcoma and metastatic melanoma.

Drug interactions

Aldesleukin will interact with other drugs:
• Concomitant administration of aldesleukin and drugs with psychotropic properties (such as narcotics, analgesics, antiemetics, sedatives, and tranquilizers) may produce additive CNS effects.
• Glucocorticoids may reduce aldesleukin's antitumor effects.
• Antihypertensive drugs may potentiate aldesleukin's hypotensive effects.
• Concurrent therapy with drugs that are toxic to the kidneys (such as aminoglycosides), bone marrow (such as cytotoxic chemotherapy drugs), heart (such as doxorubicin), or liver (such as methotrexate or asparaginase) may increase toxicity to these organs. (See *Adverse reactions to aldesleukin.*)

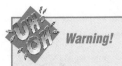

Warning!

Adverse reactions to aldesleukin

During clinical trials, more than 15% of patients developed adverse reactions to aldesleukin. These include:
• pulmonary congestion and difficulty breathing
• anemia, thrombocytopenia, and leukopenia
• elevated bilirubin, transaminase, and alkaline phosphate levels
• hypomagnesemia and acidosis
• reduced or absent urinary output
• elevated serum creatinine level
• stomatitis
• nausea and vomiting.

Altretamine

Altretamine is a synthetic cytotoxic antineoplastic drug that is used as palliative treatment for patients with ovarian cancer.

Pharmacokinetics

Altretamine is absorbed well after oral administration.

Metabolism and excretion

It's metabolized extensively in the liver and excreted by the liver and kidneys. The parent compound is poorly bound to plasma proteins.

Pharmacodynamics

The exact mechanism of action of altretamine is unknown. However, its metabolites are alkylating drugs.

Pharmacotherapeutics

Altretamine is used as palliative treatment of persistent or recurring ovarian cancer after first-line therapy with cisplatin or an alkylating drug–based combination.

Drug interactions

Altretamine has a few significant interactions with other drugs. Concomitant therapy with cimetidine may increase altretamine's half-life, increasing the risk of altretamine toxicity.

Don't mix with MAO

Use with an MAO inhibitor may cause severe orthostatic hypotension (a drop in blood pressure upon rising). (See *Adverse reactions to altretamine.*)

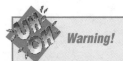

Warning!

Adverse reactions to altretamine

More than 10% of patients using altretamine in clinical trials experienced adverse reactions, such as:
• nausea and vomiting
• neurotoxicity
• peripheral neuropathy
• anemia.
Bone marrow suppression is also common.

Taxines

Taxine antineoplastics are used to treat metastatic ovarian and breast carcinoma after chemotherapy has failed. They include:
• paclitaxel
• docetaxel.

Pharmacokinetics

After I.V. administration, paclitaxel is highly bound to plasma proteins. Docetaxel is administered I.V. with a rapid onset of action.

Metabolism and excretion

Paclitaxel is metabolized primarily in the liver with a small amount excreted unchanged in the urine. Docetaxel is excreted primarily through feces.

Clinical controversy

Cultural considerations with docetaxel use

Clinical trials of docetaxel in Japanese and American patients with breast cancer revealed significant differences in the incidence of adverse effects between the two cultures.

The results

The Japanese women were more likely to develop thrombocytopenia (decreased platelet count) — 14.4% versus 5.5%. However, the Japanese women in this study were less likely than the American patients (6% versus 29.1%) to develop many of the other adverse effects, such as hypersensitivity reactions.

Other results showed fewer incidences of fluid retention, neurosensory effects, muscle pain, infection, and development of anemia in the Japanese patients. The study also indicated that Japanese patients are more likely to develop fatigue and weakness than American women.

Putting it into a plan

These results are important to consider when caring for patients receiving docetaxel. The information can provide clues for developing a plan of care and for knowing what adverse effects to expect.

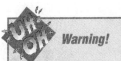 **Warning!**

Adverse reactions to taxines

During clinical trials, 25% or more patients experienced these adverse reactions to paclitaxel, a taxine:
• bone marrow suppression
• hypersensitivity reactions
• abnormal EEG tracings
• peripheral neuropathy
• muscle pain and joint pain
• nausea, vomiting, and diarrhea
• mucous membrane inflammation
• hair loss.

Docetaxel
Adverse reactions to docetaxel include:
• hypersensitivity reactions
• fluid retention
• leukopenia, neutropenia, or thrombocytopenia
• hair loss
• mouth inflammation
• numbness and tingling
• pain
• weakness and fatigue.

Pharmacodynamics

Paclitaxel and docetaxel exert their chemotherapeutic effect by disrupting the microtubule network that is essential for mitosis and other vital cellular functions.

Pharmacotherapeutics

Paclitaxel is used when first-line or subsequent chemotherapy has failed in treating metastatic ovarian carcinoma as well as metastatic breast cancer. The taxines may also be used for the treatment of head and neck cancer, prostate cancer, and non–small-cell lung cancer. (See *Cultural considerations with docetaxel use.*)

Drug interactions

Taxines have few interactions with other drugs:
• Concomitant use of paclitaxel and cisplatin may cause additive myelosuppressive effects.
• Cyclosporine, ketoconazole, erythromycin, and troleandomycin may modify the metabolism of docetaxel. (See *Adverse reactions to taxines.*)

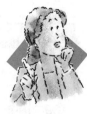

Quick quiz

1. What is the major adverse reaction that is common to all alkylating drugs?

    A.   Photosensitivity

    B.   Nerve toxicity

    C.   Bone marrow suppression

Answer: C. Bone marrow suppression is a common adverse reaction to all alkylating drugs.

2. The drug likely to be administered with methotrexate to minimize its adverse reactions is:

    A.   fluorouracil.

    B.   leucovorin.

    C.   cladribine.

Answer: B. Leucovorin is typically administered in conjunction with methotrexate to minimize adverse reactions.

3. Before administering bleomycin to a patient, why should you administer an antihistamine and an antipyretic?

    A.   To prevent fever and chills

    B.   To prevent anaphylactic shock

    C.   To prevent bone marrow suppression

Answer: A. An antihistamine and an antipyretic may be administered before bleomycin to prevent fever and chills.

Scoring

☆☆☆   If you answered all three questions correctly, extraordinary! You really mowed down the malignant neoplasms!

☆☆   If you answered two questions correctly, congratulations! You're more than competent to combat cancer.

☆   If you answered fewer than two questions correctly, give it another shot. Remember, this is your last crack at a quick quiz!

Appendices and index

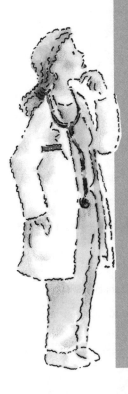

Appendix A

Common herbal preparations and their drug interactions

Herb	Drug	Interaction
aloe	• furosemide	• May increase drug effects (use together cautiously)
angelica	• warfarin	• Significantly prolongs prothrombin time when angelica is administered with warfarin (avoid concomitant use)
basil	• insulin	• May affect glycemic control (monitor blood glucose carefully)
bay	• insulin	• May affect glycemic control (monitor blood glucose carefully)
bearberry	• vitamin C	• Inactivated in urine (monitor for lack of effect)
bee pollen	• insulin	• May affect glycemic control (monitor blood glucose carefully)
betel palm	• atropine	• Reduces temperature-elevating effects and enhances central nervous system (CNS) effects of arecoline (avoid concomitant use)
	• digoxin	• Enhances cardiac effects (avoid concomitant use)
black catechu	• captopril	• Has additional hypotensive effect (avoid concomitant use)
	• verapamil	• Has additive effects (avoid concomitant use)
blue cohosh	• Nicoderm	• Increases effects of nicotine (avoid concomitant use)
burdock	• insulin	• May affect glycemic control (monitor blood glucose carefully)
butcher's broom	• doxazosin	• May reduce effects (avoid concomitant use)
	• prazosin	• May reduce effects (avoid concomitant use)
	• terazosin	• May reduce effects (avoid concomitant use)
cacao tree	• phenelzine	• May have vasopressor effects (avoid concomitant use)
	• selegiline	• May have vasopressor effects (avoid concomitant use)
	• theophylline	• May inhibit theophylline metabolism (avoid ingesting large amounts of cocoa concomitantly with theophylline)
	• tranylcypromine	• May have vasopressor effects (avoid concomitant use)
capsicum	• clonidine	• May reduce antihypertensive effectiveness (avoid concomitant use)
	• methyldopa	• May reduce antihypertensive effectiveness (avoid concomitant use)

Herb	Drug	Interaction
fumitory	• digoxin	• Enhances cardiac effects (avoid concomitant use)
ginseng	• insulin	• May affect glycemic control (monitor blood glucose carefully)
	• phenelzine	• May cause adverse reactions, including headache, tremors, and mania (avoid concomitant use)
	• selegiline	• May cause adverse reactions, including headache, tremors, and mania (avoid concomitant use)
	• tranylcypromine	• May cause adverse reactions, including headache, tremors, and mania (avoid concomitant use)
glucomannan	• insulin	• May affect glycemic control (monitor blood glucose carefully)
goldenseal	• digoxin	• Enhances cardiac effects (avoid concomitant use)
gossypol	• amphotericin B	• Enhances or increases the risk of renal toxicity when administered together (avoid concomitant use)
green tea	• doxorubicin	• May enhance the antitumor activity of doxorubicin
guarana	• adenosine	• May decrease drug's response
	• theophylline	• May cause additive CNS and cardiovascular effects (avoid concomitant use of guarana and other sources of caffeine)
horehound	• granisetron	• May enhance serotonergic effects (avoid concomitant use)
	• insulin	• May affect glycemic control (monitor blood glucose carefully)
	• ondansetron	• May enhance serotonergic effects (avoid concomitant use)
	• sumatriptan	• May enhance serotonergic effects (avoid concomitant use)
horse chestnut	• aspirin	• May increase risk of bleeding
jaborandi tree	• atropine	• May decrease drugs' effects (avoid concomitant use)
	• donepezil	• May cause additive effect and increase risk of toxicity (use together cautiously)
	• edrophonium	• May cause additive effect and increase risk of toxicity (use together cautiously)
	• ipratropium	• May decrease drugs' effects (use together cautiously)
	• physostigmine	• May cause additive effect and increase risk of toxicity (use together cautiously)
	• scopolamine	• May decrease drugs' effects (avoid concomitant use)

Herb	Drug	Interaction
jimson weed	• amantadine	• May adversely affect the function of the cardiovascular system (avoid concomitant use)
	• atropine	• May adversely affect the function of the cardiovascular system (avoid concomitant use)
	• disopyramide	• May adversely affect the function of the cardiovascular system (avoid concomitant use)
	• hyoscyamine	• May adversely affect the function of the cardiovascular system (avoid concomitant use)
	• levodopa	• May adversely affect the function of the cardiovascular system (avoid concomitant use)
	• procainamide	• May adversely affect the function of the cardiovascular system (avoid concomitant use)
	• quinidine	• May adversely affect the function of the cardiovascular system (avoid concomitant use)
kava	• alprazolam	• May cause coma (avoid concomitant use)
	• levodopa	• Increases parkinsonian symptoms (avoid concomitant use)
kelpware	• aspirin	• May increase risk of bleeding
licorice	• digoxin	• May enhance toxicity (avoid concomitant use)
	• loratadine	• May prolong the QT interval and be potentially additive (use together cautiously)
	• procainamide	• May prolong the QT interval and be potentially additive (use together cautiously)
	• quinidine	• May prolong the QT interval and be potentially additive (use together cautiously)
	• spironolactone	• May block ulcer healing and aldosterone-like effects of licorice (avoid concomitant use)
lily of the valley	• digoxin	• Enhances cardiac effects (avoid concomitant use)
male fern	• castor oil	• May increase absorption and increase risk of toxicity (avoid concomitant use)
	• lansoprazole	• Male fern is inactivated in alkaline environments
	• omeprazole	• Male fern is inactivated in alkaline environments
marshmallow	• insulin	• May affect glycemic control (monitor blood glucose carefully)

Herb	Drug	Interaction
melatonin	• magnesium	• Has additive inhibitory effects on the NMDA receptor (avoid concomitant use)
	• methamphetamine	• Enhances monoaminergic effects of methamphetamine and may exacerbate insomnia (avoid concomitant use)
	• succinylcholine	• Potentiates blocking properties of succinylcholine (avoid concomitant use)
motherwort	• digoxin	• Enhances cardiac effects (avoid concomitant use)
	• heparin	• Increases risk for bleeding effects (avoid concomitant use)
	• warfarin	• Increases risk for bleeding effects (avoid concomitant use)
myrrh	• insulin	• May affect glycemic control (monitor blood glucose carefully)
nutmeg	• clozapine	• May cause a loss of symptom control in patients taking these drugs or interfere with existing therapy for psychiatric illness
	• haloperidol	• May cause a loss of symptom control in patients taking these drugs or interfere with existing therapy for psychiatric illness
	• olanzapine	• May cause a loss of symptom control in patients taking these drugs or interfere with existing therapy for psychiatric illness
	• thiothixene	• May cause a loss of symptom control in patients taking these drugs or interfere with existing therapy for psychiatric illness
octacosanol	• carbidopa-levodopa	• May promote worsening of dyskinesias (avoid concomitant use)
oleander	• digoxin	• May enhance toxicity (avoid concomitant use)
oregano	• iron	• May reduce iron absorption (separate administration by at least 2 hours when given with iron supplements or iron-containing foods)
pareira	• lidocaine	• May add to or potentiate the effects of neuromuscular blockade (avoid concomitant use)
parsley	• dextromethorphan	• May promote or produce serotonin syndrome (avoid concomitant use)
	• lithium	• May promote or produce serotonin syndrome (avoid concomitant use)
	• meperidine	• May promote or produce serotonin syndrome (avoid concomitant use)
passion flower	• disulfiram	• May cause disulfiram reaction if extract or tincture contains alcohol (avoid concomitant use)
pennyroyal	• amiodarone	• May change the rate of formation of toxic metabolites of pennyroyal
	• cimetidine	• May change the rate of formation of toxic metabolites of pennyroyal
	• omeprazole	• May change the rate of formation of toxic metabolites of pennyroyal

Herb	Drug	Interaction
pill-bearing spurge	• atropine	• Choline may decrease drugs' effect (use together cautiously)
	• cyclosporine	• May inhibit CYP3A enzymes effecting drug metabolism (use together cautiously)
	• disulfiram	• May cause disulfiram reaction if herbal form contains alcohol (avoid concomitant use)
	• donepezil	• May have additive effect and increase the risk of toxicity (use together cautiously)
	• edrophonium	• May have additive effect and increase the risk of toxicity (use together cautiously)
	• erythromycin	• May inhibit CYP3A enzymes effecting drug metabolism (use together cautiously)
	• ipratropium	• May decrease drugs' effects (use together cautiously)
	• physostigmine	• May have additive effect and increase the risk of toxicity (use together cautiously)
	• scopolamine	• May decrease drugs' effects (use together cautiously)
plantains	• carbamazepine	• May inhibit GI absorption (avoid concomitant use)
	• lithium	• May inhibit GI absorption (avoid concomitant use)
pokeweed	• disulfiram	• May cause disulfiram reaction if herbal form contains alcohol (avoid concomitant use)
prickly ash	• aspirin	• May increase risk of bleeding
rauwolfia	• levodopa	• Decreases effectiveness of levodopa
red clover	• aspirin	• May increase risk of bleeding
	• heparin	• Increases risk of bleeding effects (avoid concomitant use)
	• ticlid	• May increase risk of bleeding
	• warfarin	• Increases risk of bleeding effects (avoid concomitant use)
rue	• digoxin	• Enhances cardiac effects (avoid concomitant use)
	• dobutamine	• Increases inotropic potential
sage	• insulin	• May affect glycemic control (monitor blood glucose carefully)
St. John's wort	• paroxetine	• May result in sedative-hypnotic intoxication (avoid concomitant use)
	• trazodone	• May cause serotonin syndrome (avoid concomitant use)

Herb	Drug	Interaction
senna	• indomethacin	• Blocks diarrheal effects (avoid concomitant use)
shepherd's purse	• digoxin	• Enhances cardiac effects (avoid concomitant use)
Siberian ginseng	• digoxin	• May enhance toxicity (avoid concomitant use)
squaw vine	• atropine	• Tannic acid may decrease metabolic breakdown (monitor patient)
	• disulfiram	• May cause disulfiram reaction if herbal form contains alcohol (avoid concomitant use)
	• scopolamine	• Tannic acid may decrease metabolic breakdown (monitor patient)
squill	• digoxin	• May enhance toxicity (avoid concomitant use)
	• disulfiram	• May cause disulfiram reaction if herbal form contains alcohol (avoid concomitant use)
sundew	• disulfiram	• May cause disulfiram reaction if herbal form contains alcohol (avoid concomitant use)
sweet flag	• disulfiram	• May cause disulfiram reaction if herbal form contains alcohol (avoid concomitant use)
tormentil	• disulfiram	• May cause disulfiram reaction if herbal form contains alcohol (avoid concomitant use)
valerian	• disulfiram	• May cause disulfiram reaction if herbal form contains alcohol (avoid concomitant use)
watercress	• acetaminophen	• May inhibit the oxidative metabolism of acetaminophen (avoid concomitant use)
yarrow	• disulfiram	• May cause disulfiram reaction if herbal form contains alcohol (avoid concomitant use)
yerba maté	• cimetidine	• May decrease clearance of yerba maté methylxanthines and cause toxicity (use together cautiously)
	• ciprofloxacin	• May decrease clearance of yerba maté methylxanthines and cause toxicity (use together cautiously)
	• verapamil	• May decrease clearance of yerba maté methylxanthines and cause toxicity (use together cautiously)
yohimbe	• venlafaxine	• Additive stimulation (use together cautiously)

Appendix B

Other major drugs

These charts review ophthalmic drugs, otic drugs, dermatologic drugs, and other miscellaneous drugs.

Ophthalmic drugs

Drug	Action	Treatment uses	Adverse reactions
Anesthestics			
Proparacaine hydrochloride Tetracaine	• Prevent the initiation and transmission of nerve impulses	• To anesthetize the cornea, allowing application of instruments for measuring IOP or removal of foreign bodies • To prepare for suture removal, conjunctival or corneal scraping, and tear duct manipulation	• Corneal inflammation • Corneal opacities • Delayed corneal healing • Eye pain and redness • Loss of visual acuity • Scarring
Anti-infectives			
Bacitracin Erythromycin Gentamicin sulfate Idoxuridine Polymyxin B sulfate Silver nitrate 1% Sulfacetamide sodium Tetracycline hydrochloride Tobramycin	• Kill bacteria or inhibit growth of bacteria or viruses	• To treat infections caused by bacteria or viruses (each drug is specific to particular organisms)	• Secondary eye infections (with prolonged use) • Severe hypersensitivity reactions
Anti-inflammatories			
Dexamethasone Fluorometholone Medrysone Prednisolone	• Decrease leukocyte infiltration at inflammation sites, causing reduced oozing of fluids and reduced edema, redness, and scarring	• To treat inflammatory disorders and hypersensitivity-related conditions of the cornea, iris, conjunctiva, sclera, and anterior uvea	• Corneal ulceration • Delayed corneal healing • Increased susceptibility to viral or fungal corneal infection
Miotics			
Carbachol Demecarium bromide Physostigmine salicylate Physostigmine sulfate Pilocarpine hydrochloride Pilocarpine nitrate	• Stimulate and contract the sphincter muscle of the iris, constricting the pupil • Improve aqueous outflow	• To treat open-angle glaucoma, acute and chronic angle-closure glaucoma, and certain cases of secondary glaucoma resulting from increased IOP	• Blurred vision • Bronchospasm • Cataract formation • Eye pain • Photosensitivity • Reversible iris cysts

Other major drugs (continued)

Ophthalmic drugs (continued)

Drug	Action	Treatment uses	Adverse reactions
Mydriatics			
Dipivefrin Epinephrine hydrochloride Epinephryl borate Phenylephrine hydrochloride	• Act on the iris to dilate the pupil • Lower intraocular pressure (IOP) (dipivefrin, epinephrine hydrochloride, and epinephryl)	• To dilate the pupils for intraocular examinations • To lower IOP in patients with glaucoma	• Blurred vision • Confusion • Dry skin • Flushing • Impaired ability to coordinate movement • Irritation • Rapid heart rate • Transient burning sensations
Mydriatics and cycloplegics			
Atropine sulfate Cyclopentolate hydrochloride Homatropine hydrobromide Scopolamine hydrobromide Tropicamide	• Act on the ciliary body of the eye to paralyze the fine-focusing muscles (thereby preventing accommodation for near vision)	• To perform refractive eye examinations in children before and after ophthalmic surgery • To treat conditions involving the iris	• Same as for mydriatics.
Other drugs to lower IOP			
Adrenergic blockers (topical) Apraclonidine hydrochloride Betaxolol hydrochloride Carteolol hydrochloride Levobunolol hydrochloride Metipranolol Timolol maleate	• May reduce aqueous humor formation and slightly increase aqueous humor outflow	• To prevent and control elevated IOP, chronic open-angle glaucoma, and secondary glaucoma	• Bronchospasm • Fatigue • Headaches • Slow heart rate
Carbonic anhydrase inhibitors Acetazolamide Acetazolamide sodium Dichlorphenamide Methazolamide	• Inhibit action of carbonic anhydrase, thus decreasing aqueous humor production	• To treat chronic open-angle glaucoma, acute angle-closure episodes and secondary glaucoma	• Hemolytic or aplastic anemia • Hypokalemia • Leukopenia • Nausea and vomiting

Other major drugs *(continued)*

Otic drugs

Drug	Action	Treatment uses	Adverse reactions
Anesthetics (local)			
Benzocaine	• Temporarily interrupt the conduction of nerve impulses	• To temporarily relieve ear pain	• Ear irritation or itching • Edema • Hives • Masking of the symptoms of a fulminating middle ear infection
Anti-infectives			
Acetic acid Boric acid Chloramphenicol Colistin sulfate Polymyxin B sulfate	• Kill bacteria or inhibit bacterial growth • Inhibit fungal growth (acetic acid and boric acid)	• To treat otitis externa • To treat otitis media (colistin and polymyxin B sulfate)	• Burning • Dermatitis • Ear itching • Hives
Anti-inflammatories			
Hydrocortisone Dexamethasone sodium phosphate	• Inhibit edema, capillary dilation, fibrin deposition, and phagocyte and leukocyte migration • Reduce capillary and fibroblast proliferation, collagen deposition, and scar formation	• To treat inflammatory conditions of the external ear canal	• Masking or exacerbation of underlying otic infection • Transient local stinging or burning sensations
Ceruminolytics			
Carbamide peroxide Triethanolamine polypeptide oleate-condensate	• Reduce hardened cerumen by emulsifying and mechanically loosening it	• To loosen and remove cerumen from the ear canal	• Mild, localized redness and itching

Other major drugs (continued)

Dermatologic drugs

Drug	Action	Treatment uses	Adverse reactions
Anti-infectives			
Antibacterials Bacitracin Gentamicin sulfate Mafenide acetate Mupirocin Silver sulfadiazine	• Kill or inhibit the growth of bacteria	• To treat infections caused by bacteria (each drug is specific to particular organisms)	• Contact dermatitis • Rash • Skin burning, itching, and redness • Skin dryness • Stinging
Antifungals Amphotericin B Clotrimazole Ketoconazole Miconazole nitrate Nystatin Terconazole Tolnaftate	• Kill or inhibit the growth of fungi	• To treat infections caused by fungi (each drug is specific to particular organisms)	• Same as for antibacterials • Pelvic cramping (with vaginal suppositories)
Antivirals Acyclovir	• Inhibit the growth of the herpes virus	• To treat type 1 herpes lesions on the lips and type 2 lesions on the genitals	• Same as for antibacterials
Anti-inflammatories			
Betamethasone Fluocinonide Fluticasone propionate Halobetasol propionate Hydrocortisone Triamcinolone acetonide	• Suppress inflammation by binding to intracellular corticosteroid receptors, initiating a cascade of anti-inflammatory mediators • Cause vasoconstriction in inflamed tissue and prevent macrophages and leukocytes from moving into the area	• To relieve inflammation and itching in topical steroid–responsive disorders, such as eczema, psoriasis, angioedema, contact dermatitis, seborrheic dermatitis, atopic dermatitis, and hives	• Adrenal hormone suppression • Stretch marks and epidermal atrophy (after 3 to 4 weeks of use)

Other major drugs *(continued)*

Dermatologic drugs

Drug	Action	Treatment uses	Adverse reactions
Hair growth stimulants			
Minoxidil	• Stimulate hair growth by causing vasodilation, which increases blood flow to the skin (exact mechanism of action is unknown)	• To treat male and female pattern baldness	• Fluid retention • Rapid heart rate • Weight gain
Topical antiacne drugs			
Keratolytics Tretinoin	• Produce antibacterial effects • Reduce inflammation	• To treat mild acne, oily skin, and acne vulgaris	• Burning • Hives • Rash • Scaling, blistering, and peeling • Skin dryness • Skin irritation • Superinfection (with prolonged use)
Counterirritants Benzoyl peroxide	• Produce antibacterial effects • Reduce inflammation	• To treat mild acne, oily skin, and acne vulgaris	• Same as for keratolytics
Antimicrobials Clindamycin Erythromycin Tetracycline hydrochloride	• Produce antibacterial effects • Reduce inflammation	• To treat mild acne, oily skin, and acne vulgaris	• Same as for keratolytics
Scabicides and pediculicides			
Crotamiton Lindane Permethrin	• Act on parasite nerve cell membranes to disrupt the sodium channel current, causing paralysis (some are also ovicidal)	• To treat scabies and lice	• Contact dermatitis • Hypersensitivity reactions • Respiratory allergy symptoms

Other major drugs (continued)

Other miscellaneous drugs

Drug	Action	Treatment uses	Adverse reactions
Nimodipine	• Inhibits contraction of vascular smooth muscle by inhibiting calcium ion influx across cardiac and smooth muscle, thereby producing vasodilation	• To treat neurologic deficits caused by cerebral spasms resulting from ruptured congenital aneurysm in patients who are otherwise neurologically healthy	• Abnormal liver function test results • Acne • Breathing difficulty • Depression • Diarrhea • ECG abnormalities • Edema • Headache • Hypotension • Muscle pain or cramps • Nausea and other GI symptoms • Rapid or slow heart rate • Rash
Pentoxifylline	• Decreases the thickness of blood	• To treat chronic occlusive peripheral vascular disease	• Dizziness • Dyspepsia • Headache • Nausea and vomiting
Sodium polystyrene sulfonate	• Causes sodium ions to exchange with hydrogen ions found in the stomach's acidic environment	• To treat hyperkalemia when urgent reduction of the serum potassium level isn't necessary	• Anorexia • Calcium and magnesium deficiencies • Constipation • Nausea and vomiting • Serious hypokalemia

Pharmacodynamics

Flucytosine penetrates fungal cells where it's converted to its active metabolite fluorouracil. Fluorouracil then is incorporated into the RNA of the fungal cells, altering their protein synthesis and causing cell death.

Pharmacotherapeutics

Although amphotericin B is effective in treating candidal and cryptococcal meningitis alone, flucytosine is given with it to reduce the dosage and the risk of toxicity. This combination therapy is the treatment of choice for cryptococcal meningitis.

Standing alone

Flucytosine can be used alone to treat lower urinary tract *Candida* infections because it reaches a high urinary concentration. It's also used effectively to treat infections caused by *T. glabrata*, *Phialophora*, *Aspergillus*, and *Cladosporium*.

Drug interactions

Cytarabine may antagonize the antifungal activity of flucytosine, possibly by competitive inhibition. (See *Adverse reactions to flucytosine*.)

Ketoconazole

Ketoconazole is an effective oral antimycotic drug with a broad spectrum of activity.

Pharmacokinetics

When given orally, ketoconazole is absorbed variably and distributed widely. It undergoes extensive liver metabolism and is excreted through the bile and feces.

Pharmacodynamics

Within the fungal cells, ketoconazole interferes with sterol synthesis, damaging the cell membrane and increasing its permeability. This leads to a loss of essential intracellular elements and inhibition of cell growth.

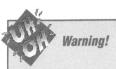

Warning!

Adverse reactions to flucytosine

Flucytosine may produce unpredictable adverse reactions, including:
- confusion
- headache
- drowsiness
- vertigo
- hallucinations
- difficulty breathing
- respiratory arrest
- rash
- nausea
- vomiting
- abdominal distention
- diarrhea
- anorexia.

Index

i refers to an illustration.

i refers to an illustration.

---

onazole usually produces fungistatic effects but
an produce fungicidal effects under certain condi-

nacotherapeutics

nazole is used to treat topical and systemic infec-
used by susceptible fungi, which include der-
ytes and most other fungi.

nteractions

azole may have significant interactions with oth-

ketoconazole with drugs that decrease gastric
ch as cimetidine, ranitidine, famotidine, nizati-
cids, and anticholinergic drugs, may decrease
of ketoconazole and reduce its antimycotic

etoconazole with phenytoin may alter metabo-
crease blood levels of both drugs.
en with theophylline it may decrease the
phylline level.
other liver toxic drugs may increase the risk
ase.
with cyclosporine therapy it may increase
and serum creatinine levels.
the effect of oral anticoagulants and can
rhage.
be given with rifampin because serum keto-
entrations can be decreased. (See *Adverse*
etoconazole.)

---

longs to a class of synthetic, broad-
azole antimycotic drugs.

netics

istration, fluconazole is about 90% ab-
buted into all body fluids, and over 80%
reted unchanged in the urine.

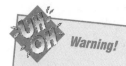

Warning!

Adverse reactions to ketoconazole

The most common adverse reactions to ketoconazole are nausea and vomiting. Less frequent reactions include:
- anaphylaxis
- joint pain
- chills
- fever
- ringing in the ears
- impotence
- photophobia.

Toxic topics
Liver toxicity is rare and reversible when the drug is stopped.

i refers to an illustration.

i refers to an illustration.

i refers to an illustration.

i refers to an illustration.

i refers to an illustration.

i refers to an illustration.

i refers to an illustration.

i refers to an illustration.

i refers to an illustration.

Notes

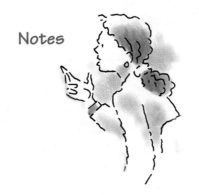

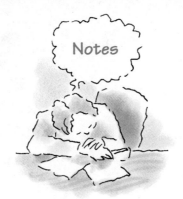